WORKING WITH TEENAGE PARENTS

Handbook of Theory & Practice
with DVD of Observation clips

for practitioners working with
pregnant teenagers,
young parents
& their children

Joan Raphael-Leff

Anna Freud Centre

First published in 2012
By the Anna Freud Centre

British Library Cataloguing in Publication Data
ISBN-978-0-9549319-3-3

Project Leader: Professor Joan Raphael-Leff

The original course was devised, implemented and evaluated from 2007 to 2009 with funds by a Department of Health Section 64 Grant. This Handbook/Trainer's Manual for the condensed training was developed independently by the Project Leader in 2009-2011 © JRL

Acknowledgements:
'Teenagers becoming Parents' came into being through a 'think tank' approach involving many contributors, some of whom became lecturers or seminar leaders on the full eight study day training course. Faculty comprised clinicians, practitioners and academics from the Anna Freud Centre, Portman Clinic, Tavistock Clinic & Centre, a variety of NHS and Voluntary Sectors. They included Drs. Carol Broughton, Anita Chakraborty, Sue Gerhardt, Zack Eleftheriadou, Viviane Green, Earl Hopper, Valli Kohon, Egle Laufer, Norka Malberg, Maggie Mills, Dana Shai, Isca Salzberger-Wittenberg, Jenny Stoker, Susan Straub, Brenda Thomas, Margot Waddell, John Woods, Marie Zaphiriou Woods. Leezah Hertzman, Helen Johnson, Natalia Stafler and Ju Tomas-Merrills led the Reflective Work Groups.
Thank you all! Your generosity of spirit was note worthy.

We are all appreciative of the eighty practitioners who piloted the first two courses. Their conscientious attendance, lively participation and evaluative feedback (questionnaires, focus group discussions and follow-up led to improvements informing this training. Special thanks to Dana Shai for collating evaluations; Laurence Dumant, for an independent qualitative follow-up study; Jan Owens of Cotelands College in Croydon, and Laura Gould for technical assistance, and the young parents at the Coram drop-in project who agreed to be filmed.

Similarly, my gratitude to the *'Pioneer' group* of practitioners Carole Grissett, Ella Jess-Reid, Laurence Dumant, Lize Course-Noel, Patsy Mounter, Sharon Singleton and Barbara Mustafa for helpful comments and detailed feedback when piloting the new condensed training course *'Adolescence as a Second Chance'*, and to Julie Stone, Gerda De Boer-Zoet and the eighteen other thoughtful professionals, who travelled from far-flung places in Great Britain and as far afield as Australia, Germany, Hong-Kong and the Netherlands to take part in the first *Training for Trainers* course. Since then, the training itself has travelled far and wide.

Finally, the section on the family was inspired by discussions in the UCL/AFC Academic Faculty for empirical, theoretical and qualitative conceptual Psychoanalytic Research. Contributors included Dr. Jan Abram, Dr. Lionel Bailly, Tessa Baradon, Dr. Tarik Bel-Bahar, Dr. Ruth Berkowitz, Prof. Rachel Blass, Dr. Minna Daum, Prof. Karl Figlio, Prof. Peter Fonagy, Prof. Jeremy Holmes, Dr. Earl Hopper, Dr. Sebastian Kraemer, Dr. Eilis Kennedy, Prof. Julian Leff, Dr. Franco Orsucci, Dr. Inge Pretorius, Mrs. Anne-Marie Sandler, Dr. Dinesh Sinha, Dr. Trudie Rossouw, Prof. Mary Target and Prof. Judith Trowell.

Adolescence as a 'Second Chance'
Training for practitioners working with pregnant teenagers,
young parents& their children

INTRODUCTION

In the current climate of budget restrictions, funding for training courses is no longer as readily available as previously. This resource, written by a specialist to enhance psychodynamic understanding of emotions, offers you an opportunity to undertake training on your own, or with a group of relevant practitioners in your own area.

We know that teenagers can be maddening!
This training addresses what happens when the identity-crises of adolescence and of parenthood coincide. We examine how practitioners are affected by working with this high-risk group, and explore the difficulties experienced by teenage mothers and fathers in meeting emotional, intellectual, social and physical needs – their own, and those of their child, which may match or clash.

Many teenagers in today's 'de-developing' Britain or elsewhere in the world, live in deteriorating no-hope communities, where apathy, escapism or violence seem the only way of tolerating a painful reality. This training offers a different way of thinking. The message is that *the emotional upheaval of adolescence and the protective forces of parenthood combine to offer a 'second chance'* – a means of enhancing self-esteem and appropriate self-assertion. With help, their increased capacity for self-reflection with greater tolerance of uncertainty changes the 'relational climate' between young parents and their child/ren, fostering resilience in both generations.

What the training offers
Adolescence as a 'Second Chance' focuses on mental health issues and provides a sound theoretical framework for understanding the maturational processes of adolescents, babies and toddlers, and interactive psychodynamics between them. It emphasises the importance of fathers, formulating ways in which practitioners can help to form a robust paternal connection with the baby, to sustain a parental partnership with the mother (even if they are no longer together).

The training addresses practical ways of engaging teen clients, and how to enhance the capacities for mentalization and self-inquiry in practitioners as well as teen parents. It identifies risk factors associated with parental immaturity and promotes early detection of emotional disturbance, neglect, abuse and trauma.

This Handbook has three parts:
- **A Theoretical Textbook,** which also includes *self-study* and *group* activities (arrowed and *italicised* in the table of Contents).
- **A Training Pack** including a DVD of clips for observation, expanded notes, handouts, reading recommendations, appendices, feedback forms and a glossary of concepts for each session.
- **A Training Manual** to enable the training to be run by a local in-house group leader for an interdisciplinary group of practitioners working in this field.

The training comprises five modules:
1. Interrelationships
2. Adolescents
3. Babies in teen families
4. Toddlers & Teen Mothers and Fathers
5. Families, Groups & Organizations

The overall focus of these different modules is increased emotional understanding. To this end, each module is subdivided into *Interactive Workshops* and *Skill-Building Seminars*, which include dialogues, small and large group discussions, interactive games and role-play. *Observation skills* are honed by viewing the relevant DVD clips attached, highlighting issues and watching the same clip again. Other skills promoted by this training include *mentalization, active listening, trust building, reflective communication, detecting disturbance, case reporting, information handling and sharing, referrals,* etc. Each module includes practical issues, recent research and clinical developments, conclusions and a detailed breakdown of the *key concepts* and *major themes* covered in each section.

Self-study has a double meaning – study of assigned films, readings and lectures that takes place without a teacher, and – *self-reflective* study.

This is quite a journey and all trainees are invited to keep a private *Learning Journal* to chart their own pathway throughout the training, expressing, clarifying and reflecting upon the feelings it has stirred up, and on the emotional impact the new understanding has had on them and their work. This remains private and for their own use alone (see p.201).

As both educational textbook and instructive manual, this Handbook also supports delivery of the interactive components in a group. **Group activities** consist of exercises and guided discussions to implement knowledge, skills and competencies that will increase effectiveness at work. For easy identification these appear in <u>framed boxes</u> in the text, providing background information and messages the leader will need in order to deliver the training. Power-point templates are available in the Handouts.

Finally, as it is used in many different countries, this training is designed with some flexibility in mind, to accommodate the particular needs of participants in different localities, and to enable each group leader to elaborate in her/his own words on the basic format as s/he sees fit.

Welcome to the training!

CONTENTS

Part 1: THEORETICAL TEXTBOOK

Module I: INTER-RELATIONSHIPS

Module II: **ADOLESCENTS**

3. <u>Interactive Workshop</u>: **TEENS: MATURATIONAL TASKS OF EARLY AND LATE ADOLESCENCE**

4. <u>Skill building seminar</u>: **PSYCHOLOGICAL PROCESSES OF PREGNANCY AND TEENS AS PARENTS**

Module V: <u>**FAMILIES, GROUPS & ORGANIZATIONS**</u>

Part 2: **TRAINING PACK**

GLOSSARY
of Psychoanalytic Terms and Concepts

READINGS
Recommended and Additional

APPENDICES

EXPANDED NOTES

Part 3: TRAINING MANUAL

EVALUATION & FEEDBACK FORMS

KEY TEXT:

HANDOUTS

Handouts for **Module I** sessions **1-2**
Handouts for **Module II** sessions **3-4**
Handouts for **Module III** sessions **5-6**
Handouts for **Module IV** sessions **7-8**
Handouts for **Module V** sessions **9-10**

Module I:
__INTER-RELATIONSHIPS__

Aims
The overall aim of this module is to enhance emotional awareness and encourage self-reflection in self and client. The first session floats some basic psychodynamic concepts of relational patterns of interaction and communication.

Learning Objectives
Training to increase understanding of the powerful internal struggles manifest in teenagers – between a contradictory sense of invincibility and fierce bid for self-assertion coupled with emotional vulnerability and a need for guidance. This training is dedicated to the idea that this very fluidity of emotions offers *a 'second chance'* – to process issues from the past and to channel these forces constructively.

<u>1. Interactive Workshop:</u>

Teen Clients - Expectations & Meaning Making

> This training workshop offers experiential activities to familiarise you with less conscious aspects of interrelationships. You can do these through *self-study* writing your feelings in your Learning Journal or in a *group setting*, exercises increase appreciation of the subtle two-way influences and complexity of interactive processes, and encourage group cohesion among participants.

Second chance
In states of transition (such as sleep or pregnancy) unresolved problems are reactivated. Both puberty and first parenting are such transitions which re-ignite previous concerns. Given good support, young parents can utilise their double emotional upheaval to address past deficits and heal old wounds. Most teenage clients will internalise good care. The experience of having their anxieties heard, and their needs understood and discussed appropriately will filter down to providing more thoughtful care for the child.

Teenagers as clients
Working with adolescents can be difficult – as clients they are notoriously difficult to engage. There are many failed appointments and late-comings. They often respond to reasonable requests with sullen silence, insolence or non-cooperative responses, and have a keen ability to pit one practitioner against another.

When anxious, frustrated, or confronted by reality pressures for which they are unprepared, teens tend to spread their anxiety around. Under stress they revert to less reflective 'black and white' forms of thinking which can be annoying. Conversely, they are also capable of great flights of fancy, questioning binary classifications (such as male versus female, straight versus gay) and engaging in creative 'out of the box' thinking, stretching boundaries to their limits, and subverting accepted ideas. These contradictions can be perplexing. We wonder why at times, a talkative adolescent will suddenly withdraw and shut people out, or become excitable or veer from charming to obstructive or manipulative. Adolescent clients present challenges: as passionate high-fliers they provoke our fears of a crash.

Their intensity, impulsiveness, risky behaviours and enactments induce strong reactive feelings in others, especially their carers. They evoke concern, bewilderment, irritation and a host of other emotions, possibly including our secret admiration and even envy...

It seems that both the 'storm and stress' and the extraordinary inventiveness of adolescence are impelled by their inner turmoil. Driven by passion, uncertainty and revived emotional issues from the past, a teenager fluctuates between child-like enthusiasm and trust, and adult-like cynicism at the sorry state of the world. How can we as practitioners help them in their search for new answers to old questions?

---

*In some of the boxes throughout this resource you will find activities and comments intended for participants in **group training**. Leader uses flipchart to note ideas.*
*If you are **self-studying** you might wish to contemplate these exercises reflectively, jotting your thoughts and feelings in your private Learning Journal- then checking out other ideas in each box. In the Group Training, the Trainer encourages interactive participation, then brings the ideas in the boxes to their attention.*
By the end of the first study-day you can be expected to –
- be more aware of your own subjective experience, expectations and prejudice.
- recognise distinctive aspects of working with teenage clients, including the importance of listening and containing anxiety.
- be better equipped to help clients to think about their own feelings and needs.
- have greater understanding of less conscious aspects of interpersonal psycho-dynamics.
- encourage the adolescent parent's own agency in decision making, with greater awareness of the effects of their choices on the baby and others around them.

Group activity: 'Secret History'
This exercise is inspired by a training module used by Dr. Simone Honikman,
Director of the Perinatal Mental Health Project, in Cape Town, South Africa. www.pmhp.za.org]
Self-study: *follow the instructions and write your reactions in your Journal.*
The group is divided into two. All members of each group are asked to 'become' one particular person – in this case, a teenager and a midwife. (30 minute exercise)
Teenager: Jane aged 17 is 22 weeks pregnant.
She missed her initial antenatal booking, and arrives 25 minutes late for the replacement
appointment, dishevelled and smelling of cigarette smoke. She seems resentful when told she will now have to wait for a gap.
Midwife's group are invited to shout out their immediate reactions
1. Members of Jane's group asked: "What is Jane **feeling**?"
They are asked to name her feelings ["frustrated; frightened" etc...]:
The leader makes it clear that there are no right or wrong answers – and that the feelings are not what she 'ought' to be feeling, but what they feel she may be experiencing. *Leader writes these on a flip chart page divided into two columns.*
2. The participants in Jane's group are asked:" what does Jane **need**?" (written in the second column on the same flip chart ["reassurance", "understanding", etc]
3. Leader now turns attention to the Midwife's group, with more information:

Midwife: <u>Rita</u> aged 38, is a divorced mother of two children aged four and six. Rita prides herself on managing her large case-load, and always arriving on time at the frequent staff meetings her staff nurse expects her to attend.

4. Members of Rita's group are asked to shout out what Rita is feeling
Then they are asked: "What does Rita need?" Responses are written on the second flip chart on the other side of the room (preferably by someone else).

<u>Leader now adds some information about Jane:</u>
There is some confusion over her address. There is a question of whether Jane belongs to the hospital's catchment area or should be sent elsewhere.

5. While writing, Leader summarises, comments, paraphrases feelings shouted out by each group ("I am feeling judged, vulnerable", etc) as they increasingly begin to comment in first person and complain openly about the other party.
6. <u>Stop after ~20 minutes.</u> Participants are asked to take a deep breath – and to physically *switch sides*, sitting in the other groups' chairs, now <u>playing the other person</u>.

Leader now adds another layer of information about Jane:
Two weeks ago, Jane told her parents about the pregnancy. Shocked and distressed that she refuses to have an abortion, her father said she is an embarrassment and can no longer live at home. Since then she was staying with her boyfriend, but yesterday, he beat her up during a row, saying he was not the baby's father. Jane slept overnight on a friend's couch. The friend lives some distance away, and the journey to the hospital took longer than expected.

7. Same procedure as previously, leader asking for feelings and needs, which are called out and added to Jane's flip-chart list:
Additional information about Rita<u>:</u>
She had a disturbed night with little sleep last night, as her youngest child woke short of breath, suffering from the croup. This has happened before, and she spent some hours with him in the kitchen, creating steam to relieve his coughing fits. Very early this morning she had to phone around to find someone to stay with him, as he could not go to his nursery.
8. Once again, her feelings and needs are added to Rita's flip-chart list.
9. Leader questions the contributors – *How do we protect ourselves and yet remain accessible, sensitive?* More details: *What kind of 'staff support?'* Etc.

10. <u>Stop after another 10 minutes.</u> Leader asks participants to take another deep breath, and go back to their *original seats* returning to their own selves, and leaving Jane and Rita behind.
Thanking participants for 'inhabiting' these people, leader asks if they are unusual cases? If not – *What was <u>new</u> in what we did today? What have you learned?*

Note the similarity of entries on both flip charts
<u>Discuss</u>: In busy work places, how can we enable clients to tell their 'stories'? How do we find out more about a client's 'secret history'?
[Helping him/her feel safe; reflecting back her/his feelings; validating these as important; listening attentively and non-judgementally, etc].

Reactive feelings
Sometimes in an encounter, there is so much going on that it is difficult to think. When the emotional upheaval of adolescence is combined with the turmoil of pregnancy and/or the responsibilities of parenting, these reactions are compounded.

Practitioners working with teen-parents often struggle to keep thinking in the presence of their clients - as young parent/s do in the presence of the infant. We may be assailed by heightened anxiety, as the teen's conflicts are pushed out into us while s/he assumes a seemingly 'unconcerned' 'devil may care' attitude. Conversely, we may feel overwhelmed by an overly anxious client. (The reactive feelings practitioners experience will be discussed later under the rubric of 'counter-transference'). We may be tempted to defend ourselves by shutting out the onslaught of feelings. But as someone said – *the mind is like a parachute, it cannot work unless it is open.*

> **Self-Study reflective exercise**: The 'secret history' gave us a glimpse 'behind the scenes' of some hidden reasons for behaving in ways that arouse negative reactions in others. We do not often get chance to appreciate what our clients might be feeling and their unvoiced needs. Can you think what lay behind some reactions your own clients aroused in you?

Expectations:

When faced with the unfamiliar, we all tend to try and dispel uncertainty by anticipating that what will happen. We approach new situations armed with expectations from past experience, as does the client. Meeting for the first time, these expectations usually operate outside the awareness of both participants. Nevertheless, unverbalised feelings infuse the emotional atmosphere of the room. Evident in our body language, inherent in our speech rhythms, tone, facial expression, posture, and even affect our body odour, they are registered non-consciously by the other, whose reaction then further affects the interchange. Based on past experience with previous carers, an adolescent client's expectations and anxieties colour the way a worker is perceived in their first encounter. But the practitioner too, brings expectations of the teen, which influence the spontaneous give-and-take. The client's collaboration or defiant withdrawal from any programme that is being offered also reflects her/his current preoccupations and resistance to change which is a desire to safeguard psychic equilibrium. The 'secret history' showed how easy it is to project and misinterpret the other's behaviour when we know so little about each other. How we meet the teen's apparent 'mindset' will set the pace. The other's mind is opaque but each teenager has a story to tell – and we must find a way to hear what lies behind the behaviour we see.

If we can tolerate not knowing, and bear to hold our own conjectures in suspense so as to remain receptive and listen rather than try to second guess – we are more likely to hear what someone is trying to tell us. And rather than a worn version, a *new* narrative may come into being, in a new situation rather than the replica of an old one repeated over and over again.

Understanding where a client is 'coming from' and what colours his/her expectations helps the practitioner to defuse anxiety about the encounter. Relying too much on information from elsewhere can also block our receptivity. By being reliable and responding authentically the worker can establish an atmosphere of trust, offering something a client may have never experienced before – the opportunity to explore their own feelings.

Actualisation:

As seen in the 'secret history' exercise, in the busy work situation, practitioners' expectations and those of young clients can clash or dovetail, as each brings their own preconceptions into contact w with the other's. We may expect the teenage parent to engage in irresponsible behaviour (or whatever) while s/he may expect us to be judgemental (or harsh, indulgent, old-fashioned, etc). We then may become the very person they expected. Furthermore, the client's reaction to our implicit criticism may then engender the very behaviour we ascribe (e.g. irresponsibility), and we ourselves may then feel justified in being critical and inclined to feel even more righteous – a spiralling process that *'actualises' expectations,* thereby reciprocally reinforcing covert images of self and other.

Most of the time we are unaware of our tendency to become caught up in these cycles of actualisation – being 'pulled' into playing out the nasty or idealised role that the other ascribes us or inducing others to play out our own expectations. It is therefore most important to recognise our own *'role-responsiveness'* to the client's unconscious wishes for gratification, so that we can work our way out of collusive participation, by understanding the part we play in it (see Sandler, 1976). And to work out what our own expectations and prejudices are, seeing how our own assumptions unwittingly affect others.

The Nature and Purpose of Role Play:

It is hard enough to monitor our own responses let alone those of another.

Role play grants us a unique experience of living in someone else's skin for a few minutes. This interactive form of engagement allows a participant to assume a role and empathically experience the feelings of the character one is playing.

It is a very powerful learning tool, as one stop the clock and examine one's feelings or 'rewind' and do it differently. Extraordinarily, when playing real but unknown cases, the role-players often display uncanny awareness of features of their characters that they have not been told. Role play can also reveal the dangers of over-identification with the client or with one's professional role. In modified form it may also be used by practitioners to get young parents to imagine what their baby is experiencing.

In the role-play situation, the Leader must give clear instructions beforehand. While still in role, players can be asked what they felt and why, and the 'audience' quizzed on their reactions. It is important to debrief role players afterwards, asking them to state their own name and to 'leave' their role behind.

Interactive systems

All encounters are accompanied by expectations and preconceptions which form an interactive field of forces. But some exchanges, especially those with a perceived authority figure, trigger very powerful unconscious feelings. In such highly charged encounters implicit memories are reactivated, including good and bad representations of our very first carers, whose presence and activities were necessary for our welfare, even survival. The intensity of these feelings (e.g. hatred, fear, clinging), in turn, has an emotional effect when we are engaged in a dialogue

---

Role Play: The First meeting Between Practitioner and a Client (10 mins)
1. *Anticipating the first appointment*
Leader asks for 2 volunteers: **A Teenage 'Client' & 'Experience'**
1. Both are sent out of the room to discuss the nature of his/her previous experience with workers. *Leader now asks for 2 other volunteers:*
2. These are the **'Referrer' who** briefly sets the scene for the **'Practitioner'**, preparing him/her for an encounter with a 'stroppy' client (1 minute). *Leader asks the group what profession both practitioners should represent, and to shout out the nature of previous behaviour and presenting problems.*
3. Those outside return, not knowing what has occurred in the room .
Actual first meeting (2 minutes of role play).
The role play proceeds with Practitioner and Client enacting their first meeting. While they are still in-role *Leader asks each about their expectations* before the encounter & what they saw, heard, felt during their meeting (2 minutes).
Stop for group discussion and comments (2 minutes)
Replay the scene taking comments into account: (2 minutes)
The Leader comments on the **new strategies** that have emerged:
"What are the first steps towards changing the culture of the workplace?"
(greeting the client; welcoming him/her with a smile; using first name, maintaining eye-contact, etc).

Teenage mothers and fathers are - teenagers!

Interim Conclusions:

This training is rooted in a theory of interaction that sees each partner in an encounter as part of **a complex system**, affected not only by his/her own feeling, thoughts and behaviour but those of the other, and by expectations based on the past and current transactions with others (which in turn reflect, modify and are modified by the intentions, expectations and mental state of that interactive partner). Hence the importance of raising our own awareness of such social pressures, through self-study or intimate small group interactions.

The training rests on an assumption that *feelings* provide a key to the human condition:

- From before birth a baby is inserted into a web of expectations and ascriptions.
- The child's internal world is constituted through early family interaction
- All mental functions (e.g. capacity for thinking, experiencing empathy or regulating our own emotional-states) arise in a relational context.
- Meanings are co-constructed in interaction with the *minds* of others within a particular culture
- Mental activity takes place on several levels at once - cognition, emotion, and imaginative fantasy coexist in our everyday life, although sometimes one or other predominates. [Note how right now, you can become aware of experiencing these]
- Different age levels continue to coexist [Just because I am 30 does not prevent me feeling like a 3 year old sometimes, or even behaving like one…]

- Unless digested, the care we received in infancy and childhood is blindly repeated with our own babies.
- The focus & timing of parental disturbance reflects the *weakest links* and residues of anxieties brought from their own childhood.
- Our defensive processes are interactive, and were co-constructed in interaction with our own carers.

[In a group situation this is a good point for a 5 minute break if necessary].

Self-study & Group exercise: without deliberating about it – complete this sentence in writing: *In Purdistan women are forbidden to…*

Intolerance

As this exercise demonstrates, we bring our *pre-judgements* even to imaginary people and situations. Many of us behave in ways that are inconsistent with our professed conscious ideals of 'liberty' and 'equality'. Prejudices have been called 'viruses' of the mind. When we respond 'instinctively' we are repeating unquestioned ideas and value systems we have imbibed from others since childhood. Clearly, our relational encounters are influenced not only by expectations, attitudes and reactions, but by these basic beliefs that are built into the ways we act and speak, yet by-pass thinking. Our values may be contradictory, or apply to some groups but not others who remain idealised, invisible or unworthy in our scheme of things.

As we identify groups by labels - 'men', 'women', 'adolescents', or ethnic categories, religious minorities, etc - *false hierarchies* begin to take on a social reality of their own, giving rise to inequitable or potentially oppressive practices. Some omissions are thoughtless but social arrangements perpetuate discrimination: For instance, breastfeeding access is still restricted in many public places. Wheelchair users and parents pushing double-buggies find access through narrow doorways impossible. Other forms of discrimination are less obvious. For instance mental health problems. See: http://www.youtube.com/watch?v=4tiYbhVBjTk

---

Group/Self study: *Are young people unfairly discriminated against?*

Prejudice

Prejudice is not something esoteric. It affects every area of our everyday lives and WE drive it. A New York grafitti at Ground Zero states: *'Fear is our common enemy'*. Ageism, Racism, Sexism, Religious fundamentalism and all other forms of prejudice are inherent to *systems of belonging* – in which we tend to see ourselves as 'good' and project what is strange ('alien' and 'bad' or needy, greedy, mad…) within us into another group. Awareness of 'in' and 'out' groups begins in infancy, as 'stranger anxiety' attests.

We often find ways of elevating ourselves by putting others down. Thus generic categories are not political givens but reflect our own irrational beliefs and weaknesses externalised onto others. And we each are guilty of prejudice. How often have we said: "you can't trust 'those people'" (whether we meant bankers, teenagers, colleagues, Jews, doctors…)

Adolescence as a 'Second chance'

Our own intolerance does not take account of *personal* attributes of people within the despised or 'dangerous' group but lumps them all together, 'depersonalising' them – and sometimes, 'dehumanising' too. Anxiety drives barriers to keep each other out, especially those who seem different to us. The Berlin wall, and the Israeli' fence' are examples of physical barriers but there are psychic ones too.

Clearly, any form of group labelling is *a social act.* Bigotry can be personal or institutionalised, even legislated (as in apartheid South Africa or homophobic societies). It can be disguised or blatant: from Victorian times until recently many bars or clubs declared themselves: 'Gentlemen only'. In the 1950s, signs on London Boarding Houses could openly state: 'No children, no dogs, no coloureds'.

> *In addition to perpetrators, and victims, there are supporters and bystanders.*

Courage and Collusion

Silence about known injustice is an act of compliance. It takes courage to stand up and oppose it. With hindsight we know that Whistle-blowers or heroes who oppose discrimination can change history. When Jews in Denmark were forced by the Nazi's to wear identificatory yellow stars, the Danish King adorned one himself, followed by the rest of his subjects – which defeated the signifier's specificity. But often ordinary people can have amazing effects. By defiantly refusing in 1955 to give up her seat for a white person on a segregated bus in Alabama, Rosa Parks triggered the movement for civil rights for African-Americans in the USA. Subsequently, white Freedom Rider supporters also needed courage as their integrated buses were fire bombed by angry mobs. Similarly, the many demonstrators who marched during the Arab Spring. Even small acts can have an effect.

> **Dialogue**: Think of a racist joke.
> *What you do when someone tells one?*

Prejudice can take subtle forms, often appearing to be based in physical, sexual or genetic differences. The Greeks assumed that because women have wombs they are *'hysterical'* and behave irrationally. But only 100 years ago women were regarded as intellectually inferior due to their smaller brains. And until recently 'unwed' mothers and their 'illegitimate' children were ostracised. Today in the UK over 45% of births are to unmarried women (vs. only 12% in 1980). [We must remember though to read statistics with a critical eye: for instance, of 34 EU countries surveyed, the highest unwed birth rates occur in France, some Eastern European nations (Bulgaria, Estonia, Slovenia) and Scandinavia (64% in Iceland, 55% in Sweden and Norway, and 46% in Denmark). These figures reflect not only reduced stigma but complex demographic vectors, such as different rates of cohabitation. Likewise, single motherhood: in countries with low divorce rates like Spain, Portugal, Italy and Greece increasingly, women choose to remain both unmarried and childless, and the general fertility rate is very low indeed. with only 6% of mothers unmarried (Eurostat Yearbook, 2010)]. Statistics can be manipulated and although information may be caged in scientific language, we must read critically, and review our own assumptions and challenge generalisations which tend to perpetuate dominant values but obscure individual needs and different choices.

Teenage mothers

Young mothers are often pathologised for deviating from the 'norm' of older, better educated, and/or married mothers. It is true that immature not-fully developed bodies can lead to obstetric complications, yet it is unjustified to generalise from this to inadequacies in mothering. All of us have encountered emotionally mature adolescents who manage to fulfil their chosen role as well as many older mothers or fathers do. Equally, we have all met disturbed older parents. It is not *age* per se that creates problems but the juxtaposition of incomplete developmental tasks with high parenting demands, and often, detrimental social conditions. Similarly, single mothers may do as well (or as badly) as partnered ones. Research all over the world shows similar findings: *What counts most is whether mothers have support and a friend in whom they can confide.* Sweeping statements about the need for marriage may sound convincing; but social conventions do change.

> **Large group discussion**: Do children need fathers? [3-5 minutes]

In societies-in-transition like ours, we can no longer advocate one 'correct' life-style. *What is important is the quality of relationships.* But nor can we afford to be unquestioning. We have tended to marginalise fathers but much research shows the detrimental effects on children of their absence.

Similarly, an association exists between low educational attainment and economic adversity. This is a socio-political problem. With adequate child-care facilities and financial grants, teen parents can be helped to complete secondary school while their children are young, and/or can train vocationally, or go on to tertiary education at a later stage, when older women are interrupting their own career paths to have babies (or fertility treatment). But such decisions are influenced by social conditions, including job availability, for young people.

> **Reflective thinking:** Ask yourself: <u>We were blind to sexism not long ago. What might be our blind spots today?</u>
> *[Self-study: use Journal. **Group:** 3 minutes discussion. Leader uses flipchart]*
> <u>NOTE</u>: Be bold!! The aim of this training is not only to raise self-awareness, but to generate a capacity for critical and creative thinking.

Socially constructed representations

The UK today seems more like a pluri-cultural society rather than an integrated multicultural one. This detracts from a potentially enriching cross-fertilisation. In London, one of the most ethnically diverse cities in the world, over third of the population belonging to minority groups, and about 300 languages are spoken. As a practitioner you may have many clients from ethnic groups different from your own. Although we overtly express commitment to cultural diversity, behind PC sounding pledges our non-conscious prejudices often remain operative behind the scenes in unprocessed 'us' and 'them' feelings. Our selective focus, jokes and thoughtless comments tacitly endorse common beliefs about specific groups – 'Gypsies steal'; 'the Irish drink too much', 'the Scots are mean', 'the English are… fair/ brutal/ cold/ welcoming/ stiff-upper-lipped/ eccentric', etc. Such assumptions not only brand a whole group but colour our own expectations of how individuals will behave – which

> *Internalisation is the process whereby something becomes incorporated as part of self identity*

as we have seen, can invoke the very behaviour we anticipate.

In our busy daily lives, many of us rarely pause to wonder what it feels like to be marginalised. Nor do we acknowledge that an 'outsider' view may include a candid perspective of 'us'. Worse still, these prejudicial conceptual networks (whether age, sex, race, religion or class related) not only dis-empower people, but can come to be taken in and internalised, affect a person's self-image, behaviour and actual performance. The converse is true, too. A before-and-after study at Vanderbilt University in the USA, revealed that black students gained 20 points on previous exam results when tested again shortly after Obama's election!

We tend not to question the origins of prejudice. The socially constructed hierarchies we encounter are not givens, but 'man made' (patriarchal?), and differ cross-culturally. But whatever they are - in common, the prejudiced person or group feels superior to those designated as inferior, whose subjectivity and 'sameness' is denied, which in turn, gradually affects the *self-concept.* However, with conscious effort, this process can be reversed: as Women's Lib put it: *'We are not 'beautiful'! We are not 'ugly'! We are angry!'*

Or in the words of Steve Biko: 'Being black is not a matter of pigmentation – being black is a reflection of a mental attitude. Merely by describing yourself as black you have started on a journey towards emancipation, you have committed yourself to fight against all the forces that seek to use your blackness as a stamp that marks you as a subservient being' [Steve Biko, the 'father' of Black Consciousness, 1971. *I Write What I Like*, Picador, Africa, p.52).

Socio-Cultural Competence:

This is the ability to understand and interact effectively with people of different cultures. It entails an awareness that one's own worldview colours what we see. And that our potential bias can be overcome by an *open mind* – suspending our own beliefs in a receptive attitude towards difference (age, gender, ethnicity, etc), listening and being willing to question our assumptions.

This is a circular tactic: by making a conscious decision to become more 'culturally competent' and treating each encounter as <u>unique</u>, we listen differently and can dispel some of our own automatic racist, sexist, ageist reactions and discriminatory beliefs and practices. However, we need to remember that as practitioners, our theoretical conceptualisation too, primes our sensitivity and interpretive orientation.

> **Self-study and group participants** are reminded to use their Journals to record thoughts and feelings after this workshop so as to honestly re-examine some preconceived ideas about ourselves and others. And to continue doing so, on an ongoing basis, privately and in peer groups.

Healthy Ambivalence

Prejudice can be disguised. We express it in seemingly neutral but generalised formulations. For instance the statement: 'All mothers love their babies' does not take account of different bonding rates, healthy ambivalence, circumstances of conception, variation in the desire for intimacy, and a temporary breakdown in a mother's capacity for empathy. A psychoanalyst-paediatrician once listed 18 good reasons why mothers feel hatred towards their babies (without acting on it) (see Winnicott, 1947). Similarly, practitioners may dislike their clients' behaviour at times. However, when ambivalence is *denied* by parents (or practitioners) they tend to feel compelled to relate in a 'sentimental' way – idealising the baby (or client), and/or projecting their negative attitudes elsewhere, and similarly, we may treat our teenage client as a dependent or monstrous 'alien', rather than acknowledge similar human frailties in themselves.

When we are with young clients, the asymmetrical power relationship adds clout to our pronouncements. Our advice may be followed unquestioningly; or some small criticism we make may be experienced as an accusation leading to shame and confusion. Conversely, a simple helpful suggestions may be taken as an attempt to 'rule' their lives and our attempts at reassurance are often seen as 'patronising'. How do we get it right?

Threesomes' Exercise: <u>Superstition</u> [*5 minute discussion in threes]*:
A client says that her partner's mother insists that she hang a chicken-bone above her (mixed-race) baby's crib, to fortify his bones. *What do we say?*
<u>The Post-Exercise Message:</u>
It a painful experience when we discover that our thoughts, feelings and interactions are riddled with prejudice.
But, we need not remain bound to social intolerance. *What can we do?*

Emotional 'literacy'
A non-judgemental self-aware practitioner can better establish an *authentic relationship* which accommodates a mixture of feelings in herself and the client. We become more aware of the many factors driving emotion, including a striving to repeat and/or repair emotional damage. We know that having a baby retriggers many intense uncontrollable feelings of disappointment, frustration and rage, especially towards carers.

A young mother in the throes of trying to differentiate herself from her own mother while dealing with the powerful contradiction of herself becoming a mother while still so close to her own childhood yearnings is likely to arouse complicated feelings. Ironically, recognising our irritation and resentment helps us to behave more respectfully towards others. Owning our own destructive impulses and fantasies without acting on them harnesses our emotional understanding. If we take *responsibility for our own feelings*, including hostility, even and especially towards the people we care for, genuine *empathy and concern* can arise. This applies not only to the individuals in our care - but to disparate gender, racial, religious or ethnic groups in whom we project aspects of our own idealised or repudiated selves.

Summary:
This first workshop can be summarised through three concepts:

<u>Meaning Making</u>
- We try and make sense of new situations.
- In times of uncertainty and threat we revert to old *expectations* and solutions, 'transferring' feelings from previous situations to new ones.

- In a 'dialogue' there is pressure to *'actualise'* the other's non-conscious expectations and fantasies (through our 'role responsiveness').
- However, personal encounters are about getting to know another person's mind.
- If the practitioner remains open to the client and gains his/her trust, receptivity to new experience is boosted, with willingness to grow.

'Co-Creation'
- Meanings are *'co-constructed'* in interaction with others, partaking of the particular sub-culture in which we are each embedded.
- When two people interact, each brings in their own forces, mutually regulating the interaction between them.
- In close relational encounters, especially emotionally charged ones, the strongest habitual responses of each partner are activated (including presumptions and prejudice).
- If engagement is ongoing and frequent, the exchange between them increases in complexity yet 'settles' into a recognisable reciprocal pattern.

Intersubjectivity
- For practitioner (or parent), inter-subjective recognition means taking the client's (or child's) subjective perspective into account as well as their own.
- An intersubjective approach that holds the client's feelings in mind, offers her/him a chance to learn about minds.
- If we can accept each other as a subject – our respective subjective meanings, influence and are influenced by the other's mind – thus co-creating a *new* situation.
- New understanding destabilises old relational patterns, generating a shift.

Conclusions:
The mind of the other is opaque as long as we are unaware of their secret histories and unspoken thoughts. Relationships are co-constructed by the expectations of both partners, which may be actualised as each puts unconscious pressure on the other to exemplify what they anticipate. As practitioners, we have to develop emotional awareness of our own contribution to the 'co-constructed' relationship with our clients. Similarly, we must develop socio-cultural competencies, learning to question prejudice and detrimental procedures, and to identify our own idiosyncratic or negative reactions.

Key Concepts:
Expectations; Actualisation; Role Responsiveness; Collusion; Prejudice; Co-construction; Internalisation.

Major Themes**:**
Difficulties in engaging teenagers as clients.
Reactive arousal of practitioners' feelings, including contributions of our own resonating adolescent experiences, biases and blind-spots.

Module I:
INTER-RELATIONSHIPS

2. Skill-Building Seminar:

The inter-connectedness of minds:
Co-Constructions and Mentalization

Learning objectives:
This seminar develops the practitioner's interpersonal skills to engage teenage clients, to activate their own and the client's capacity for mentalization, including curiosity about her/his own feelings, and those of the baby.

Effects of Past Relationships on Relationships
We have learned that supportive practitioners who '*contain*' their own emotions can do so for their teenage clients. In turn, through gradual internalisation of the care they receive, young parents can begin to provide this 'containment' for their babies. But, as noted, teenage clients are difficult to engage.

Exercise: What are successful methods of engaging teenage clients?
Self-study – *write a list in your Leaning Journal;*
Group discussion - *Use whiteboard, power-point or flip chart to write suggestions. If the following points do not arise spontaneously, include them:*
- A non-judgmental approach
- An informal invitation (texting reminders)
- yet maintaining upfront and clear boundaries
- Make it fun! Capitalise on their curiosity
- Focus on the teen NOT the baby
- Providing a familiar setting for the first meeting (café?)
- Establishing a support network of other teen mothers,
- Befrienders, advocates, etc.
- Engaging fathers? Other family members?
- Encouraging responsibility; understanding; empathy

Through respectful engagement young parents can begin to take responsibility for their own mixed feelings. By learning from the practitioner they become better at accepting, processing, and empathising with 'difficult' emotions of the child (or partner), while simultaneously maintaining a clear boundary between self and other.

This becomes noticeable in more agential descriptions of feelings: 'I feel afraid', 'I am angry, sad, confused, guilty...' rather than victimised depictions: 'I feel persecuted, manipulated, neglected, rejected'. 'S/he makes me feel mad...'

When early in life a person has been subject to inadequate or damaging care with little understanding of her/his emotional needs or even recognition of major preoccupations – this not only creates negative expectations of care, but leaves deficits: whole areas of exchange that have become closed off cannot be explored or communicated.

In encounters with the 'caring professions' young people whose principle carers have let them down may be wary of intimacy and unable to form close relationships.

Wounded people guard against being hurt again.

Adolescence as a 'Second chance'

Building up trust will require extra sensitivity, reflection and tact on behalf of the practitioner. How do we do this?

Skills: Building trust and a good relationship

*[**Group:** Use flipchart to write participants' ideas. Introduce the issues below. Self-study: write in Learning Journal]*

- Be honest; set boundaries; maintain values
- Ask the teen-client what s/he would want in their 'ideal world'.
- Acknowledge *difficulties of motherhood* [unpatronising praise; build on positive strengths; offer a role model]
- *Do not offer solutions* to family problems and 'baggage', but empower the client to stay with the pain, and consider how his/her thoughts, feelings and behaviour are conveyed and interacted within the family.
- Help teen evolve *reasonable expectations* about the child, to enable her/him to respond to emotional cues, to offer encouragement, set limits and foster awareness of consequences.
- *Name* conflictual feelings and help the young parent to think about her/his own inner experiences, and possible sources of repetitive patterns of behaviour.
- Help the young person *take responsibility* for his/her own feelings, becoming aware how language both expresses and shapes our self-concept as agents or victims.

Each new intimate encounter evokes a medley of old expectations and anxieties

---

Here are some psychoanalytic concepts may help practitioners understand why certain clients behave towards them in ways which may feel incongruous:

Co-Construction: Transference & Counter-Transference:

Freud noted that all findings are re-findings. *Asymmetrical situations of dependency* (such as the power-differential between an older practitioner and a teenage client) are particularly charged. These encounters arouse old feelings of vulnerability, frustration or distrust derived from care-situations in childhood. In therapeutic exchanges in which the client feels freer to voice whatever arise, feelings transferred from the past are more in evidence: a living, changing expression of internal 'working models' (as Bowlby called our expectations of care). Impulses, conflicts, and defences arise as undigested residues of primary relationships, now 'transferred' into the present relationship.

These unlaid 'ghosts' from the past are transferred onto us which explains why sometimes our clients treat us as other than who we are (as a 'saint', a traitor, fairy godmother, monster or omnipotent persecutor...). The emotional experience may be enacted with us. It forces us to experience what the client is experiencing thus providing a sense that their feelings can have an impact.

Transference changes over time, such that the same practitioner is at times experienced as a withholding 'witch' or a generous mother; a strong or weak paternal figure; a helpful or rivalrous sibling and so on, depending on heightened feelings at different points in their exchange. The emotional quality of transference provides us with a glimpse (rather than a full accurate picture) into the past. What materialises in the client's mind client to be projected onto us gives us an inkling of their own experience with caregivers in childhood and possibly, what is possibly now being projected onto the baby in their own care. What is transferred is a *'relational climate'* – an overarching internal representation of different attachment experiences with varying degrees of security.

> **'Transference'** — is a set of intense feelings, unresolved emotional issues and relationships from the past which are unwittingly transported into new situations.

But it is even more complicated. A practitioner who is depicted as a loving, omnipotent, neglectful or rejecting parent may also be treated at times in the way that parent treated the child, for instance with a tirade of criticism about never getting anything right. We suddenly feel what it was like to *be* the child of that benign or malevolent parent. And as we now know, expectations and internal representations can actually *induce* responses, bringing about the anticipated reactions – so the practitioner may in actuality begin to get things wrong, like the child of that critical parent!

Understanding transferred feelings is very intricate as the same emotions can stem from different motivations or simultaneously express different anxieties. For instance, the client who constantly heaps praise on the practitioner may reflect a wistful yearning for praise, indicating of how s/he would have liked to be treated. But it might also constitute a form anxious placation of a potentially critical and frightening figure – or both. The important thing is to recognise this complexity – and that you can never fully understand your client. But you can explore the feelings through those that are aroused in you.

Counter-transference:

Luckily, we can get a 'feel' for what is happening as the client's unconscious relational expectations activate specific feelings in us. The psychoanalytic term 'counter-transference' refers to feelings that include your intuitions, 'gut reactions', and non-conscious impressions of the client's emotional gestures, bodily stance, tone and delivery which are registered somatically, as well as our conscious responses to her or his expressed attitudes and anxieties, and unconscious pressurising projections.

> **'Counter-transference'** feelings — are the 'totality' of the practitioner's emotional reactions, fantasies and feelings evoked in relation to a particular client.

Affecting the practitioner, these feelings also provide subtle hints of denied or suppressed feelings in the room. In fact, sometimes, the unspoken desires and feelings we pick up in this way are at variance with what is being consciously verbalised by the client. For instance, when s/he chatters on but the usually articulate practitioner finds herself tongue-tied and/or unable to 'name' what s/he is hearing, it may be indications of unmentionable feelings in the client.

But – the practitioner must also consider that for she is worried for reasons of her own, about the feelings this area of discomfort may arouse in her.

> CAUTIONARY NOTE: This is sensitive stuff. It is important to convey that the work-interchange is 'muddied' by a practitioner's own unresolved 'baggage' and reluctance to learn something about him or herself. Likewise, workers, and indeed whole teams, can be hampered by their unacknowledged counter-transferential responses to the client's suffering, or 'stirring'.

Co-constructed systems

Our counter-transference feelings enable us to *experience* emotional aspects of the client's early care situations – not only how s/he felt, but what their carers felt about them. Sometimes we resonate to the client's feelings. When our sensations feel 'strange' to us, we recognise them as reflections of the client's non-verbal communications. For instance, a sudden feeling of breathlessness or chest pain may be somatic reflections of the client's sense of emotional suffocation or 'broken-hearted' suffering. Our counter-transference feelings can also help us to build up a picture of some of the teen's silent expectations which unwittingly lead to repeatedly responding to practitioners (or others) like someone from the past. Exploring this with the young person can be relieving, if s/he feels listened to and believed. *Evoking the client's curiosity in their own feelings is crucial.* However, our interpretations of their behaviour must be tentative, and respectful of mental states. But, the emotional pull can be strong, and ideally, the practitioner can empathise with the adolescents' anxieties and dilemmas, yet retain a separate and distinctive view. Feelings that cannot be thought about tend to be enacted. Putting them into words helps makes sense of the psychic pain, and may help to grasp avoided or unremembered experience. Teenagers' attitudes to the past can change through having a 'second chance' to stop and think about, rather than enact feelings. The capacity to find one's own psychic experiences *meaningful* leads to better emotional understanding, affect regulation, impulse control, self-monitoring, and the experience of self-agency.

Small Group Discussion: The Practitioner's 'baggage'
[5 minutes]. *Participants form small groups of 4 or 5, with those sitting either side and/or immediately behind them, to discuss:*
What is personal 'baggage' and how does it affect interaction with clients?
Stop the discussion and ask for ideas [2-3 minutes].*Write these on flipchart.* [Elaborate on the metaphor of 'baggage' – suitcase full of fancy stuff, treasures, dirty washing, torn clothes…needs sorting]. Now ask for individual feedback about feelings during discussion – awareness of internal/interactive pressures and expectations [5 minutes]. *[**Self-study**: write your thoughts in the Learning Journal]*

Monitoring our own feelings

We all have our own 'hang-ups' and need to become aware of them. Freud, for example admitted that he was discomforted by being treated as the mother in the transference. In our own work, memories of being an adolescent, and how we ourselves were treated by carers affect the situation, as do our unexplored feelings about sexuality, aggression, drugs and the myriad other deeply stirring issues teenagers bring. We may feel seduced or turned off by the excitement, or get intensely involved in 'dramas' the young client brings. Close encounters are co-constructed in the subtle give-and-take between transference and countertransference, often without our conscious knowledge. As we have learned, interaction is a two-way process and we infuse our own listening to the client's utterances with our own subjective ideas.

In an asymmetrical exchange, it is important to recognise that we are there to try and understand our *client's* mind. The relationship between practitioner and client is vital because in helping clarify some underlying issues it can enable the teenage parent to find meaning in her/his own and other people's behaviour, including the child's.

Therefore we must monitor our feelings. Sometimes, when these *resonate* with those of the client, it is difficult to know to whom they belong. Again, we ask ourselves: 'Why am **I** feeling this now?' adding – *'I wonder what I make the client feel?'*

> ...*'it is an extraordinary thing that the Unconscious of one human being can react upon that of another, without passing through the Conscious.'* (Freud, 1915.p194).

Knowing one's self, a practitioner may recognise 'strange' feelings that are clearly evoked by the adolescent's unconscious desires, for example the need to be punished or indulged. Various specific responses in us such as boredom or irritation may be created by the teenager's defences against their own unbearable feelings of anger, fear or anxiety which they find too hard to think about or to express. When the young person defensively disowns anxiety, and denies feeling it in what is clearly an anxiety provoking situation, this may be because the anxiety is all projected into the practitioner, who feels over-anxious as a result. But — we too transfer feelings and expectations from the past. The source of anxiety may lie in our own reluctance to address an issue, not because of concern over the client's vulnerability but due to our own fearfulness, prudishness or distaste.

At times it can be difficult to distinguish between impressions which derive directly from the *client's* contributions and those which emerge from our own troubled past experience. Whereas the former can serve the practitioner as an intuitive instrument to better understand the teenager's feelings, the latter may form a powerful intrusion, or an impediment to the unfolding interaction.

When, rather than picking up on the client's unexpressed feelings, a practitioner's 'baggage' leads to defensiveness, it inevitably impairs our ability to remain receptive to the client. It is therefore important that each worker reflects on unresolved personal issues which might be impeding their work.

> *Peer or individual supervision is helpful in seeing one's blind-spots.*

We must consider that our counter-transference response may be based on *identification* (as opposed to *empathy*) with the teen-client. Her/his transference may 'needle' us or push a 'button' relating to unprocessed issues from our own adolescence which arouses our anger, anxiety or hostility.

There may also be *an unconscious correspondence of fantasies* between a particular client and us, such as the teen's wish to be rescued and our own wish to rescue. Conversely, the practitioner may be so identified

> *The crucial aspect is our capacity to think about such feelings.*

with the teen's baby or toddler, seen as deprived or maltreated, that it leads to one-sidedness and lack of empathy for the young parent/s own difficulties. If *an impasse* in communication arises it is important for the practitioner to determine whether it is evoked by resistance in the client or in her/his self. Difficult counter-transference feelings should be monitored and elaborated on in one's private Journal or brought to supervision (for further understanding of the role of the Learning Journal in Self-study, please see p. 201 of the Training Manual).

Team work

It is an interesting observation, that *agencies,* too, can have their own counter-transference responses to clients' transference. A disorganised client who expects the worst can cause chaos among a variety of workers, with loss of a coherent work strategy. Likewise, some types of problems posed by particular clients can create over-zealous or competitive responses or a sense of 'drift' in the system that manifest in delay, with avoidance of urgency, or even a form of 'paralysis' among professional teams.

Sometimes, a young client may *split* the transference between professionals – with one regarded as 'bad', intrusive, bossy or hostile, and another seen as the sole source of 'good' stuff. The temptation for a worker to angrily refute or try to live up to these transference expectations, or for one to brand the other is a good reason for practitioners to meet to try and pool their information and respective opinions when dealing with a shared client. Open communication can help them to examine different ascriptions, and to resolve potentially contradictory responses.

> Cautionary Note to the Leader:
> The workshop is not a therapeutic session. It is therefore necessary to protect practitioners from self-disclosure in the large group. Encourage participants to reflect at home in their private journal about their emotional responses to the issue of counter-transference. The message is that in working with clients, it is up to each of us to carefully observe and monitor our feelings and to ponder the origins of particularly strong or unusual emotions. Hopefully, through self-reflection such reactions can be better understood, contained and not enacted in the exchange with the client. More difficult issues with particular clients should be taken to supervision. This message is reinforced in small Reflective Work Groups, where personal accounts are more permissible.

It is important to remember that in any encounter, expectations participants bring to an interaction affect the other. Each dialogue is *co-constructed* and influences are *bi-directional*. Emotional involvement can feel scary, and past expectations are powerful deterrents. However, past feelings are not just 'transferred' into the present interchange hoping to be actualised. They are also affected by the actual experience. The contact with you may be the first time the client experiences an *authentic* caring relationship.

A practitioner who understands some of the client's anxieties can draw on the reality of their 'here and now' relationship to explore and co-create new ways of being together. Thus, in addition to positive or negative, transference and counter-transference feelings, a practitioner who builds up trust can count on a work alliance with that part of the client that wishes to bring about a healthy change.

> *A 'work alliance' introduces a respectful and ethical sense of joint purpose.*

If Reflective Work Groups are set up they offer a place for the practitioner to explore in detail how the young person may be encouraged to think about emotional causes, explanations, and solutions to their problems to help reduce their victimised feelings of grievance, anger and/or self-blame and sense of need to be punished ['the price of sin'].

Interactive Skills: Exploring unknown territory
These strategies may help you engage your client in a 'work alliance':
- Help the client to create a coherent life story.
- Tentatively name and summarise some recurrent problems and anxieties.
- Help the client to think about these and to seek her/his own solutions.
- Identify and strengthen the young client's strengths.
- Provide a *model* of thinking about feelings
- Try to understand misunderstandings and admit your mistakes.
- Don't collude with the client's desire to please you.
- Increase the client's confidence to endure uncertainty, frustrations and obstacles.
- Stress that the client's new capacities can help her/him to think about the baby's feelings too.

'Here and Now'

We have learned that like any other intimate encounter, the exchange between practitioner and client engenders complex *interweaving* feelings. Transference and counter-transference are interactive processes, which importantly, relate not only to the client's past but to the *'here and now' meeting*. When things go wrong, the practitioner must ask her/himself what s/he might have done to stir up these intense feelings at this moment, and must acknowledge mistakes.

We keep the young person's mind in mind, and try to help her/him to keep the baby's mind in mind, thinking of the child's needs as separate from her/his own.

We reflect back what we see. This reflective process is activated by exploring the client's ideas about what is happening between us and them self, and giving some feedback on these. This can be an effective way helping the young person to understand and cope with feelings, by recognising the connections and differences between one's own perspective and that of somebody else. Acknowledging that others have their own emotional reasons for doing things enhances the client's capacity to 'mentalize'. When issues can be addressed honestly, this authentic form of relating provides opportunities for growth, for the practitioner as well as the client. But we must recognise that each partner in the exchange experiences an internal struggle between *a desire to understand the other and resistance to such new understanding.*

Interim Conclusions:

Interaction is systemic. A client's expectations are rooted in previous experience of other carers, and are transferred into new situations, colouring how you are related to and emotionally perceived. Understanding where these perceptions come from lessens the effect on your own behaviour towards the client. Furthermore, your own unresolved feelings ('emotional baggage') informs the way you approach *this* teenager which in turn influence the client's give-and-take and collaboration with, or resistance to, whatever is being offered.
- Together, you and the client *co-construct* an emotional 'relational climate' which consists of the 'here-and-now' as well as your respective preconceptions (including expectations, prejudices and childhood experiences of being care for).

- As practitioners, we try and contain our feelings, and avoid imposing an emotional agenda.
- We reflect back, drawing on our counter-transference responses to better understand (rather than meet) the client's feelings and desires.
- But empathy and reflective capacity are impaired by over-identification.
- To minimise collusion, we aim to be realistic about what we can offer given our own personal limitations, our caseloads and restricted resources.
- Our reflective thinking about why a young mother behaves as she does, and why we react as *we* do, may enable us to help her to reflect about herself and her infant.

Mentalization

Mentalization is a form of imaginative mental activity: the ability to perceive and interpret human behaviour in terms of mental states: emotions, needs, goals, intentions

As human beings, we all have the potential to 'mentalize' – to become more aware of our own feelings, and to try and 'read' the mind of the other, and understand their behaviour in terms of underpinning beliefs, hopes and desires. This capacity is honed already in infancy through interaction with carers who believe that the baby possesses a mind. Their awareness that internal experiences guide the infant's behaviour is inextricably interwoven with an appreciation of his or her own feelings and thoughts, as well as a capacity to reflect upon the baby's feelings – and to 'mirror' them back.

Psychological understanding develops through the perception of oneself in the other's mind, as a thinking and feeling person.

Reflective Function:
By 'mirroring' and naming the child's emotions, the parent sharpens the child's awareness of his/her own feelings, and of the mental states that guide human behaviour. The mother or father's reflective capacity pivots on their ability to think of the child's needs as *separate from their own* – and hence, on the carer's ability to take a different perspective. Parental 'reflective function' – holding mind in mind– means having the capacity to think about the baby's desires, intentions and vulnerability – and to cope with these without becoming overwhelmed by the infant's feelings or by one's own unintegrated anxiety or hostility. This in turn enables the carer to soothe the distressed baby, regulating fear or anguish without frightening or causing further disruption.

Even parents who had insecure attachments and traumatic events in childhood, can promote security in their children, if they are able to evolve a coherent and insightful understanding of their past. Conversely, when even a reflective mother or father is too stressed, s/he moves into 'survival mode' (Allen, 2006) and anxiety inhibits their capacity to mentalize or soothe the infant. *Stress engenders negative assumptions.*

Attachment and Mentalization

Clearly, reflective functioning is affected by both current stressors as well as negative experiences in the past. However, it is rooted in procedural memory and usually operates automatically and outside of consciousness. The way parents act with their child is predictive of the quality of attachment and of the child's capacity for mentalization. *Secure attachment* is linked to high parental reflective function – to the mother or father's recognition that their infant's behaviours are meaningfully linked to underpinning mental states. Through their interchanges the child gradually evolves a *'theory of mind'* – a dawning understanding that s/he and others possess 'minds'.

Insecure mothers (and fathers) who are low in reflective functioning disavow not only the child's internal experience, but their own! A carer who does not believe that an infant *has* feelings cannot mirror these. Parental inaccuracies or failure to reflect back feelings deprives that child of the building blocks for understanding the *meaning* of emotional reactions, his/her own and others'. In adulthood s/he may still lack the capacity to articulate these feelings. Conversely, a secure child begins to recognise that others may have different views, and that one's own behaviour influences that of others towards us. As we learned, how we come to perceive others and behave towards them is shaped by their behaviour towards us which in turn influences our ongoing mental representations of both self and others. In babyhood, body-image too, and knowledge of one's own appetites and sensations are also shaped by others, through their touch and physical baby-care – the intimate handling which includes feeding, bathing and the 22,000 nappy changes in the first year of life!

Thus, a parent's emotional responsiveness greatly influences the child's capacity for mentalization, and the extent to which s/he can finesse understanding of his or her own feelings and behaviour and that of others in terms of 'mental states' - thoughts, moods, motivations and beliefs about each other and the world. As practitioners, we too, differ in our capacity for mentalizing – from simple to complex awareness of the subtleties of our own and the client's states of mind.

However, under conditions of stress this reflective capacity is reduced in all of us. Our anxiety leads to controlling behaviour, prejudice and set expectations which in turn leads the client or child to perceive the carer as hostile and unsupportive.
Unaware of our defensive feelings or the motivation for them it is easier to deny that such feelings exist than to admit our fears, mistakes or 'weaknesses'. But through self-monitoring we can hone our own capacity for reflective function, and promote emotional understanding in our clients.

> Mentalization which begins to develop in babyhood, has implications for interpersonal relationships in childhood, and particularly, for intimate relationships in adolescence, and for parenting practices when that person becomes a parent. This training aims to enhance the capacity for reflective functioning in the

Adolescence as a 'Second chance'

Summary

'Mentalization' means interpreting our own behaviour and that of others in terms of underlying mental states, feelings, thoughts, beliefs and desires. It forms the basis of our capacity for human relatedness and 'mind mindedness' consists of

- Holding the other's mind in mind
- Understanding and repairing misunderstandings
- Attending to mental states in oneself and others
- Feeling curious about the feelings behind behaviours
- 'Seeing oneself from the outside and others from the inside'.

Large group discussion: <u>What does a teenage parent client need from the practitioner.</u> *These are some answers which may come up:*

- be trustworthy and reliable
- remain engaged without an agenda
- listen non-judgementally, igniting curiosity about interactive processes.
- be empathic but not intrusive. [Neither under-involved nor over-identified]
- be fair and not 'take sides' in external conflicts, or in the young person's own internal dilemmas but rather *voice the core issues*

The practitioner reflects back the client's feelings, validating their importance and remaining 'uncorrupted' (especially if the teen's world view is delinquent).

- identifies some of the underlying *anxieties* rather than becoming punitive
- clarifies *consequences* (e.g. of risk-taking) which the adolescent is unable to see, or succumbs to peer pressure in his/her decision making
- is attuned to the teen's own questions of *'who am I/what am I becoming?'*
- emphasises the importance of recognising feelings, in the baby too
- presents realistic options (return to education; acquiring vocational skills, helping the toddler make friends, etc.)
- helps the client out of poverty by increasing self-confidence, aspirations and agency (teaching the adolescent 'to fish' rather than feeding him/her)

Conclusions:

Interpersonal stress militates against mentalizing. When we practitioners have time and space for reflection we feel 'held' (by the trainer, line-managers, etc.) increasing the accuracy of our own reflective functioning, which enables us to provide better containment and understanding for clients. Parents tend to recreate the emotional atmosphere of their own babyhoods. By helping teenage mothers and fathers to think about their own feelings and to wonder what is happening in their child's mind, we can improve the quality of interaction between them, with better conditions for growth.

READING for next module: Waddell, M (2009) 'Why teenagers have babies'. This book, p. 216.

Key concepts:
Resistance;
Regression; Idealisation; Denigration. Mentalization, Reflective Function.

Major Themes:
An emotional interaction is bi-directional and co-constructed. Past feelings, expectations and emotional conflicts are transferred into the present interchange. Transformation occurs through reflective functioning.

Module II:
ADOLESCENTS

Aims:
The overall aim of this module
- to become more aware of subjective experience, yours and that of teenage clients
- to have greater understanding of the developmental tasks of adolescence
- to encourage mentalization and promote life-course improvement in teen parents

Learning Objectives
This module hones your capacity for mentalization and tools for promoting healthy fulfilment and reducing risks by timely detection of signs of emotional disturbance
.

3. Interactive Workshop:

Teens: Maturational Tasks of Early and Late Adolescence

This workshop explores maturational processes in adolescence and the ways pregnancy and parenting derail these. Participants can expect to
- become more aware of the complexity of the teenage client's emotional experience in reworking old issues while developing new capacities
- see the young parent's perspective in the struggle to accomplish her/his own developmental tasks while fostering the baby's
- be equipped to promote emotional understanding, coping skills and resilience

Adolescence as a 'Second Chance'

In the West adolescence is regarded as a *transitional period* between childhood and adulthood, extending way beyond the teen-age years. It offers opportunities for exploration, experimentation and play – a chance to re-engage with the past while consolidating adult interests, and time to question given assumptions and expand boundaries. The adolescent quest is to discover one's 'unique self' - but paradoxically, inhabiting a fixed identity is resisted and its actualisation postponed. It is socially accepted that during this prolonged period of reappraisal the young person will not be expected to take on full adult responsibilities. But clearly, for teenage parents, this is not the case!

In Anna Freud's words, *adolescence offers a 'second chance'* – to rework earlier issues and to find new solutions to old problems (1981:247). This potential for making healthy use of the emotional turmoil of adolescence underpins your work. With puberty, adolescents experience fluctuating moods which is one reason they seem so puzzling to their parents, and others. These include conflicts between exciting daydreams about autonomy and sadly relinquishing being the parent's responsibility.

Mentalization: What lies behind these contradictions of adolescence?
- Silence, need for privacy and sensitivity to external intrusions
- Talkativeness, loud music to block out internal intrusions
- Preoccupation with own feelings and lower attunement to those of others
- Social withdrawal yet deep concern about relationships
- Moodiness, irritability, unhappiness, intense reactions
- Confusion, impulsiveness, sadness, resentment, some acting out
- Panic attacks and lack of confidence coupled with ideas of 'invincibility'.

Adolescence as a 'Second chance'

Progress in adolescence does not occur in a linear developmental path, but is often marked by the return to old and familiar childish patterns of behaviour, needed to deal with anxieties related to loss of childhood, and the fantasies accompanying new sexual and aggressive feelings (Laufer & Laufer, 1984).

Mentalization: What lies behind these typical manifestations of early adolescence? [age ~13-16]

- Preoccupations with bodily changes, somatic experience & physical appearance
- Tension between exploring new ways and regressing to old familiar patterns
- Intrusion of infantile processes into more adult behaviours
- Boundary testing and search for control: struggle with parents/authority figures over limits and rules
- Mild antisocial behaviour peaking in mid-adolescence.
- A craving for excitement which may involve relatively benign means such as dance, music, competitive sports or more worrying risk-taking activities.

*[In a **group training**, for each of the following text-boxes, the Leader asks participants for their ideas, including examples. **Self-study:** expand these entries].*

Family alliances and the balance of power shifts as adolescents seek more independence yet paradoxically, as new bodily and cognitive changes disrupt previous hierarchies, confidence in competing with peers or succeeding intellectually at school, the young adolescent is driven back to needing parental reassurance. Challenged parents may feel bewildered by the contradictions. Those unable to provide age appropriate boundaries either over-intensify their control or abandon regulation altogether, thereby increasing the teenager's sense of abandonment or defiant rebellion in his/her search for adequate limit-setting coupled with warmth and support). A growing body of literature indicate the benefits of parental limit-setting, with poor parental monitoring clearly linked to negative outcomes in adolescence, such as antisocial behaviour, substance use and sexual risk-taking. One specific characteristic of early adolescence is that 'danger' is felt to be located both within - in impulses and fantasies, and without - in the very existence of the loved ones of her/his childhood, raising anxieties and a need for to differentiate from them. Young teenagers try to remove themselves from the parental presence physically by slamming doors, and emotionally by expressed indifference and/or opposition. At the same time they do want their involvement, sometimes secured by arousing concern.

The wish to leave home is openly expressed as a desire or threat, and sometimes,

---

Role Play: Task: to discuss a point of conflict *[5 minutes]*

1. Room is divided equally between – *'early' and 'late' adolescence.* Participants cluster in threes: an Adolescent, Parent/main caregiver and Observer/reporter.

2. The 'Reporters' inform large group of what they observed during the role play [maximum 10 minutes of brief summaries]

Message: Lability of teenage emotions indicates a creative search for *change.*

Self-reappraisal, the upsurge of feelings and tendency to question authority and progressive 'out of the box' thinking all offer teens a 'second chance', both to work-through emotional deficits and conflicts belonging to the past, and to achieve healthy authenticity in the present. But teenage parents have a double dose!

Practitioners must be able to identify disturbance in teenage parents who need referral to specialist adolescent psychotherapists for more intensive work.

precipitously acted upon. Conversely, the economic climate means a prolongation of dependence, with many people in their thirties still living in the parental home, unable to afford accommodation elsewhere!

Previously professionals advocated that ideally emotional detachment from early carers take place through a gradual mourning-like process, allowing for a period of reaffirmation of their relationship before the young person actually leaves home (A. Freud, 1938). The average age of menarche has dropped from 16.6 years in 1860, 14.6 in 1920, 13.1 in 1950 12.5 in 1980 to 11.7 in 2010!

Mass media intervenes: Internet,

> *Rapid engagement with sex short-circuits the slow processes of grieving the loss of childhood, and acclimatising to the pubertal body.*

television, music video and sexually explicit lyrics all contribute to the adolescent's individuating self-image and attitudes to sexual activity. Earlier puberty, peer pressure and glorification of precocious sexuality also impacts on pre-teens - 'tweenies' – further lowering the age of first sexual contact in western cultures. The adolescent who is hurriedly pushed through these developmental processes will bypasses the psychologically painful but necessary experiences of leave-taking (Blos, 1976; Laufer & Laufer, 1984). This has implications for teenage parents which places extra demands and heavy responsibilities on the young person.

Mentalization: What lies behind achievements of Late Adolescence? [~16-24]
- Interpreting one's feelings and finding one's own 'voice' and value
- Separating from the parents while recognising them as complex people.
- Trust in one's own creative capacity (not having to prove fertility)
- Confronting differences and similarities between the sexes and genders; and confronting the meaning of one's own sexual feelings
- Finding an appropriate position in peer-group hierarchy (or gang)
- Making more realistic plans for future

Maturational Processes

The prolonged learning phase of adolescence is both disrupted and accelerated by pregnancy and parenting, no longer allowing for gradual maturation in terms of fulfilling emotional, intellectual, social and sexual tasks – and achieving a balance between these. While separated here, these maturational (or developmental) processes are clearly intertwined. Precocious development in one area may jeopardise or enhance another. Interference with the usual trajectory of adolescent development necessitates extra help from family and practitioners to encompass both adolescent and parenting goals.

Mentalization: What constitutes teenage Emotional Development?
- Maturation involves increased mentalization vs. acting-out
- Greater capacity for tolerating frustration due to enhanced self-reflection
- Achieving a relatively stable sense of self
- Balancing tensions between dependence and a desire for self-sufficiency
- Achieving mind-mindfulness and management of own feelings
- Developing realistic self-esteem, acceptance and integration of mixed feelings and of multiple fluid complementary aspects of 'identity'.

Adolescence as a 'Second chance'

Camaraderie

Bodily changes in puberty mean that actual fertility and greater physical strength render childhood fantasies of impregnating or becoming pregnant, or beating up the withholding parents a real possibility. This feels alarming as internal controls are still labile. Timing of puberty has sex-linked effects: early puberty in girls may be a source of embarrassment and lack of emotional maturity to handle sexual advances while late-maturing boys suffer lower confidence and have a poor body image compared to their taller and stronger friends. Emotional instability and mood swings are typical and in vulnerable teens, reawakened childhood conflicts may be frightening, leading to escapist solutions and intensified risk-taking: eating disorders (anorexia, compulsive binging or bulimia), substance abuse and alcohol addiction, promiscuity, as well as self-mutilating, dramatic suicidal bids or aggressive tendencies. These often reflect difficulties in differentiating from the parents.

The *peer group* offers a new 'home' and feeling of belonging, a mainstay, especially for young people whose sense of identity is less than robust. A teenager's conscious self appraisal is bolstered by solitary and joint rumination, and participation in local group activities and a wider variety of youth culture. After puberty, spontaneous imaginative play may feel too dangerous, and to avoid the risk of inadvertent self-revelations, free play is replaced by structured pastimes such as computer games or boisterous group activities. Competitive sports or marshal arts also provide intellectual challenges and safe outlets for testosterone- boosted aggression. But like childhood play, roles are rehearsed and a variety of social stances and attitudes explored through dance; drama, social play; humour, mass media, and the many 'disguises' of popular youth culture including the vicarious emotional revelation of rapping or subversive song lyrics. http://www.youtube.com/watch?v=k6EQAOmJrbw

Internal conflicts and deliberations about 'identity' may find partial relief in email, blogs, Face-book, or other discussion groups. These time-consuming internet modes of virtual communication flourish, sometimes eclipsing face-to-face

> **Mentalization:** <u>what does Social Development entail?</u>
> * Openness to exploring the wider world (beyond family and school)
> * Reassessing external and internal self-other relations
> * Gradual disengagement from dependency on parents and elaboration of more complex relations to them
> * Learning to control aggressive/ sexual impulses
> * Moving towards intimate relationships
> * Gaining awareness of other perspectives

contacts. Today's UK teen-agers are estimated to spend nearly eight hours a day talking or texting and communicating electronically with others, of which only eight percent is directed at adults. Direct engagement may feel more formalised, and few teenagers find the internal emotional resources to free themselves from the binding social demands and gender stereotypes of their peers. Some invest their passion in religious or political groups, informed social activism or spontaneous youth activism, like those in Paris in 1968, the youth Intifada and recent Middle Eastern uprisings, or London street riots.

In the absence of transitional rites of passage, Western youth may generate inventive forms of group initiation with rituals of their own making, including endurance tests, and solidarity activities. Contemporary markers in establishing a common identity are clothes, hairstyles, tattoos and piercings. Local slang and accent simultaneously signify a contradictory message – a *subversive* provocation to adults, and a *conformist* declaration of belonging to a teen counter-culture. For many adolescents, a sense of identity is heightened by physically excelling - at bike stunts, break-dance, skateboarding, surfing, vaulting and other skills including rooftop leaping (Parkour or PK) which raise 'street cred' among peers. Engagement in extreme sports or delinquent acts and vandalism capitalises on the teenager's propensity for risk-taking, usually conferring higher status.

Commonly, as each generation of teenagers pulls away from the previous one they indulge in their own form of 'outrageous' shared experience. With extraordinary Flappers in the 20s, Hippy extravaganzas in the 60s, flamboyant Punk styled-hair in the 70s and the jet-dyed Goth hair, zipped clothes, distinctive body-piercings and tattoos of the 90s, each generation of teenagers creates their own style, new visual art and revolutionary musical forms as a creative challenge to parental culture. Across generations of teens, the dynamic attraction of specific kinds of music oscillates between tension and release. But there are ironies. At this very time of seeking 'autonomy' and 'grown up-ness', the pace and regularity of the rhythmic beat and repetitive tempo echo that of the (intrauterine) maternal heartbeat (see Rosenblum et al, 1999). Once a girl becomes pregnant and a mother she is rapidly excluded from these activities. Despite needing friends more than ever, she becomes increasingly isolated after leaving school, as her mates continue to celebrate their leisure-time in ways that preclude her unless she has family support or can afford a baby-sitter.

The second growth spurt
Until very recently there was a common belief that the brain stopped developing around age five. But with new techniques, neuro-scientific studies at University College London and elsewhere show that with the onset of puberty (and continuing right through adolescence and into the late twenties) the brain undergoes a massive wave of developmental changes. Rapid growth in the pre-frontal area is similar to that of the first two years of life, but is incomplete until the early 20s. But the limbic system of pleasure seeking and emotional reactions is highly activated, as in toddlerhood.

Mentalization: Thinking about thinking: how does teen Intellectual Development occur?
• Through mentalization and a search for meaning
• Taking responsibility for own thoughts, actions, beliefs
• Becoming aware of the consequences of decisions
• Self-discipline, beginning to consolidate work patterns
• Establishing interests, acquiring adult skill/knowledge, assessing future prospects. Making realistic plans

This very significant reorganisation is an adaptation which gradually helps the teen to develop the intellectual 'machinery' for meeting specific demands of his/her particular social environment in a changing world. Structural and functional changes gradually increase the ability to synchronise emotion and cognition. But in early adolescence, parts of the brain that deal with reward processing, and fight and flight are more easily aroused, and those that deal with harm avoidance and self-regulation are still comparatively immature (Steinberg, 2009) accounting for the high level of risk-taking, impulsive over-reactions and distractability. Higher and lower regions of the brain operate simultaneously, and taking responsibility for decision-making is complicated by the incomplete process of cognitive development (Patton & Viner, 2007). Needless to say, the developing brain is vulnerable to toxins including alcohol, drugs and even, nicotine –which are taken as hedonistic stimulants.

The adolescent's *mind* is also in a state of upheaval as anxiety-laden issues resurface, revitalising old preoccupations with sexuality, birth, male and female differences, and issues of love, rivalry, aggression, and death, first examined in toddlerhood. The turmoil is such that for many adolescents, previous defences prove inadequate to cope with the rapid alternation of focus between internal and external, upbeat and despondent feelings, and interpenetration of rational and erratic behaviours. Bunking off school, delinquent acts and extreme risk taking may seem to offer escape routes from internal conflicts as well as obligations In anxious insecure teenagers, tension arises between the thrilling yet frightening possibilities the future seems to hold, and both nostalgia and grief about losing the comparative safety of childhood. Because of these conflicts and the rapid hormonal driven mood swings, adolescence can be a frightening time for young people, who sometimes fear they are going mad.

The fundamental change of puberty
Heralded by appearance of secondary sexual characteristics and the onset of menstruation/nocturnal emissions, the main features of adolescence are *potency* and *power* – the potential realisability of desires and aggressive impulses. With menarche specific body issues predominate, associated with a female sense of fertility, sexual vulnerability and periodic cycles. A girl is forced to reappraise her body-image. Her familiar corporeal identity is disrupted by the disconcerting 'otherness' of the changing body. Self esteem is vested in physical attractiveness, and appearance becomes a central measure of selfhood, dominated by hormonal swings which affect

---

Physiological changes

Body: New capacities: physical strength, changing body shape and signs of virility/fecundity (menstruation and emissions). *Brain*: Gradual development of the medial prefrontal cortex [of reason, planning and executive function] with reversion to more 'primitive' brain areas inducing impulsive decision making.

---

her complexion, girth and mood. She sprouts breasts, pubic and underarm hair; her sweat smells different; the unknown interior of her reproductive body forces itself into her awareness, making its presence felt in aches, secretions and menstrual blood. The bodily enclosure, its monthly fluctuations and leakages, and ultimate restrictions of a 'biological clock' have to be incorporated. But some girls, unable to accept their new female identity, repudiate the change through anorexia, bulimia or binge eating, hysterical symptoms, self-harm and other attacks on the newly fertile body. These disturbances often reflect difficulties in differentiating from the same-sex mother. Cutting or self-burning can be a disguised attack on the maternal body, or on the pubertal body that seems to still 'belong' to mother. Premature pregnancy, too, delivers an unconscious communication to the mother, or a means of refusing adolescence. However, these problems are now so commonplace among western teenagers that practitioners may see them as a social trend rather than bodily expressions of identity confusion, depression, persecutory disorders, anxiety states and/or PTSD following childhood insecurity, deprivation or abuse. Similarly, for a teenage boy. The experience of uncontrollable bodily emissions, embarrassing erections and sexual impulses must be accepted, owned and managed. Male embodiment involves embracing a 'grown up' physique, with mental mastery over erotic fantasies and the physical strength to do damage. Sexual urges, and fears about loss of bodily control intensify with concerns about abnormality, accompanied by (often compulsive) masturbation and sexual experimentation. Vivid daydreams can also heighten anxiety, blurring the boundaries between imagination and the world of reality, as if thoughts and fantasies will be expressed in action.

> *Hormones:* kick in with puberty resulting in
> * Difficulty in concentrating/ emotional hypersensitivity
> * Altered sleep patterns – teens need up to 12 hours of sleep, beginning late at night until noon (some secondary schools now begin later to accommodate the teen's changed body clock)
> * Altered appetite: rapid growth. 80 percent of growth hormone is released during sleep and on awakening, like a young baby, the teen is very hungry.
> * Difficulty in affect-regulation and self-soothing
> * Many teenagers experiment with smoking, alcohol and illegal drugs although few use them regularly.
> * Experimentation among friends is less worrying than when alone.

Note: The Royal College of Psychiatrists notes that while Cannabis was previously believed to be relatively harmless, there is now good evidence that what is currently available is stronger, and can intensify mental health problems during adolescence, doubling the risk of developing schizophrenia.

Agency
The idea of becoming an adult and a 'subject' in one's own right, involves *agency* – disengaging from parental care and appropriation care of one's own body; making decisions and accepting the consequences. This involves shifting the family power structures which reverberates systemically within the family constellation. Part of the storm-and-stress complexity of a young person's mission lies in its *contradictory nature* — the dual task of both separating from the parents while maintaining identifications with them, when they themselves may have difficulty relinquishing their authority and recognising the young person's new capacities. As cognitive abilities grow, a sense of competent agency is crucial to the adolescent's self-esteem - in making choices, undertaking self-directed action, and feeling in control.

Ironically, in their own struggle to achieve 'self sufficiency', some adolescents may feel rightly or wrongly that they are being abandoned by the family. Disappointment in the parents during adolescence is inevitable, and accompanied by a sense of loss, loneliness and disillusionment (Blos, 1976). Indeed some parents may try so hard to grant their teenager autonomy that they renege on their responsibilities. An adolescent often has to look elsewhere for support - finding surrogate mentors and extra-familial authority figures as role-models, such as teachers, pop-singers, celebrities or – gang leaders, with peer pressure to bully or scapegoat others.

Sexual development
In girls anxieties proliferate, about bodily ownership, gate keeping and coping with sexual harassment, coercion or even rape. Popularity is linked to 'sexiness' and peer social pressure may induce girls to engage in sex before they are ready to do so, stirring up unconscious fantasies of illicit activities

> **Mentalization:** what is teen Sexual Development?
> * Achieving a coherent body image and sense of sexual identity and pride
> * Becoming aware of sex as an intimate encounter (vs. a physical activity)
> * Self-respect and responsibility for sexual body

and exaggerated dangers of skin permeability and threats of damage to the body interior or vulva during sex; fears about infections, genital abnormality or sexual aberrations. Crucial sex differences and universal similarities between the sexes, genders, and sexualities are endlessly debated. Simultaneously, there may be little information or reassurance and sex may be an embarrassing, even forbidden conversational topic at home. As in toddlerhood, in adolescence once again incestuous desires and aggressive impulses must be renounced, but now, precisely because such fantasies have become *actualisable* which increases the prohibition on discussing worries of a sexual nature, with parents or siblings.

Part of the confusing excitement is that when a fecund teen becomes sexually active, the Oedipal triangle is triumphantly rotated. Rather than excluded, the young person now is an *active* participant. The teen's security of attachment, and the solidity of his/her generative identity (confidence in a capacity to be creative rather than needing to procreate) will determine whether she or he succumbs to sexual excitement as addictive. Adolescents who have suffered violence at home, may fantasise they are the product of an aggressive parental coupling. In vulnerable adolescents, reawakened anxieties may lead to misguided escapist solutions. Some girls may confuse sexual arousal with anxiety, while boys might respond to anxiety with sexual and/or aggressive behaviour (Welldon, 2011). Combining imagination and bodily activity most teenagers utilise masturbation as 'trial action'. In health, *sexual experimentation* (another form of play) takes precedence over uncontrollable acts such as promiscuity, compulsive theft, self-harm or neglect of the body. However, when body ownership fails, hatred of the sexual body and its enticing forbidden desires may be enacted in suicidal attempts, risk taking behaviours and addictions, including gambling, alcohol and substance abuse, and violence (see Ladame & Perret-Catipovic, 1998).

Unconsciously some of the confusion of adolescence lies in an internal conflict between the wish to cling onto vestiges of having a child's body for which the mother is responsible, and an opposing sense of depression and self hatred for these longings. These vie with urgent feelings of excitement in possessing a body that is sexually alive, ripe for new experiences. The new body image means giving up the fantasy of idealised perfection of the pre-pubertal body looked after by the mother (Laufer & Laufer, 1984). Teens must now incorporate a sexually functioning penis or clitoris/vagina/ovaries and uterus.

High-risk sexual issues:
More than half of young people in the UK have their first sexual experience before the age of 16. Ironically, peer pressure to engage in under-age sex may be fuelled by bravado and false bragging by school friends about sexual experiences. Some teens are driven to promiscuity by pre-conscious yearnings to be popular, loved, stroked and needed. Apart from the risk of pregnancy, the significant threat of sexually transmitted infections (STI) may not register in the young adolescent's consciousness, especially during lovemaking.

Inconsistent use of contraception is due not only to ignorance or casualness. Despite awareness of the dangers, unprotected sex is often justified by reluctance to 'spoil the mood', the male preference, disillusionment with the pill or an invincible sense that 'it won't happen to me'. But it does, and teenagers are more likely than other age groups to use emergency contraception; failing to start regular contraception after this, they are repeat users. While many North American programmes emphasis *abstinence* as the only 'foolproof' way of avoiding pregnancy, the British advocate sex-education, and are currently trying to emulate the Netherlands which has the lowest teenage pregnancy rate in the West, starting sex at an average age of 17.7 years, with very low abortion and STI rates among young people, 93% of whom use contraception, compared with 53 per cent in Britain. The Dutch programme begins SRE with five year olds and sex is much discussed at home.

There are inconsistencies among studies which highlight various social demographics as disproportionately represented in high-risk groups for teenage conception, pregnancy, and STI. As noted previously, generalisations must be treated with caution as social stereotypes can skew research, obscuring cultural factors and individual differences within groups. For instance, statistics citing elevated rates of teenage pregnancy among particular ethnic minorities may include refugees from dangerous war situations with systematic rape. Or, by contrast to previous research, a recent London study showed that although black British and Caribbean young men do report earlier sexual activity, contrary to popular myths, they are at least as responsible about contraception as other groups. Furthermore, the same findings may have different implications. In a study in Hackney, amongst black African youth, high perception of parental disapproval was associated with *increased* risk of unprotected sex. By contrast, parental condemnation influenced young men and women from Bangladeshi, Pakistani and Indian ethnicities to start sexual activity *later*, but their use of contraception was no different from that of white British teenagers. See: http://www.education.gov.uk/research/data/uploadfiles/rw42b.pdf

An important conclusion is that *all* young people irrespective of their ethnic origins, require information, open sex and relationship education and access to contraception and sexual health services and practitioners who are supportive, sympathetic, culturally sensitive but receptive to their own personal needs. Needless to say, apart from contraceptive ignorance and bravado, there are many conscious and unconscious motivations for conceiving during adolescence, as we shall see.

Gender and Generativity

More than 100 years ago Freud proposed it is not anatomy, but psychic interpretation of one's body that determine aspects of our sex and sexuality. In keeping with his pioneering work today we accept that gender is not a direct expression of the female or male biological body but resides in a set of social and personal subjective beliefs— *how the mind perceives the body.* Gender is a highly personalised construct made up of various constituents. These components may be integrated or disjunctive, and change in salience and centrality at different life phases and in different contexts.

Self-study or group discussion: <u>What are the components of gender identity?</u>
1. <u>Sexual Embodiment</u> - gradual acquisition of a sense of *maleness/femaleness*
2. <u>Gender Representation</u> – of a *masculine or feminine* self-concept and psycho-social expectations of appearance and performance of roles and activities
3. <u>Erotic desire</u> – revisions of *hetero/homo erotic attraction*, including fantasies which may or may not be enacted in sexual activity and peer-defined expectations according to permissible parameters of the desire to love and be loved by a member of one's own or the other sex.
4. <u>Generative Identity</u> - self representation as a *potential pro-creator* which may find expression creatively or through actual reproduction (Raphael-Leff, 2007)

Gender formation is *a lifelong process* which emerges through primary relationships, bodily sensations and sociocultural experience. Gender identity undergoes revisions at life's transitional points including toddlerhood, adolescence, pregnancy, infertility, menopause, etc. when generative anxieties and meanings of gender are reinterpreted.

> *The experience of sexed subjectivity relates to psychic meanings not anatomy*

Reappraisal of Gender and Generativity in Adolescence
Sex, which reflects chromosomal status at birth, is distinguished from *Gender as a self-categorising psycho-social construct.* Gender's potentially fluid self-ascription also contrasts with the factual fixity of anatomical sex (although today sex-change operations mean that that too can now be changed).

One's gender begins to be established through early identifications and internalised potentialities which are consolidated during toddlerhood, when, heightened by *oedipal conflicts,* identification with gendered aspects of significant others peaks. Exciting fantasies about sole possession of one parent or sibling, and elimination of all rivals must be relinquished in favour of one day finding a mate of one's own outside of the family. With puberty, gender is re-evaluated with arousal of bodily excitations and myriad thrilling possibilities. The young person may feel the need for hetero and homo-sexual experimentation before allowing a sense of gender identity to consolidate.

In adolescence, the four constituents of gender (embodiment, representation, desire and generativity) are reinterpreted in the light of the new reality of actual potency. Virility inserts a boy as a potential link in the genealogical chain, as does menstruation for the girl. Retrospectively, childhood's expectations, appetites, identifications, feelings of 'omnipotence' and oedipal fantasies are revised. No longer a pre-potent child, the adolescent is now bound to another round of anxiety provoking reappraisal of sex, sexuality, gender, now including reproductive possibilities. Equally troubling are painful issues of *finitude*—consciousness of mortality, irreversibility of time, arbitrariness and the unfinalisability of identity.

Emotional Disturbances in Teens
Not surprisingly, adolescence is by definition a state of emotional turmoil, and four out of ten teenagers experience mild depression. Importantly, there is *a spectrum of distress*, between normality and severe disorders. We all experience various degrees of mental turbulence at different times in our lives, particularly under conditions of stress which mobilise deep anxieties. Disturbance is triggered by traumatic situations which rupture our psychological defences. These may be life-threatening or highly arousing events, including contagious arousal, such as caring for a baby and/or exposure to primal substances, or unmitigated close proximity to someone with mental illness [see p. 113].
Recent studies suggest that often severe emotional disorders in adolescence often go unrecognised, even by concerned family and friends. Several websites (for instance the Royal College of Psychiatrists or YoungMinds) are aimed at teenagers with advice on seeking help. In the UK, more than one in five teenagers feel that life does not seem worth living! Because of their tendency to impulsivity and risk taking, such

feelings must be taken seriously in teenagers as suicide is a real (if unintended) possibility, especially following breakup of a relationship

NICE guidelines advocate referral paths following detection and risk-assessment. Australia has set up a preventive network organization called 'RU OK?'

Suicide attempts may also relate to a dread of growing up. Hatred of body changes which have catapulted them out of the security of childhood may lead to furious or despairing attacks on the body which has betrayed them. Others loathe and punish themselves. It is estimated that one in five girls aged ten to eighteen self-harm in secret, using razor blades to cut their arms or thighs or matches to burn themselves. Some tear out their hair. Such attacks may not only self-mutilations, but a punishment to the mother who gave birth to this body. Some even succeed in stopping the processes of puberty, through anorexia. Practitioners must be able to identify adolescent disorders, including severe anxiety, repeat abortions; relational failures, reluctance to grow up, risky behaviours and depression and its attendant raised risk of suicide. Girls undergoing puberty at a very young age are particularly vulnerable to disturbance, as are immature teenage parents who have to cope with double predicaments of adolescence and pregnancy/parenthood. [Antenatal and Postnatal disturbances are detailed in modules III and IV].

The indicators below can help practitioners identify distress:

> **Skills**: Some Common Signs of Emotional Problems in Adolescents:
> * over-eating, or strict dieting, anorexia or bulimia
> * excessive daydreams, sleepiness and disturbed sleep patterns
> * a persistent over-concern with appearance
> * cutting or other forms of self-harm
> * severely fluctuating moods
> * prolonged periods of rage
> * severe anxiety with panic attacks or phobias
> * incapacitating obsessional rituals and defences. ·

Also see:www.rcpsych.ac.uk/mentalhealthinfoforall/youngpeople/adolescence.aspx

When disturbances are severe and beyond the remit of the practitioner, tactful negotiation with the teenager and referral to appropriate therapeutic services is crucial, especially when a baby is involved.

Gender Differences in Developmental Disturbance:

One way of identifying disturbance is to see it in terms of *failed social regulation* of sexuality or aggression. This may lead to uncontrollable acts (excessive daydreaming, vandalism, compulsive theft, eating disorders, violence or suicidal attempts) and/or risk-taking behaviours or addictions (gambling, alcohol, substance abuse and promiscuity).

In cases of *failed body ownership*, hatred of the sexual body or its enticing forbidden desires is enacted in self-harming attacks, self-neglect or compulsive sexual and other bodily activities reflecting unconscious fantasies (such as a search for authenticity, described above). Promiscuity or sexual contact with older men may reflect a search for the absent father (Waddell, 2009) or to some girls, cuddling, foreplay and heterosexual sex may unconsciously offer a chance to re-experience the most primitive contact between mother and child (Pines, 1988).

In many cases adolescent girls tend towards *'internalising'* (including secrecy, withdrawal, depression, anxiety and somatic problems) and boys towards *externalising* behaviours (anti-social behaviour, vandalism and aggression).

Why is this so?

Gender differences may be linked to the fact that most primary caregivers are female. The same-sex aspect of girls and their mothers/carers may account for greater female sensitivity to the social environment on the one hand, and a much higher rate of *somatised* bodily expressions of unbearable feelings, on the other. As we have noted, the early carer's misperceptions, disapproval, demands or rejection during the child's early use of her mind, are retained as procedural rather than cognitive memories. These are expressed psychosomatically. Maternal shame and/or anxious fantasies about her own feminine corporeality may have been projected onto her baby daughter's body to be unconsciously absorbed by her, which increases the child's difficulty in differentiating and possessing the changing pubertal body-image – a girl's attacks on her own body may be disguised attacks on her mother. Importantly, psychic representations of femininity and female sexuality are not merely 'all in the mind' but can impact directly on physical development. Adolescent girls, who resist growing up may actively deny their move to adulthood by becoming amenorrihic or anorexic, thereby avoiding the secondary characteristics of a fertile female body, such as breasts and menstruation. Conversely, triumphalism and a precocious desire to usurp the mother may result in premature pregnancy.

Others become addicted to NSSI (Non-Suicidal Self-Injury). Compulsively self-harming from a very young age, not in a state of depression but as a search for *authenticity* – getting to what lies 'under the skin'. Some seek the sense of control. Others get a 'rush' from seeing the skin rip or their blood drip. Yet others cause themselves physical pain to blot out psychic pain, or to feel 'real', to get relief from anger or find out who they are. Sadly, despite these poignant feelings and scars, their secrecy is such that they do not get help as the disturbance may not be obvious to others. see http://self-injury.net/resources/articles/general/why-are-so-many-teenage-girls-cutting-themselves

In recent years neuro-scientific advances that allow researchers to watch the brain in action have produced findings showing some differences between the sexes in brain function and connectivity. However, sex determination is not over by birth, and there are critical periods of development when the sexed features of a child's brain is particularly malleable. It is now clear that the effects of hormones and genes interact, and the contribution of genes is modified by experience, with implications for the wiring of the brain and, ultimately, for behaviour. Meanwhile, it is important to *avoid sexual stereotypes*. The crucial aspect in contemporary rethinking of gender is consideration of the needs of individuals, and for practitioners to help them to find ways to negotiate positive solutions.

[re 'neuro-myths' see: www. neuroeducational.co.net].

Mentalization skills: Self-reflection applies to the practitioner as well.
Ask yourself as well as your client: *'What were you thinking when that situation arose?' 'How did it make you feel?' 'Would you have wanted this scenario to work out differently? In what ways?'; 'Does this make you think of anything similar you might have experienced in the past?'*

Family Dynamics around Teenage Pregnancy

The average teenager is engaged in trying to evolve an authentic sense of identity by differentiating from other family members, especially parents. This process is affected by the emotional inter-relationships and feelings circulating within the family. Older parents, especially menopausal mothers, may unconsciously envy their daughter or son's youth and budding sexuality. Life stretches ahead for the teenager, laden with thrilling opportunities, just at the point when the mother feels herself to be unattractive and on the wane. This may lead to competitive activities (including the parent's affairs with much younger partners) or harsh restrictions, and sometimes, envious attacks on the teenager's creative ventures. Younger parents who feel that their pubertal child no longer needs them may choose this point in time to launch a work project or social activity that leaves the child feeling deserted. Some parents may decide to separate from each other and/or find another partner, or even conceive another child. It is not uncommon for daughters and their young mothers to be pregnant at the same time.

Although most young people tend to cultivate a feigned indifference to family happenings, *teen-age conception* often occurs in response to significant life events in the household (such as those mentioned above), or within the broader context of extended family and friends. The pregnancy may offer an opportunity for renewed closeness however, some parents resent premature grandparenthood and the extra demands on their time and resources: http://www.parentchannel.tv/video/becoming-young-grandparent-0 While teen pregnancy may constitute a family pattern, slotting the girl into four or even five generations of supportive mothers, other families find the stigma too much to contemplate, and if the girl refuses an abortion, relations with her nearest may sour.

Clearly then, excluding specific cases of contraceptive failure or ignorance, non-consensual sex or rape, there can be multiple conscious and unconscious motivations for conceiving. The propensity of young people *to enact what cannot be symbolised* may lead to a fantasy of omnipotence, and the bravado of teenage fatherhood and motherhood as a means of bypassing the emotional work of adolescence!

Large Group Exercise or Self-study *[jot down thoughts in Learning Journal]*:
<u>What are usual motivations for teenage conception?</u> (5 minutes)
Group: *call out motivations [5 minutes] writing ideas on flipchart.*
Self-study: *write in Journal — then explore the ideas below:*
- a desire to prove his/her fertility (vs. 'getting' a baby)
- seeking identity, purpose, value
- loneliness, low self-esteem, disillusionment
- to find 'someone to love'/ 'someone to love me'
- peer pressures/sanctioning or social rejection
- 'invincibility' or 'dicing' with fate: denying consequences of unprotected sex
- to keep a failing relationship
- to become 'fully adult'/ to emulate mother
- a means to get out of home, or to find a home (get a home?)
- an unconscious 'message' to her own parents
- to flesh out a fantasy baby
- a desire to recapture lost aspects of her [baby-]self
- to repair or renegotiate incomplete developmental tasks
- to create the 'perfect family'/rewrite history
- to cheat Death (especially in cases of life-threatening illness

Unconscious Motivations for conception

Pregnancy seems a means of establishing femininity in identification with the fertile, powerful mother who can create life (Pines, 1988). To others, identification with the pregnant mother is more narcissistic, a fantasy return to one's own origins by embarking on a journey like that her own mother undertook when pregnant with her daughter. To yet others, unprotected sex, like other forms of risky behaviour, contains a message to the mother, a bold declaration of body ownership. Like anorexia, cutting and self-harm, pregnancy may constitute a form of unconscious revenge on her mother – by attacking the body she used to look after or staking a claim of rights to do as she wishes. It may also signify a form of guilty reparation, giving the mother a baby to compensate her for past losses or for attacks the girl feels she once made on the mother, and on her babies born and unborn. She may wish to prove her fertility, to reassure herself of her intact body, undamaged by maternal retaliation (Klein, 1932).

The unconscious motivations for pregnancy are many and varied. Conception may represent a defiant act of becoming like the mother when this feels rivalrous and forbidden. Pregnancy may seem to offer a way to differentiate herself out from her mother while at the same time it unconsciously serves to preserve the connection - *'becoming'* the mother so as not to lose her. Conception may also be motivated by unconscious yearning for paternal love, by creating an 'Oedipal' pregnancy with an older man, in the hope of being looked after herself. Similarly, a teenage boy may wish to prove his virility, or become the father he never had.

Family Reactions

Emotional reactions to the news of the pregnancy by mother, father, brother, sister, step-siblings, grandparents, friends and the wider community, have a profound effect on young people's attitude towards it, including whether or not to terminate. Who they choose to tell about the pregnancy and anxieties around it says a great deal about family relationships. However, in most cases, the decision about outcome ultimately must rest with the young person. See: http://www.parentchannel.tv/video/pregnant-teens-and-young-fathers.

We know that around half of all teen pregnancies in the UK end in abortion. This may be a coerced termination when the prospective baby is rejected by the family. However, family disapproval can also lead to the teen's defiant retention of a possibly unwanted baby.

The relationship of her own parents to their unexpected grandchild can feel empowering, or healing to an insecure adolescent. However, at times it may retrigger an intense experience of 'sibling rivalry' if the young mother feels deposed by her own child and envious of the attention s/he receives, especially from her parents. Even if she lives apart from them, an adolescent mother may treat the child as a same-generational sibling in competition with her for scarce resources, needing intervention of a third person to provide care for her so that she can do so for the child.

In turn, the family of origin may already feel overwhelmed by having to handle the difficult contradictory mix of their daughter's bid for independence and adulthood, coupled with her clinging and regressive trends, with increased financial dependence and need for emotional support at this time of taking on responsibility for another dependent little person. Given the need for family support during this period of intense needs and prolonged growth *family therapy* may be indicated. This is urgent when decisions about termination are involved, particularly where there are powerful intergenerational conflicts, or religious or cultural counter-forces operating within the situation.

Teenage Pregnancy – a double crisis

The viability of an adolescent pregnancy is often a topic of extended family debate, and as such it becomes a receptacle for the expectations, wishes and projections from all family members. If it is decided that she continues with the gestation, she faces a **dual crisis** as the *emotional turmoil* of pregnancy occurs at the same time as that of adolescence. And the younger the girl, the more acute the double upheaval.

As noted, adolescence is almost always a time of disequilibrium. Some of the aroused emotions of pregnancy dovetail with teenage turmoil. Other needs are contradictory, and the double demands may push some vulnerable adolescents to their limits:

- On a physical level, some girl's view the newly *pubertal body* with anxiety or even repulsion. Menstrual blood may have raised confusions about inner-body intactness and fears about leakage and loss of control. Her bodily hair and vaginal secretions may be seen as puzzling, gruesome or dirty.
- Conception now introduces new physical sensations, discharge, tiredness, nausea and vomiting.
- Most teenagers are concerned with physical appearance and normality. The bodily signs and symptoms of pregnancy may seem 'gross' in the context of comparison with classmates.
- Nausea, unexpected vomiting and the uncontrollable growth of her belly and swelling blue-veined breasts are especially troubling, as are stretch-marks etched on her smooth skin, and new vaginal and nipple secretions, and areola discoloration marring pride in her fresh young body.
- Given the degree of stigma, a pregnant girl may experience dilemmas about maintaining total secrecy, telling a few carefully selected friends and/or dissociating and ignoring her symptoms while hoping it will 'go away'.
- At the very time of trying to assert her own *bodily ownership*, she is invaded by another, with blurring of boundaries between self and other which she may experience as pleasant 'communion' or competition over shared resources.
- Similarly, past and present cohere as she carries the baby within her as she herself was carried by her mother.
- While engaged in the quintessentially feminine experience – doing what only females can do – there is some confusion, as the process was triggered by a sperm, and her fetus may be male.

She thus lives with a state of internal contradictions and external uncertainty and unpredictability, hoping for and/or dreading a miscarriage. And if it occurs, may feel guilty, punished for her wishes, and frightened by the experience.

- If pregnancy continues, at a time when she is still sensitive about sex and sexuality – her *sexual activity* is disclosed by her swelling body.
- Then, with unruly *fetal movements*, anxiety is heightened by the idea of two people inhabiting her body. She fears that the stranger who now lives inside her and feeds off her resources knows her inside-out, and once born, will disclose her innermost badness and hidden feelings.
- In cases of girls who have experienced *sexual abuse* the sense of enforced intimacy during pregnancy reactivates issues of bodily invasion, loss of autonomy, bodily privacy, and sensual hyper-sensitivity.

- As she grows heavier (and feels 'fatter'), there may be both a desire for, and a dread of, *separation*. She may experience the idea of birth as loss – feeling she will never be closer to her baby than she is during pregnancy. Worries about damaging the baby during labour may lead to panic attacks. Anxieties about vaginal or internal damage and fantasies of bursting, being torn apart or emptied out are common.

Note to antenatal practitioners:
Teenagers are particularly vulnerable during pregnancy and anxious about the birth. The higher incidence of complications due to physical immaturity and emotional disturbance during pregnancy cause concern. *Teens need special attention* - antenatal information, support and continuity of care throughout pregnancy, labour, birth and at least the first six weeks postnatally. If the baby is to be given up for adoption, the matter needs to be addressed and worked through during pregnancy rather than sidestepped. If she wants to keep the baby it is important to foster a positive emotional relationship with the unborn child, if possible, hopefully involving the baby's father before the birth, even if they do not have a relationship. *Supportive work* with the wider family, the partners, or individual therapeutic work during pregnancy will influence the nature and degree of postnatal involvement. *Young couples* may benefit from joint perinatal counselling to help them through the transition to parenthood.

Conclusions
- During transitional states (like dreaming, adolescence, pregnancy and early parenthood) old unresolved/unprocessed issues are reactivated, raising acute anxieties about uncertainty, helplessness and annihilation, and primitive defences against these.
- Adolescence involves a regeneration of previous themes, now reworked in the context of realisable fantasies. The juxtaposition of adolescence and pregnancy raises the likelihood of complications due to the teenager's physical immaturity and emotional vulnerability.
- In pregnancy and postnatally the unknown baby becomes a *receptacle* for the family member's desires, anxieties and projections

Key Concepts:
'internalising' and 'externalising' behaviours; unconscious reactivations.

Major Themes:
Adolescent maturational processes - emotional, intellectual, social, sexual development and gender reappraisal. Unconscious motivations for conception, family reactions to pregnancy;

Module II:
ADOLESCENTS

4. Skill building seminar:

Psychological Processes of Pregnancy
& Teens as Parents

Leaning Objectives

> - Skill building to foster insight, awareness of difficulties and recognition of emotional disturbances during pregnancy and early parenthood.
> - To promote relational skills in practitioners and resilience in clients

'Disequilibrium' in pregnancy

Many women experience a high degree of emotional receptivity during pregnancy. This heightened experience is one of psychic permeability to pre-conscious impressions. Such close contact with the unconscious may feel quite weird. Qualitative studies of pregnant women's emotions have found a range of 'symptoms' such as mood swings, vivid dreams, magical thinking and 'premonitions', as well as more disturbing depressive reactions and primitive anxieties, intrusive thoughts, introjective and projective mechanisms (see Glossary). Mixed feelings and elaborate day-dreams are not uncommon, as the pregnant woman 'plays' imaginatively with all the possible scenarios of her future baby and motherhood.

> *The many months of pregnancy provide an opportunity for the young mother-to-be (and her partner?) to get to know the baby in her womb – to notice patterns of sleep and waking, movement styles, to learn more about the amazing capacities of the fetus and to think about the impact their own life-style and intake decisions have on the unborn baby.*

Expectant Fathers

We tend to forget that the partner of a pregnant woman also may need attention at the time when so much is focused on the expectant-mother. In fact GPs find that co-habiting fathers-to-be tend to visit the surgery more frequently than usual for them, and with parallel ailments (back ache, nausea, weight gain, food cravings, insomnia etc). These 'couvade' symptoms, recognised in many societies, are usually disparagingly referred to as 'sympathetic pregnancy'. However, only recently several biocemical studies have revealed that potential fathers too, are affected by pregnancy, including *hormonal changes*! Like other primates who share hormonal changes during pregnancy these may play a role in priming males to provide care for their offspring.

Hormonal shifts in expectant parents

- Expectant fathers and mothers have similar stage-specific changes in hormone levels, including higher concentrations of prolactin and cortisol in the period just before the birth, and lower postnatal concentrations of sex steroids (testosterone or estradiol) seemingly to optimise baby-rearing.
- The stress hormone cortisol levels spike about four to six weeks after men learn they're going to be fathers, subsiding as the mother's pregnancy progresses. This

is assumed to be a 'wake-up call' to the impending reality of the new baby, alerting the man to think about the future.

- Male elevated levels of prolactin echo the high levels in pregnant women (it stimulates breast milk production); cortisol is found to be higher in mothers who bond more responsively, are better able to recognise their own infant's odours, and are more sympathetic to his/her cries.
- In the three weeks after the baby's arrival, levels of testosterone (the 'male hormone' associated with competitiveness, aggression and sex drive) drops by roughly a third, seemingly to enable the new father to focus on the baby.
- It may also serve an adaptive response with a reduced desire to have sex just prior to the birth as well as the decreased need to engage in 'fight or flight' behaviours, or extra-marital affairs.
- Social factors also intervene: in 1959 only 4% men attended birth; now 94%. Animal research has shown that exposure to the birth reduces the propensity to attack newborns, or even increases maternality.

Hormonal shifts in cohabiting men seem to be sparked by exposure to the pregnant woman's hormones and may similarly prepare them for parenthood. A father's testosterone levels creep back up as the child grows and becomes less vulnerable but there are suggestions that the stimulation fathers experience wile interacting with their children (even if they do not live with them) may elevate prolactin levels. *Researchers stress that hormone levels are not predictive of fathering behaviour and there is no 'normal level' of paternal hormone change.* However, alteration in hormone levels have now been well documented in North America, and recently, in East Africa, Jamaica and China. More study is required to establish if a similar response occurs in non-biological fathers.

[For more details see:
- http://www.mayoclinicproceedings.com/content/76/6/582.short
- http://www.sciencedirect.com/science?_ob=ArticleURL&_udi=B6T6H-403W3KX2&_user=10&_coverDate=03%2F31%2F2000&_rdoc=1&_fmt=&_orig=search&_sort=d&view=c&_acct=C000050221&_version=1&_urlVersion=0&_userid=10&md5=2f824d6efdb861b129d2a701ba9818ec]

Even for those young men who plan to participate in a 'hands-on' way with baby-care, finding a way to be involved during pregnancy may seem daunting. A common experience is one of being marginalised by professionals and the girl's family alike. A teen father often feels left out in antenatal clinics, with no role in labour other than as a 'coach' rather than a loving partner and expectant father. There may be subtle put-downs in parent-craft classes as though men need to learn what comes 'naturally' to women. But given a level 'playing field' are equally sensitive in interpreting and responding to baby cues.

Both sexes are equally capable of baby-care

Sex distinctions

Far from the blissful period usually imagined, pregnancy triggers many emotional issues which may aggravate the situation between previously amicable sexual partners. Initially these may relate to the conception as unwanted by one or both of them. The young man may express doubts about the baby's paternity. He may envy her capacity to gestate his baby or resent her bodily control over their fetus. Conversely, she may envy his intact body and nausea-free transition to parenthood. He might resent her sexual inaccessibility, her

Even in the most egalitarian couple pregnancy dramatically highlights the difference between the sexes.

tiredness and the emotional changes of pregnancy and her inability to participate in 'fun' social events or to fulfil household duties to his satisfaction. On the other hand, his sense of exclusion or jealousy of her closeness to the fetus and later breastfeeding the baby may mirror her envy of his relative freedom compared to her own.

Other scenarios of conception may be the result of unwanted sex or even rape. *International and UK evidence find that at least of 4% of teenage conceptions are due to non-consensual sex*, with a history of sexual abuse as a precipitating factor as well as current intimate partner violence. Indeed, studies exploring teenage motherhood as a consequence or legacy of childhood sexual abuse have noted the disruption to young women's lives and their increased vulnerability to revictimisation, substance misuse, mental health issues and poor school attendance. Understandably, there is also a decreased likelihood of using contraception while under coercive partner control which inhibits a young woman's ability to retain autonomy over sexual intimacy, including condom use (see Coy et al, 2010).

Clearly there is a need for therapy, but this is also an issue for *sex-education* among young boys, including emphasis with teenage youth about a continuum from macho expectations to non-consensual sex, dispelling bravado, exaggerated masculinity and myths of 'uncontrollable' male sexual urges, as well as female drunken incapacitation and susceptibility to sexual coercion, etc.

In some cases the baby's father may not know about the pregnancy or impending birth. Or may be uninvolved due to his disinterest, or problems with drink or drugs. Some may be in custody or live far away. Some are older men. Indeed, in the USA, of pregnancies to an adolescent mother only 30% to 50% involve a father younger than 20 years at the time of the child's birth. So in a high proportion of cases, the baby is fathered by a much older (often married) man, who may refuse contact or has minimal input after the conception. For a variety of reasons, some men may be excluded completely by the pregnant teen or her family.

Mentalization: <u>What underpins the subjective experience of pregnancy for both partners?</u> *[5 minute Debate]*

Pregnancy is a function of an interactive effect between 3 intertwining systems:

- *Physiological experience***:** new sensations, symptoms, antenatal tests and ultra-sound scans, physical complications, etc - which are interpreted in the light of
- *Personal representations***:** fantasies, hopes, fears and wishes within a representational set of complex connections that may include imagery of the sexual partner, changing body image, the unborn baby, emotional relationship with own parents and attitudes to parenthood - coloured by
- *Socio-cultural expectations* about pregnancy, maternal and paternal identities, collective beliefs, and the actual experience of emotional/social support systems and teen interactive networks.

Adolescence as a 'Second chance'

Pregnant adolescents

<u>Preoccupations during the three phases of Pregnancy:</u>

1. During the initial phase, the girl is usually preoccupied with the new experience of **pregnancy** – its emotional meaning for her, her physical symptomatology and unwanted effects of hormone production (e.g. initially high nausea-inducing progesterone), and changes in her body shape. If she is not in a state of denial, there may be deliberations about termination or remaining pregnant.

2. By the second trimester her focus centres on **the fetus** as her inner world changes with the increasingly defined movements of inside her. Any sense of body ownership she has achieved is now disturbed by her unruly occupant. To some there is a sense of close bonding, to others a feeling of being exploited. Social relations alter too, as the pregnancy now declares itself to all and sundry, and abortion becomes more complex. Negative and positive self-attributions and a view of the fetus inside her as benign or malevolent are woven from the stuff of her fantasies and past emotional experience. These representations are highly influential and if they persist unchanged until after birth, will colour the primary relationship from the start.

3. In the third trimester preoccupation revolves around the idea of a **real baby** - with birth anxieties, and concern about what kind of baby she will be 'getting', the many changes in her life and how she will measure up in becoming a mother. There is often intense rejection of the idea of breastfeeding - fearing that her newly grown erotic breasts will be commandeered by the baby, as well as anxieties about indistinguishable uterine and orgasmic contractions (Raphael-Leff, 1991, 1993)

Mentalization Group or Self-study: <u>what preoccupies the mind of a pregnant teenager?</u> *[debate or explore your own thoughts, then examine the ideas below]*

- Confusion as pregnancy superimposes physiological transformations on her already unfamiliar pubertal body image
- Anxieties about her appearance as 'obese'
- Shame (and/or pride) at being shown up as sexually active
- Alarm at the uncontrollable nature of hormonal fluctuations, emotional lability and the baby's movements inside her
- Pressure to make realistic preparations for the baby while feeling so uncertain of her own identity and emotional resources
- School work demands while preoccupied with the pregnancy, or if she leaves school, exclusion from ordinary peer-group activities and social isolation.
- Anxieties about coping with labour pains, and vaginal stretching
- Doubts about her ability to mother a baby

Skill building: <u>Fostering bonding:</u>

The pregnancy months offer a chance encouraging the young woman to *cultivate a relationship with her unborn baby*. Anxiety relates to feeling out of control: Supportive specialist midwife or social worker can explain the preparatory changes occurring in her body and mind, focusing on her processing and working through *feelings that need resolving before the birth*. Reduce anxiety that her body feels no longer within her control *relaxation and breathing techniques* to decrease panic attacks during pregnancy, help her fall asleep despite discomfort, and assist in labour. Learning to recognise signs of imminent labour and what to expect during the birth reduce uncertainty. Information about who she can have with her during antenatal classes and labour, and knowledge about different kinds of pain relief and their availability during labour, and provision of a doula can all make the difference between an anxiety ridden third trimester and a relatively calm one.

Antenatal Representations

Research has found that postnatally, adolescent mothers' representations of their babies at one month are related more to their antenatal ideas than to the infant's actual behaviour (Zeanah et al, 1986).

During pregnancy, when for many months the woman is actually joined to her baby through the umbilical cord, her feelings about their two-way connection involve both giving out and taking in: her own contribution to placental 'feeding' and her absorption and dispersal of fetal waste products through her own body.

Placental Paradigm

The various positive and negative permutations of a pregnant woman's representations of this *placental coupling* of her unborn baby and herself as container/mother are influenced by her own conscious ideas and unconscious fantasies about her baby-self in relation to her own archaic mother. Different notions about the placental exchange conjure up different emotional climates in pregnancy (Raphael-Leff, 1993).

Skills: Detecting emotional disturbance during pregnancy

Placental Paradigm

Self-as-mother	*Fantasy baby*	
R e p r e s e n t a t i o n s		
(archaic mother)	*(baby-self)*	Manifestation:
Mixed ideas: +-	+-	healthy mixed feelings
Fixed ideas: +	+	idealisation
−	+	depression
+	−	persecution
−	−	anxiety
+|−	+|−	obsession
+/−	0	detachment

A teaching model for identifying antenatal disorders: '+' & '-' signs indicate positive or negative representations; ['+|-' = obsessional separation of 'good' and 'bad']. © Joan Raphael-Leff, Psychological Processes of Childbearing, pp.55-9; Anna Freud Centre, 2005

Most pregnant women experience healthy mixed feelings which alternate and change even in the course of an hour (due to the baby's movements, her own mood, activities, social interventions, tiredness, hunger, sexual desire, etc.). Other women have 'fixed' ideas. If these remain unmitigated, they augur badly for the future relationship. For instance, a woman who idealises the baby and herself as mother will be disappointed in the ordinary one she gets and the good-enough mother she will become. One who sees herself as empty or bad and unable to provide what the vulnerable, perfect being inside her needs, will feel guilty and depressed. Another who regards herself as benign but feels invaded by a parasite feeding off her resources, feels persecuted. A belief that she and the baby are incompatible, and bad for each other raises acute anxiety which might lead to abortion, or months of suffering. One who has breakthrough ideas about harming the baby will have to spend an inordinate amount of mental energy to obsessionally keep bad thoughts, images, doubts or ruminations away from the 'good' aspect of the baby in her mind.

A young woman may protect her fetus by defensively projecting 'badness' elsewhere – developing phobias about certain foods, places or cosmetic substances as dangerous during her pregnancy, or paranoid anxieties about her midwife or other carers. If she talks about these, we may recognise repudiated facets of her own internal world projected outwards. It is worrying when the baby who is both part of her yet separate is regarded as a source of danger. However late in the pregnancy, she may become determined to have a termination to rid herself of the 'bad' thing inside her. If the pregnancy continues and her baby-phobia is not mitigated, this results in fetal abuse, hitting her belly or starving the baby inside, or even planning infanticide. Despite the shame involved, hopefully, she will confide her worries to trusted relatives, friends or practitioners.

A woman's representations of this placental connection define *the emotional climate of pregnancy* which may involve a great deal of suffering for the woman, and can affect the unborn baby as well.

Note for antenatal practitioners:

The 'Placental Paradigm' (above) is a schematic model that helps us to conceptualise different disturbances. + and - signs signify positive or negative feelings, irrespective of the specific content of the fantasy (this means the model can be used in different cultural contexts). Specialist midwives and other practitioners who see the young woman during pregnancy or health visitors can address the inflexible nature of fixed representations, suggesting that if troubled by it, the pregnant teen may wish to understand the origins of her all-enveloping feelings. *Rigid mono-thematic ideas during pregnancy* justify referral for perinatal counselling with the aim of mitigating the need for such powerful defences to prevent them becoming incorporated in the relationship with the baby postnatally.

SELF-STUDY HOMEWORK: read: http://birthpsychology.com/free-article/ unraveling-our-beginnings-embryonic-science-fetal-psychology

Antenatal risks
There is now evidence that the expectant mother's affective states during pregnancy – particularly depression, anxiety and elevated life stress are associated with subtle alterations in the neurobiological substrate of the fetus' emerging affect regulation system (Bergner et al, 2008). Apart from biochemical transmission a pregnant woman's emotional state may also have an indirect effect on the unborn child through the distressed young woman's poor clinic attendance or unhealthy lifestyle. Depression, persecution, anxiety and childhood abuse are associated with unhealthy eating and smoking, alcohol, drugs, self-harm; risk-taking behaviours including suicide and enactments. Adolescent consumption habits and erratic lifestyles as well as bodily immaturity raises the incidence of complications during pregnancy and of preterm delivery. Babies born to teenage mothers have an increased risk of low birth weight and 60% higher rates of infant mortality.

In studies conducted around the world, *maternal diet*, especially during the early months of pregnancy has been found to have a profound effect on the child's future health, and research into pertubations of the materno-fetal supply line shows that offspring are more vulnerable in later life to the effects of a variety of diseases if their mothers were malnourished when pregnant (Burton, Barker & Moffett, 2011).

Intimate partner violence also tends to increase during pregnancy, with at least 10% of pregnant women affected [Also see Module IV, skills based seminar 8]. Domestic violence includes 'any incident of threatening behaviour, violence or abuse (psychological, physical, sexual, financial or emotional) between adults who are or have been intimate partners or family members, regardless of gender or sexuality (DH 2005) during pregnancy puts the woman and her unborn baby in danger. It increases the risk of miscarriage, infection, placental abruption, fetal fractures, ruptured uterus and physical disability, premature birth, low birth weight, fetal injury and death. In fact, domestic violence has been identified as a prime cause of miscarriage or still-birth, and according to the report on confidential enquiries into maternal deaths in the United Kingdom (CEMACH) many of the women who died during or immediately after pregnancy had reported domestic violence to a health professional during the pregnancy.

Demographically adolescents are more susceptible, especially with an unintended pregnancy, tendency to delayed antenatal care, smoking, alcohol and drug use, lack of social supports and STI/HIV/AIDS. Nonetheless, as we know domestic violence can arise within any religion, ethnic/ racial group, at any socioeconomic level, educational background or sexual orientation. Apart from the direct effects of spontaneous abortion, fetal injury or death from maternal trauma, indirect effects of maternal stress are increased smoking, alcohol or drug use due to anxiety. There is an elevated rate of maternal postnatal depression and physical risks for children in the household, and to the baby once born.

The ubiquitous nature of antenatal care offers opportunities for screening and advice, and when questioned in 2011 many British pregnant women agreed with instituting a policy of monitoring. Health care professionals, especially midwives will receive special training in identification and care of women experiencing domestic abuse, including formulating sympathetic responses to disclosure; clear local protocols and

> A US project's Acronym RADAR:
> **R**outinely screen every patient
> • **A**sk directly, kindly, nonjudgmentally
> • **D**ocument your findings
> • **A**ssess the patient's safety
> • **R**eview options and provide referrals
> (Massachusetts Medical Society, 1992)

referral pathways with continuity of midwifery support, flexible appointment times and if necessary, venues, and providing more than one opportunity for women to disclose. http://www.midirs.org/development/MIDIRSEssence.nsf/link/ 757181624A03A2D38025783B00502D7A?

Their duty of care towards the fetus indicates that with or without disclosure by the woman, if a midwife suspects there is harm or potential harm it should be raised with the Supervisor of Midwives. Apart from obvious injuries or unexplained missed appointments, a practitioner may be alerted by psychological manifestations of fear, anxiety and depression, flat affect, dissociation and other symptoms of PTSD with startle responses and/or over-compliance to the partner, who may present as overly solicitous, hostile or demanding, or very controlling.

Disclosure is very difficult because of shame, threats, economic dependence and other sensitive reasons. It is most important that they are believed and the response to their admission is received warmly. It is often hard for practitioners to know what to say under such stressful conditions. An obvious spontaneous response is tell the client you are sorry she has been hurt and that it is not her fault. She did not deserve to be treated this way but help is available.

Antenatal emotional disturbance

A longitudinal study of over 10,000 women found that *maternal anxiety* is transmitted in pregnancy through high levels of cortisol passed to the baby through the placenta during gestation, and retained in abnormal cortisol levels after birth. These are found to be linked to behavioural problems, anxiety, attention deficits, hyperactivity and behavioural problems in the offspring, at age seven. If the mother had been stressed during the third trimester an effect was still found even when the children had reached the age of ten (O'Connor et al, 2002).

Clearly, antenatal practitioners are in a prime position to identify a woman who is highly anxious, depressed, feeling persecuted or troubled during pregnancy, to support and prepare her for referral for psychotherapy asap. Therapeutic treatment before the birth is advantageous in alleviating the mother's condition before it becomes established in the relationship with the infant.

Naming Perinatal Emotional Disturbances

Manic states	*[masked by pregnancy 'elation']*
Depression	*[risk of suicide]*
Persecution	*[risk of infanticide]*
Anxiety	*[panic states; risk to fetus]*
OCD	*[rumination/intrusive ideas]*
Detachment	*[as if not pregnant- risk:neglect]*
PTSD	*[flashbacks, nightmares, emotional numbing and/or heightened arousal]*

The Royal College of Obstetrics estimates that up to *one in seven women experience a mental health problem* at some point in pregnancy or after the birth.

- Depression and/or anxiety are the most common antenatal mental health problems, affecting up to thirty out of every hundred pregnant women.
- Some 20% of pregnant women suffer depression by 32 weeks antenatally, of whom 6% are still depressed at 8 weeks postnatally; others who were well during pregnancy develop PND after the birth.
- 20-40% of depressed mothers also report obsessional thoughts of harming baby.
- Some 30% of pregnant women suffer anxiety, as many do postnatally.

Skills: Screening Statements for fixed reps.

Depression: *During this pregnancy I've had thoughts of hurting myself*
felt quite sad without knowing why
Anxiety: *During this pregnancy I have felt anxious or had panic attacks with out knowing why*
Persecution: *The baby seems as intruder or parasite inside me*
A battle goes on inside me between what I need for myself and what the baby wants from me
Obsessional thoughts:
Strange ideas come into my mind about hurting or molesting the baby
Detachment
Pregnancy will not affect my life one bit
[JRL, 2011]

Many emotional changes fall within the normal range of pregnancy *'disequilibrium'*. These become worrying only if associated with 'fixed' feelings and/or behavioural risks to the woman herself or her unborn child. For instance, suicidal fantasies, severe eating disorders, substance misuse (nicotine, alcohol or drugs), incapacitating compulsive behaviours, phobias, panic attacks, self-harm or elevated risk of intimate partner violence. Where these are identified, the client should be referred rapidly for perinatal counselling or psychotherapy. 'Talk therapies' are popular during pregnancy as they do not involve drugs and evidence on their efficacy [see *Scientific American*] demonstrates that psychodynamic psychotherapy not only works, but keeps working long after the sessions stop. http://www.scientificamerican.com/article.cfm?id=talk-therapy-off-couch-into-lab&page=2

Positive supportive relationships help foster *resilience* – the ability to cope effectively with stress, to adapt to change and to recover from adversity.

Note for practitioners:
Offering your young client your emotional support during pregnancy can free her to overcome some trepidation and defensiveness. However, if she has fixed ideas that are not responsive to reason, you must help her accept a referral for professional help. The argument that perinatal therapy can alleviate future problems in the relationship with the child is a good incentive.

Teen Mothering

"Don't do that!" shouts the young woman on the bus at the young baby on her lap, slapping the little hand that pulled her earring.

Caring for an infant is an incredibly demanding task. Continuous close physical proximity and exposure to 'primitive' feelings open an unexpected trapdoor to one's own sub-symbolic reactions. To remain responsive, a closely attuned empathic carer has to keep her/himself receptive to the baby's emotions, galvanising all his/her own mental capacities to fathom the non-verbal non-conscious communications. Many new parents find this defenceless open state very threatening. Single parents who cannot share their minute to minute ordeals with a concerned partner feel even more susceptible if they are *unable to debrief*. Very young parents are further hampered by lack of experience and emotional immaturity. While some are exceptionally able, most teenager parents feel overwhelmed by premature full-time responsibility for the physical welfare and emotional needs of a dependent infant while still feeling dependent and confused about identity.

Practitioners working with teenage parents have at least two clients in need of empathy whose diverse wishes and developmental processes can coincide or clash.

In the West, where adolescence is acclaimed a carefree period, it is difficult for a young parent to give up the activities of their contemporaries. As we've noted, their capacity for empathy and competent reflective functioning are undermined at times of stress and adolescent self-absorption. Feeling harassed and afraid the baby's demands might escalate, they lash out angrily in self-defence. Lacking sufficient guidance and unable to put these anxieties into words, they impose rigid routines or clutch at false certainties to reduce their trepidation and panic states.

They are not alone. Studies find that most new mothers of whatever age and in a variety of cultures find parenting difficult. A cross-cultural study of eleven countries find some form of morbid unhappiness after childbirth is widely recognised, and associated with crying babies, feeding difficulties and baby health concerns in the context of isolation, lack of emotional and practical social support, poor relationships with partners, family conflict and tiredness (Oates et al, 2004).

In societies-in-transition such as our own, where extended families are dispersed, and childrearing traditions have been eroded, it is a daunting task, even for older women. to remain attentive and attuned to the needs of preverbal baby for whom one has total responsibility. Difficulties in a mother's capacity to respond empathically to her child's needs derive from ongoing current stressors as well as issues in her own developmental history.

A young mother who has not yet achieved self-determination may feel caught between conflicting loyalties. Still emotionally entangled with various members of her family of origin, she may feel embroiled in their concerns. This may impede her full emotional investment in the new family of her own making. In fact, on an practical and economic level it may be impossible for her to extricate herself, and she may feel unable to take decisions for her baby who is simply incorporated into her own mother's realm. Conversely, a young mother who (of choice or necessity) is living separately from her family may not have sufficient emotional support to maintain her independence from them.

> *The practitioner's awareness of the separate needs of adolescents and their babies, and of the complex dynamics of inter-relationships is crucial in her work.*

Mentalization Exercise: What characterises teenage parents' reactions? *Group: Use flip chart. Small groups (2-5) discussion, 5 mins+5 mins total report-back to large group.. Self-study: record your answers in Journal. Then check these out:* Shock at the irreversability: "what have I done?"
- Discrepancy between fantasy expectations and reality of parenting
- Daily struggle – re housing, money, sleep, relationships
- Putting their own needs first; or treating the baby as an 'extension'
- High self-expectations and fear of being judged as failing in parenting
- Deprivation – feeling they have 'no life'

When the transition to parenthood conflicts with the ordinary preoccupations of adolescence, a young person needs some *'time out'* to contemplate away from the baby, and to do her own teenage thing, while the all-consuming responsibility of looking after her baby is reduced.   Otherwise, the unmitigated demands of caring for the child will inevitably generate resentment in the young

Reflective thinking: positive features of teen mothers:
- Flexibility, spontaneity, 'going with the flow'
- Enjoying the moment – pregnancy and parenting are not 'projects' to be studied
- Less sentimentality: can be brutally honest about experience ['Breastfeeding is gross'…]
- Keen to learn
- Playful: treat child like a sibling

person, leading to defences, distortions and a desire to escape. Her good-enough mothering of the baby may alternate with benign neglect, or guilt-ridden defensive over-involvement or an impulsive flight from accountability. It is essential that *respite* is built in as a provision for young parents, with support or even co-parenting when possible. A repeat or second pregnancy occurs in 35% of adolescent mothers within 2 years of the first birth, with 17% of those adolescents going on to deliver a second child in that time frame.

Self Study: Watch the Oscar winning short film 'Wasp' directed by Andrea Arnold and write your reactions to it in your Learning Journal

---

In my view this is essential viewing for anyone involved with young parents, giving a 'behind the scenes' view of what it feels like on a day to day basis.

Information: The film is available for download or to watch online from various urls. At the time of writing the ones below seem to operate.
- http://www.imdb.com/title/tt0388534/
- http://www.download-finished.com/archive/andrea-arnold-wasp-uk-2003-23min-s16mmavi.html
- http://www.youtube.com/watch?v=jKPg7-GbK8Q

If you wish to purchase the DVD it can be obtained from Amazon as part of the Cinema 16 series of Cinema16: World Short Films and Cinema16: European Short Films (US Special Edition) DVDs, and as a bonus feature on the Fish Tank DVD in the UK. Also see European Films: http://www.cinema16.org/dvd.php?dvd=4Wa

---

Group Training: The **Oscar winning film 'WASP'**, produced & directed by ANDREA ARNOLD, 2002. *[23 minutes]. Leader: allow 30 minutes for large group discussion/debriefing.*

After the screening allow for few moments' silence after this very shocking film, then encourage a group discussion [15 minutes] asking:

What feelings did film arouse in you?

Once many have spoken, emphasise these aspects:

Countertransferential anxiety: her impulsiveness; sense of impending disaster;

Anger at mother; **Sadness** for both mother and her kids: The oldest as a young carer; streetwise; reflective; empathic. Others - exposed to adult-world exposure; survival skills; symbolic play;

Empathy for the Mother caught in a TRAP
- Her many sacrifices – lack of education; living in a state of limbo since school-days; few social and intimate relationships; sexual needs;
- Incomplete adolescent developmental tasks
- Her affection; maternal joy, love, care, spontaneity, play alongside benign neglect

4. Towards end *ask some leading questions*: Should kids be in care? [if not]

What could we have done to help?

[support during pregnancy; continuity of care; respite; sustenance; utilising her own network; encouraging asking for help; involving child/ren's father/s? And other family members]

Relational Skills for Practitioners - How can we help young parents?
- **Be authentic.** Empathising with parenting difficulties can help a young mother (or father) to confront their own limitations and human frailty. This in turn may enable them to 'forgive' some grievances towards their own parents.
- **Be creative:** foster attentiveness by asking the teen parent to remember what it felt like to be a child.
- **Be positive**: encouraging insight into developmental issues and the complexity of their own mixed feelings, can help the teen withdraw negative projections from the baby.
- **Be empathic**: enrich their emotional vocabulary by helping the teen convey what s/he appreciates about what the child is feeling and doing.
- **Be sensitive:** use your counter-transferential reactions to identify and understand emotional distress in teenage client/s and their children.
- **Be aware**: when alarm bells ring or ordinary support does not bring relief, it suggests a more deeply rooted disturbance that needs specialist help.
- **Be knowledgeable** about local resources for Perinatal or Couple Counselling or Parent-Infant therapy. Get client's permission for a referral

Skills: Increasing resilience in young parent/s and child:
- Offer trustworthy support and care to help teen replenish their resources
- Encourage teens to use their own special skills and capacities creatively
- Help the teen to develop a sense of agency by achieving realistic goals
- Help the teen to learn from ongoing experience, and to take a long-term more flexible view of stressful and frustrating events.
- Enhance the teen's capacity for mentalization and self-inquiry
- Invite the parent to try and think about what the child may be feeling.
- Arouse her/his curiosity about the baby's capabilities and ways of communicating needs so as to establish a more meaningful relationship.
- Provide constructive feedback to improve the parent's self-esteem.
- Assist the teen to assume responsibility for his/her own feeling
- Help promote the child's agency by commenting positively on behaviour, encouraging self-help, explaining intentions, repairing misunderstandings.

Summary: Precipitants of Distress in Teen Mothers:
- Lack of emotional support
- Preoccupation with own developmental issues
- Difficulties controlling own aggression and/or establishing limits
- Vulnerability of lone mother to the child's ambivalent feelings towards her
- The child is more exposed to maternal depression, intrusion and/or control when there is no partner or confidante to mediate between mother and baby
- Sleep deprivation: a fundamental necessity (dangers)
- A sense of 'induced guilt' in the child who curtails a young mother's freedom.
- Partner disappointment/jealousy/envy. Chaotic management and/or violence.

SELF-STUDY HOMEWORK:
Read: A. Joyce in Human Development pp 23-71 (see Google Books);
Also: Fraiberg, Tronick, Trevarthen in *Parent-Infant Psychodynamics*.
Watch: http://www.channel4.com/programmes/help-me-love-my-baby/4od#2918381

Conclusions:
Pregnant teens and young parents still undergoing emotional, intellectual, social, sexual developmental processes of their own. Practitioners can mitigate the emotional vulnerability of lone mothers and their children by being an empathic listener, legitimising the teen's needs (which can be at odds with those of their child/ren), arranging regular respite, and promoting an improved way of family life.

Key Concepts:
'Disequilibrium; Placental Paradigm; Antenatal Representations, paternal hormones.

Major Themes:
Sex distinctions and emotions in pregnancy; Intimate partner violence. Perinatal emotional disturbances. Teens as parents.

Module III.
BABIES IN TEEN FAMILIES

Aims

To foster greater insight in practitioners about teens as parents, and the emotional experience and needs of the babies in their care.

By the end of this third module you will have a greater understanding of the psychodynamics of co-constructed processes between babies and their carers, through which the infant's mind is constituted. Also increased knowledge of :
- Attachment patterns (Secure; Insecure Anxious; Avoidant, Disorganised)
- Mentalization
- Parenting orientations – Facilitator, Regulator, Reciprocator and Conflicted styles of interaction

---

5. Interactive Workshop:

Attunement, Attachment & Affect

Learning Objectives:

Interactive exercises will promote practitioners' theoretical understanding of components of the primary interchange to include
- attunement, communication and repair of disruptions
- empathy, containment and reflective function
- affect regulation (including self and mutual regulation)

Self Study/Group Exercise: *'Home is where we start from'* (Winnicott, 1986):
Each person writes down 5 words associated with *'home'*. The Leader asks for examples of these – writing them on flip chart and asking for a show of hands for the most common of these – usually security, predictability, warmth, comfort, etc.

A 'secure base'

We can think of a home like a hothouse in which we have a feeling of belonging. A home is where we start from as Donald Winnicott stressed, and inherent maturational process flourish if it is a 'facilitating' environment. A welcoming home provides a safe place to freely express emotions. Many confident infants find in their home what John Bowlby (1988) called a 'secure base' for experimentation – from which to venture out into the wider social world. For others, where traumatic circumstances or parental unpredictability impinge, home is filled a sense of danger necessitating vigilance.

Primary interrelationships at home usually involve a mother and/or father or other primary caregiver, and sometimes siblings, grandparents or other relatives. A baby's sense of self comes into being through intimate exchanges with others, at first at home, or carried on the mother's front or back, or a pushchair, Emotional understanding and cognitive learning take place through *interactive processes* which are so much part of ourselves that even our most private thoughts are a product of social interaction. From the language we speak to the imagery of our fantasies. Further mental growth occurs as toddlers venture out into the wider world, with the confidence to expand their social network as they carry the 'home' inside themselves. Insecurity is a form of homelessness.

Primary Interaction

Developmental research has now established that not only babies but even newborns are far more capable and discriminating than previously suggested, endowed with exquisitely sensitive feelings, curiosity about others and an innate need to be close to those who look after their needs. Interaction begins from the earliest hours and if the older partner pauses to give the baby 'space' to respond, a *proto-conversation* emerges, even in some premature babies, with 'turn-taking' statement and reply (Trevarthen, 1974). A warmly responsive playful companion, who enjoys their communications is of prime importance in infants learning to think, play and recognise emotions through give and take.

Mothers, fathers, siblings, relatives, other babies and even strangers can resonate to what babies communicate because every one of us has been a baby. Parenting itself is rooted in our babyhoods, in 'procedural' knowledge that comes from having been parented in particular ways. This is what is meant by *'transgenerational transmission'* – the unthinking activity by which a mother or father recreates the 'relational climate' of their own infancy, doing with their baby what was done for and to them by their own carers. This type of 'relational knowing' which begins to develop from the first weeks of life precedes symbolic verbalized knowledge, and remains implicit into adulthood (Lyons-Ruth, 1999). When looking after an infant up pop non-conscious representations and emotional enactions from one's own infancy (Raphael-Leff, 1991; Beebe, Lachmann & Jaffe, 1997).

Play

As much of caregiving is intuitive and never reaches consciousness, many carers may be unaware of their own tremendous influence - that their baby's *mind* is being constituted within that amazing powerhouse of interaction between them. Gradually, as the baby's sense of self grows, 'reciprocity' of the early months gives way to a 'dialogue' (Joyce, 2003, p.62). This manifests from the middle of the first year when, showing interest in special toys and objects, the infant invites the carer to participate in their shared reality (Trevarthen, 1974). To be most enjoyable, play routines are to be repeated again and again, but with some variation and joint elaborations.

The child's growing awareness that the caregiver continues to exist even in their absence is played out in 'peek-a-boo' type-games, reflecting loss and the joy of reunion - a joy that is enhanced by the responsive enjoyment of others:

> Seated on her mother's lap in the garden, baby Z [aged 5 months, 3 weeks] avidly watches out for return of the football her father has tossed up in the air. She greets it excitedly as it descends back into her line of vision. Infected by her delight her parents laugh with her as catching the ball, daddy exclaims "oooh" and she tenses with suspense as he makes it vanish again. . . .

With growing mobility, the crawling infant often looks back at the carer's face to check whether s/he is safe, indicating awareness of the m/other as a protector with a different perspective. Such is the power of the glance that around eight months the baby will inhibit an action s/he has begun if the parent says 'no'. Relishing the special quality of each intimate relationship is counterbalanced at this time by an *emergent fear of strangers*. Unknown people will be viewed with suspicion and the familiar carer is ardently sought. The baby may now create a *'transitional object'* – a teddy, 'security blanket' or piece of fluff that imaginatively represents the temporarily absent protector, and under the infant's control it can help him/her manage the painful gap of absence, of falling asleep or negotiating a parting (Winnicott, 1953). This ability to create a home-laden creature marks beginning of imaginative creativity. However, it has been noted that when there are too many changes of carers and/or their inexplicable and permanent loss, it might be problematic for the child to even develop the inner sense of constancy that allows for such self-management.

These maturational features also reflect the child's growing *'theory of mind'* – a dawning awareness that s/he and others have thoughts and feelings through, a mind which understanding is distilled. From affect resonance with carers in the early months, the infant now develops a more developed capacity for empathic sensing and responding to the moods of the other.

Mirroring

Most carers of young babies intuitively speak a form of 'motherese' – a high pitched, repetitive, rhythmic baby-talk. They spontaneously match the baby's prevailing emotional 'mood', and then tend to *'mirror'* it back. What is interesting is that they do so in an exaggerated way, thereby providing 'social biofeedback' which gradually enables the baby to recognise his or her own emotions, and to differentiate these from the carer's feelings, which are not overstated (Watson & Gergley, 1996). An adolescent parent is as capable as anyone else of doing this. But s/he may feel embarrassed to do chat with the infant in public, or sometimes is too engaged with internal feelings to have the mental space to consider the baby's.

> *Receptivity feels risky if it threatens to arouse uncontrollable feelings.*

Attunement

Sensitive responsiveness to the infant's needs depends on the carer's 'openness' to emotion. Many young parents find it difficult to maintain the kind of unstructured free-flowing attention necessary to fathom the baby, and the first year before speech evolves seems extremely frustrating. Articulating the infant's needs can seem like a mammoth task for a young person, struggling to verbalise their own. The alarm-bell pitch and persistence of a baby's cry arouses a fierce desire to restore quiet. Some parents harden themselves to ignore persistent crying, dismissing it as 'noise' or a form of 'emotional blackmail'. Others feel devastated by the sound of crying which really 'gets to' them. Exhausted by the strain of making a concerted effort to fathom the baby's desires, around half of all new mothers confess to having wanted to throw to baby out the window or smother it (see p.113). When the preverbal baby cannot 'tell' them in words what s/he needs the wail – *'What d'you want!?'* is a common irritable refrain among young mothers.

Well, what *do* infants want? A simple answer is that much of the time babies want to be *recognised* and *enjoyed*. Teenage parents can be very good at this – spontaneously seeing the amusing side of things, creating fun situations and stimulating their infants. However, during the day babies have many different levels of consciousness, from contented alertness to fretful sleepiness. At times there may be a mismatch between the degree of interaction the infant wants and the carer's desire to engage in fun and games. Practitioners can sometimes help carers improve their understanding of what the infant needs by showing them how to observe more closely – watching the baby's gestures and body language; listening to the tone and gist of his/her communications. Being able to step back and *re-run'* the sequence of a failed encounter can be useful. Sometimes a few minutes of interaction are filmed and the videoed material can be shown and discussed with the young carer (see Handout 3).

---

2 minute **Pre-observation Exercise** in pairs: the first one gives her/his watch or cell phone to the partner who queries details about the shape of hands, numbers, etc.

Training in Observation

The exercise demonstrates that observation is different from 'seeing' and you may not have registered the details, even of something you look at many times a day. Observing objectively is impossible, as we always imbue what we see with our own meanings. However, we can become aware and monitor our own biases, striving to suspend assumptions while observing (see Appendix 5). It takes time to acquire the skill. As this training course progresses if you practice observation you will achieve a greater understanding of what the experience of developing an *'observational stance'* entails – an impartial, non-judgemental attitude, and capacity for tolerating anxiety and resisting being drawn into inappropriate engagement or prematurely making judgements. If you decide to undertake a disciplined observation, try for one that is 'naturalistic' rather than a contrived situation – an encounter that affords a glimpse into an emotional interchange between a client and practitioner, or a baby and some significant other, that provides some insight into the quality of the relation.

Group/Self-study Observation Watch DVD material of a mother and baby on a sofa.
1. *What have you seen*?
2. Try and focus your observation: *What does the baby do? How does the mother respond? ...then what happens? ...What does the baby seem to need from the mother at this stage of development?*
3. Watch the same clip again – this time be aware of your 'counter-transference' feelings
4. Leader: facilitate a **group discussion,** emphasising an *'observational stance'* - issues of maintaining neutrality, respectfulness and curiosity. Raise the potential implications for the parent/child of being observed, and the intrusiveness of a tape-recorder, camera, etc. Boundaries, cultural differences, diffidence, compliance, etc.
5. Wonder with the participants what they might have *said* in the situation.

A Dialogue
Clearly, for the child, social interaction has a structuring role. Ongoing interpersonal engagement promotes a particular understanding of the world. But again, it is a two-way process. As babies and carers learn to know each other they develop *reciprocal patterns of reaction.* Cumulative evidence shows that, in conjunction with genetic endowment, the quality of early social inter-connections with the carers actually provides the *organising framework of the infant's brain.* The more any particular interaction pattern is used, the more it fires that same pattern of neural activation, thereby reinforcing some pathways and inhibiting others (Schore, 2001).

Towards the end of the first year, the baby has evolved greater complexity of symbolic thinking. Understanding of language will depend on the amount, quality and style carer of communication. Conversational speech with frequent questions and explanations expands the infant's comprehension, refining particular *meanings*. A carer who recognises the importance of a dialogue to achieve *mutual* understanding rather than just imposing their own view) furthers the child's sense of agency. Through appreciating different points of view the child develops a greater understanding of perspectives, and complex distinctions between appearance and substance, between false and true beliefs, presence and representation, pretence and truth… The particular pattern of exchange into which each carer inducts the infant, rests on his or her perceptions of the baby: as an intriguing communicative little partner, a noisy nuisance, a wise saviour, a 'whinger', a chatterbox, a 'blob'…

Their interactive processes determine what it feels like for each partner to *be* with the other, and contributes to the child' self representation, at every developmental level.

Modes of communication

From birth it is clear that newborns vary in their degree of alertness, readiness to respond and the clarity of cues they provide. So, understanding the baby's needs is not only a function of parental orientations and capacity to recognise minute indicators, but is also influenced by the neonate's constitutional and temperamental factors. However, carers also *modify* the baby's disposition by their irritation or patience, receptiveness or dismissal, disinterest or a true wish to understand. We have long known that infants whose communications are not responded to promptly or ignored during the first few months, *cry more in subsequent months*.

Recent research explains the mechanism by which this escalation occurs. Saliva swab tests show higher levels of stress hormones in distraught babies whose cries elicit no response. Neurobiologists find that when chronic, high levels of cortisol are 'toxic' to the developing brain. By comparison, in those neonates whose carers do respond promptly, 'happiness-making' endorphins are released to counteract the stress hormone cortisol, thereby establishing a basis for future self-soothing. [Clearly this has implications for the 'controlled crying' system].

> *Secure attachment is the firm expectation of distress being met by comforting.*

Disruption and Repair

A secure emotional bond evolves when a baby feels safe, and kept in mind by a carer who recognises s/he is a little person with needs and feelings. However, this does not mean being perfectly understood. Even in the best circumstances carers often miss or misinterpret subtle clues to what the baby is feeling. We have seen how complex human interaction is, and inevitably, there are always misunderstandings, disruptions and mismatched responses. But infant research shows that *the crucial aspect of communication is 'repair'* – the carer's desire to really understand the baby's state of mind, their willingness to admit mistakes, and wish to try and learn from them. Amazingly – babies too, engage in repair!

Expectancies

If the child's interactive desire to understand and to restore meets a carer's wish to clarify and repair, not only does the infant feel understood but influential. A young child whose *opinion* is sought feels able to affect others, be they parent/s, siblings or others. Carers who are emotionally accessible and have faith in the child instil a sense of *agency*—the belief one can bring about a desired state (Raphael-Leff, 2010b). This capacity for self-help begins very early. In addition to their specific gifts and unique sensitivities, neonatal research has established that <u>all</u> babies have an amazing pre-symbolic type of intelligence involving *'expectancies' of action sequences.*

An infant develops that sense of agency and causality when s/he realises that certain behaviours will have consequences in the environment (e.g. crying brings the carer or banging the cot can operate the mobile). Micro-tracking shows that from moment to moment an infant learns to anticipate certain sequences between his own actions and those of the interactive partner. If these expectancies are suddenly violated, the infant shows surprise, puzzlement, rage or confusion.

This is clearly demonstrated by the perplexed, then distressed responses of a baby when an experiment is conducted instructing the carer to keep a 'still-face'. The infant expects a certain type of *'contingent' response* as a reaction to his/her own call or contact. When the reply is incongruous with expectations, it is disturbing.

Influences are 'bi-directional' – the baby's response to the carer's facial expression, or the carer's response to the baby's night-waking or, on a more subtle level, to gaze avoidance or babbling, is affected by his/her own moods and needs, but also influenced by the other's reaction to his/her response which sets a dynamic interlocking pattern of *'expectancies'* of being together.

The specific dynamic interplay within each pair creates *expectations of exchange*, including matching patterns of affect, arousal and timing with mutual as well as self-regulatory consequences (Beebe et al, 1997). If this sounds familiar, it is because (as we saw in the first module), we continue to operate this way in our adult relationships too. But the more 'rigid' our 'expectancies', the less resilient we are in the face of the unexpected.

Interactive repair and repeated mis-attunements followed by re-attunements contribute to the infant's growing capacity for self-organisation.

When a mother-baby pair show a positive balance between disruption and repair it is predictive of secure attachments later on, around one year. Successful pairs show typical sequences of *match-mismatch-rematch* within a fraction of a second (Beebe et al, 1997).

Gradually, this type of sequence expands the complexity and coherence of their *'dyadic consciousness'* - the interweaving of co-constructed processes between the infant and the carer that is unique to <u>that</u> particular relationship (Tronick, 1989) and different with other carers. Conversely, chronic failure to recognise and repair misunderstandings and to 'reconnect' has long term negative effects. By three months patterns of interaction are set. As seen in observations over time, a baby whose moments of frustration are met by a generous carer willing to repair, becomes resilient, establishing trust in his/her own agency. S/he gradually develops a capacity to self-soothe, and copes well even when the anticipated response is not

> Practitioners can help new parents to become more observant - to recognise disappointed expectancies in the baby, and to provide better repair when they have misunderstood these *['Oh! You wanted X'...]*

forthcoming. Babies also engage in mutual and self-regulation with other babies.

But in chronic situations of unremitting mismatch and aggravation most infants give up and become listless and/or withdrawn, Others seek 'escape routes' from overstimulation. The baby of an unresponsive postnatally depressed mothers learns to match her toned-down response while an infant whose mothers has a persecutory disorder (paranoid beliefs) may defend against the carer's hostility or intrusiveness by 'switching off', but not before the malevolent projection has become embedded in the self-image.

Nature/Nurture
Recent research shows that the carer's responsiveness to communications not only affects the baby's behaviour, but actual brain development! The innate core-brain is the seat of automatic responses of survival, but the 'social' brain is the seedbed of the ever-evolving mind - and this is constituted interpersonally, between carer and baby. In the first two years after birth neural networks proliferate at the extraordinary rate of 1.8 million new synapses per second. These are activated, reinforced or pruned within primary relationships (see Karmiloff-Smith, 1995). Neuro-imaging shows that during this critical early period of prolonged dependence, enduring patterns of 'connectivity' in brain circuits are thus shaped by interactive engagement with carers. The infant's neuroplastic malleability calls both for protective care and lively playful emotional responsiveness from others in order to promote healthy flexible connections (Balbernie, 2001). Conversely, emotionally damaging

> *Endowment is activated, modified or inhibited by the specific emotional-social environment of interaction*

effects of parental depression, abuse and neglect are associated with *permanent* maladaptive 'wiring' of neural response patterns affecting neurobiological stress systems (Pollock, 2005; Watts-English, 2006).

In teen parents caregiving reactions are affected by the fact that they themselves are undergoing further brain development triggered by puberty. Younger mothers do not show the same patterns of increased heart rate and cortisol in response to a baby cries that older mothers do. Some researchers attribute this diminished attunement to adolescent neural immaturity while the medial prefrontal cortex (the brain region important for planning and executive functioning) is still developing (Giardino, et al 2008). However, the very malleability of their own brain circuits makes adolescence a 'second chance' opportunity for changing and repairing defective patterns.
This exciting new evidence of interactively responsive growth seems to resolve the old 'nature or nurture' debate by showing that developmental processes are a complex product of the combination of both genetic disposition and childrearing patterns (see Music, 2011; Gerhardt, 2004; Balbernie, 2001 pp. 152, 154, 157 in the Readings).
Also see: http://www.sciencemaster.com/columns/wesson/wesson_early_01.php

Attachment
John Bowlby, the originator of Attachment theory proposed that like all helpless young primates, human babies seek proximity to their carers as a means of protection against danger. They do so through a series of innate evocative behaviours - sucking, crying, smiling, following, and clinging. Over the first year of a baby's life, the parent's availability and attentive responsiveness will contribute to an internal feeling of security. This boosts confidence and an ability to tolerate incrementally greater separations by using the carer as a *'secure base'* from which to explore the world. A test procedure called the *'Strange Situation'* is used as a standard measure of such security, looking at the response of one-year-olds to a brief separation and reunion with mother or father and interaction with a stranger under replicable laboratory

conditions. A helpful link for theory and research related to attachment theory: http://www.psychology.sunysb.edu/attachment/   Also see Expanded notes, p.178.

When distressed, an infant who is **'securely attached'** actively seeks contact, and feels rapidly comforted by closeness with the carer. This sense of safety is made possible by caregivers who feel *secure* in themselves, holding the infant's experience and needs in mind, without discharging their unresolved anxiety or guilt onto the child.

By contrast, an **insecure 'avoidant' attachment** develops when a carer is *dismissive* of the child's emotions, and is controlling, inconsistent, rejecting or neglectful. At one year this baby shows little unprompted affection towards,, or preference for that carer over a stranger. The toddler has defensively 'deactivated' the need for attachment. Cultivating pseudo-independence, the child seems indifferent to the carer's whereabouts and responses, and may actively avoid her/him after a separation. However, when their heart rate is measured, it belies this indifference.

Parents who are inconsistently both *enmeshed or withdrawn*, have toddlers who exhibit features of insecure **'anxious'** (ambivalent) **attachment,** including heightened vigilance in relating to that carer, and little spontaneous exploration in his/her presence. When separated the one year old tends to become very distressed and on reunion shows mixed approach-avoidance responses – both seeking and resisting contact.

Children of parents who are preoccupied with unresolved issues of trauma or loss in their own pasts have **'disorganised' attachments** with disoriented behaviour such as freezing, rocking, head-banging, dissociative states, and disorientation in response to the carer's frightening and often abusive responses. While rare in the general population, this attachment pattern can be seen in almost two-thirds of disturbed families (for a more detailed elaboration, see Expanded notes for Module III).

Once again what is apparent is *the two-way interactive exchange.* Security lies in learning gradually to manage one's own sadness, anger and anxieties in a safe context with a carer who responds sensitively and 'survives' rather than collapsing, retaliating or attacking. In later life, this secure inner core offers protection during periods of high stress.

The quality of early care can predict attachment status of the child at one year.

- Thus infants who will later become **'avoidant'** tend to have mothers who are over-stimulating, intrusive and intense. They tend to look at the mother less, unless they can self-sooth by fingering their clothing while gazing.

- Infants who will later become **anxiously attached** have mothers who are under-involved, detached, or inconsistent; who fail to respond; or who attempt to interact when the infant is not available.

- **Disorganised attachments** are related to escalating bouts of parent-infant over-arousal that spiral out of control. And mothers who are significantly more likely to display frightening (or frightened) behaviour toward their infants.

This is an illustration of different emotional *'relational climates'*, which will also differ with other caregivers. And indeed, the same child will respond with different degrees of security according to the particular carer. However, when cumulative experience is very intense and largely takes place with one significant primary carer, the child evolves an inner representation of that attachment figure – an *'internal working model'* [IWM] that forms an *expectation* of future experience with carers (Bowlby, 1969).

Attachment in Adulthood

Early patterns persist. Research suggests that adolescents' 'romantic' experiences are primed by their attachments in babyhood, with secure teens developing a 'higher quality' of intimacy based on their parents' perceptions of love relationships (Roisman et al, 2005). Importantly, studies show that practitioners too, are influenced by their own attachments, with insecure workers tending to work better with people of the same defensive 'strategy' as themselves, as opposed to secure practitioners who can contrast with their clients. Case managers who are involved intervene with their clients in greater depth than case managers who were more dismissing (Dozier et al, 1993). The Adult Attachment Interview (AAI) enables researchers to get an idea of our past attachment. It can not only gage how an expectant mother views her own childhood but whether this has been processed, and how this already informs her future relationship with the unborn baby. Attachment patterns of a one year old can be predicted already during gestation from interviews with the pregnant woman about her own early attachments (Fonagy et al, 1993). Similarly, a further study by that team showed that the way fathers recall their own childhood attachments is predictive of their infant's attachment to them by their first birthday.

Observation: <u>Young father putting his baby son's trousers on.</u>
What did you see? What are the differences did you note between this mother and father? Is the baby securely attached?

Interim Conclusions:

- A baby is born with an innate capacity for interrelatedness, and his/ her identity is formed through emotional responses of the specific carers s/he interacts with.
- Like a seismograph, the infant baby resonates to emotional 'vibes' and rumblings of hidden 'earthquakes' far below the surface. Also picking up on absences or rejection by other key players within the wider constellation, and their effect.
- On the basis of these each baby comes to evolve an 'internal working model' of key relationships and uses these representational systems to expect (and bring about) certain responses in a given situation.
- Secure attachments shape a coherent representation of the self-with-carer.
- Insecure attachment involving inconsistent experiences with caregivers is underpinned by *split* unintegrated persecutory and idealised representations of the relationship/s.
- Secure attachment facilitates confident exploration of the external world, and also enables exploration of the internal world – that is, psychological awareness of mental states and feelings in self and others, and hence, 'emotional literacy' and a reflective capacity.
- By contrast, insecure attachment involves either a defensive ignoring of the mental contents of the other's mind (avoidant attachment), or over-involvement with the mind of the other (anxious-ambivalent attachment), or a hyper-attunement to the mental states of the other to the neglect of understanding one's own mental states (disorganised/disoriented attachment).

Different Orientations to Parenting

Attachment reveals the quality of the connection to the carer – which can be transmitted across generations. Orientations describe the beliefs and reasoning that motivate what mothers do and what is happening 'behind the scenes'.

Societies in-transition, such as our own have no set traditions of parenting. Each mother and father is freer to follow their own inclinations (subject to socioeconomic conditions). When, in parallel to the inception of attachment research I set out to investigate styles of parental interaction, my observations delineated three 'orientations' which differ according to personal beliefs and underpinning representations about self and babies. Cross-culturally, independent researchers have since replicated my model of orientations. The modes of parenting - *Facilitator, Regulator and Reciprocator* – all fall within the normal range (except for the extremes and a 'conflicted' group), and their attributes cluster statistically.

You may recognise them from your own observations of clients and friends.

A 'Facilitator' adapts to her baby; a 'Regulator' mother expects the baby to adapt

---

Before going into further detail, *try and guess the answers to these questions* (either writing these down in your Learning Journal, or in group training, on the flip chart).

Self-study or Group: Orientation guessing game:
 1. How would each mother feed?
 2. What about weaning?
 3. How would each mother treat crying?
 4. What about sleep?
 5. What would constitute 'security' for the baby?
 6. Who is the primary unit?

Maternal Orientations

A 'Facilitator' enjoys pregnancy, feeling this is the pinnacle of her feminine identity. She 'communes' with her unborn baby and hopes for a 'natural' birth, to provide a smooth transition to their reunion. Postnatally she believes that her baby knows what s/he needs, and that because of their intimate contact during pregnancy, she, the biological mother is especially attuned to deciphering his/her needs. As exclusive carer, she adapts herself to following the infant's initiative in order to provide the perfect babyhood she wishes she had had. This means keeping the baby close at all times, including at night as any gurgle is regarded as a communication. Her involvement is total, she relishes being a mother, and she feels remorseful about 'lapses' from the bountiful ideal of mothering that she tries so very hard to uphold. She feels very strongly that she constitutes the baby's security. In time, as the infant engages with others or prefers exploring without her she may feel somewhat rejected, meeting temporary disengagement with persuasive efforts to reengage.

What is happening unconsciously? Denial of her own ambivalence increases her anxieties about the baby's vulnerability, and may result in over-protectiveness. As the growing infant begins to separate, the mother's own separation anxieties may lead to her over-involvement with the toddler or to another pregnancy.

A Regulator mother finds pregnancy disagreeable and plans to use whatever medical aid is available, including epidurals or Caesarean, aiming for a 'civilized' birth. The newborn feels like a stranger and the parturient needs time and space to recuperate before bonding. Once home, fearing her brain will turn to 'mush' if she loses her grip on her familiar identity, she works hard at back as soon as possible to her pre-pregnant self and shape. As she regards her baby as pre-social she sees her role as promoting *socialisation* by getting him/her to adapt to the household. Wary of being emotionally aroused, she introduces a routine which both increases predictability and reduces the need for too much intuitive involvement. Somewhat alarmed by being solely responsible for meeting the baby's total dependency needs, she aims to share care. And since she believes that at first the baby does not differentiate between people, she brings in the co-carers early, and hence, even if breast-feeding, introduces bottles in the early weeks. Shared care also enables her to go out on her own, returning to fun activities or non-domestic work place as soon as is feasible, and the routine provides continuity across carers. Her identity in invested in being a 'person' rather than just a mother. Feeling she needs adult company to keep her sane, she maintains a degree of detachment so as not to become 'sucked in' to the 'yummy-mummy' thing. So that she can resume her sex life, from the start the baby sleeps in a separate bed, and preferably another room, and is quickly conditioned to go back to sleep unaided when s/he wakes at night. Because she distinguishes 'real' crying from 'noise', she can institute 'controlled crying' at night, and by day, ignore or discipline unjustified demands. Encouraging independence, the Regulator mother applauds physical advances, such as crawling, and dismisses 'clinging'. While liable to become depressed in the early months of home-bound 'slog' with a 'boring' baby, mothering feels much more rewarding in later months, once the baby is mobile, interesting, affectionate and beginning to talk. Most play tends to be stimulating, but with an educational goal, and verbal interaction involves instructions and a sometimes sarcastic commentary that emphasises their difference. *["No way! that's my chocolate! Touch it and you'll self-destruct!'].*

'Behind the scenes' there is an anxiety about the 'thin end of the wedge'. The representation of the infant as pre-social, with untamed urges and insatiable appetites signifies that any lapse in the routine could result in an outbreak of wild impulses, sleep refusal, unending feeds, incomplete toilet training and escalating exploitation of her goodwill. She also recoils from contagious arousal of her own dependency needs and weaknesses.

Finally, the *Reciprocator* mother who manages to simultaneously hold both sides of the equation in mind – the baby as both *similar* to herself in having (mixed) human emotions, yet *different* from her in being a baby. She follows the baby's lead but also initiates, offering comfort but fostering affective self-regulation; giving feedback, and negotiating each moment separately, with the infant and others in her life. However, this kind of mothering is hard going as unlike the Facilitator who adapts, or the Regulator who expects the baby to adapt, there are no rules to follow. This capacity for thoughtful interaction rests on a mature ability to tolerate uncertainty and ambiguity it herself as well as others.

Understanding is based on *empathy* (rather than identification like the Facilitator or dis-identification like the Regulator). Close relatives or friends may be enlisted to cover her when she works from home, or part-time elsewhere, but she tries to hold her baby in mind at all times, and whenever they are together, her exchanges with the baby tend to be conversational, playful yet emotionally attuned, and verbal content is informative: a mixture of matter-of-fact explanations and plans, with direct emotional feedback as well as imaginatively improvised ways of relating to the baby's state of mind (Raphael-Leff, 1991). She is truthful about hardships, and aware of her mixed feelings, and those of the baby, too, and tries to make a clear differentiation between what belongs to whom.

Studies show that Facilitator/ Regulator/ Reciprocator parenting orientations are easily observed during pregnancy, long before their actualisation with the birth. These orientations are based on unconscious representations of self and baby during pregnancy (remember the 'placental paradigm'?) reflecting the degree to which difficult care-experiences from the past have been 'metabolised', and how ambivalence is tolerated or denied in herself and others.

In their extreme form idealising Facilitator mothers and persecuted Regulator mothers are unable to tolerate the idea of coexisting good/bad emotions in themselves or in the baby – and hence, tend to cut off from one or other aspect of their own mixed feelings about their baby, about them selves, their own mother, partner and others.

Many a Regulator finds it hard to tolerate the baby's emotional neediness which reminds her of weaknesses she has suppressed or overcome with effort. She may feel hostility towards the baby who seems able to express these cravings so openly while draining her resources. Faced with a crying baby her first response is to look at her watch, and if a feed or nap is not due, assume some other physical cause – the baby feeling too hot or cold, cramped position, teething, needing a nappy change, or experiencing colic, etc.

Factors in changing orientation
Psychological
Psycho-historical & current variables
Motivation for conception of this baby
Degree of emotional support/ confidante
Socioeconomic
Age, employment/career status
Number of children & gaps between them
Partner? Social/economic pressures
Cultural expectations
Life events (bereavement, loss of job…)
Physiological
Pregnancy/birth complications
Postnatal health, hormonal swings/sleep
Emotional experience of parenting the previous child

Whilst a Reciprocator might wonder if the crying baby is lonely or bored, seeking interaction or a change of scenery, a Facilitator tends to put the distressed baby straight to her breast. Vicariously indulging her own baby-self through unlimited gratification of the child's needs (and a desire to be needed) she may find it difficult to tolerate the growing baby's separation, and the toddler's open expression of negative feelings and desire for independence.

Under stressful conditions, Regulators 'loom' over the baby, becoming more controlling and/or dismissive of dependency and emotional outpourings, berating themselves for not having applied a more rigorous regime. Anxious about the baby's unhappiness, Facilitators 'hover', guilt-ridden, experiencing the infant's distress as a personal failure, and a criticism of their not-bountiful enough mothering.

Interestingly, these orientations are not fixed like personality traits – they can and often do change with subsequent pregnancies. Many teenage mothers are in a state of rebellion against their own mothers, or denying difference, emulate their orientation trying to 'be' them. But as internal conflicts are resolved, and the inner world alters with maturation and greater acceptance of their own healthy ambivalence, many Facilitators and Regulators to veer towards Reciprocation.

However sometimes a Regulator may change towards facilitation, feeling the need to indulge herself and the next baby. And vice versa, a stay at home mother who finally resumes her education or takes up a career and then finds herself pregnant, may opt to regulate this baby. Clearly colleges with a crèche reduce the stark choices for teenage mothers. It is also very difficult to facilitate a baby born very soon after the last, which may nudge a would-be Facilitatir towards reciprocation. A fourth group of mothers, *conflicted* between facilitating and regulating, alternate inconsistently and unhappily during the first two years, feeling frustrated with their own confusion.

Links with Attachment

Research associating these orientations to attachment theory shows that maternal orientation (assessed when the baby is six months old) predicts security as measured later by the Strange Situation at one year. As expected, moderate Facilitators, Regulators, and Reciprocators all raise secure toddlers while extreme (enmenshed) Facilitators breed ambivalent babies, extreme (dismissive) Regulators have avoidant babies, and those who are 'Conflicted' and chaotic, veering inconsistently between the two orientations have disorganised offspring (Scher, 2001). Conflicted carers feel compelled to simultaneously reject and heighten the infant's attachment-related affects and behaviours.

Fathers' Orientations

Fathers too have their own orientations which range from *Participators* who wish to take part in primary care to *Renouncers* who feel they may become involved at some later date, but see the early nurturing as 'women's work'. Already during pregnancy, male *Reciprocators* hope to share care (Raphael-Leff, 2008). Recent research has shown that cohabiting males are also affected by hormonal changes. Fathers exposed to newborns experience various degrees of testosterone reduction and increased prolactin which appear to enhance the paternal capacity to nurture. Both their own orientations and *'maternal gatekeeping'* will determine the actual postnatal division of responsibilities in parenting, especially where teen parents are concerned.

> **Role Play:** Facilitator and Participator discussion as bathtime approaches

A 'Ladette' may decide to 'go it alone', possibly not even telling the baby's biological father about impending fatherhood. Conversely, having rejected his involvement during the pregnancy she may need him to share the daily care of their infant; or she may even want him to look after her. Thus her attitudes and actions (and those of various family members and practitioners) will promote or impede the father's engagement with the baby.

The particular combination of orientation styles in each couple can create or mitigate distress. For instance, if a Facilitator and a Participator both desire exclusive care of the infant, they may find a way to cooperate and share care. But some such couples actually compete jealously over the baby's attentions. Likewise, if a macho Renouncer refuses to offer any help, and in addition insists that his Regulator partner is a full-time mother, she is likely to become distressed, needing to share-care and have time off. Work outside the home has different connotations - a Regulator who is unemployed or a Facilitator who *has* to go out to work are both likely to become distressed, for their respective reasons (see Raphael-Leff, 1985a, 1991; Scher & Blumberg, 2000; Scher, 2001; Sharp & Bramwell, 2004; van Bussel et al, 2009). And likewise for fathers, who as we will see, also suffer from postnatal depression and

> *Timing and the nature of postnatal distress is triggered by specific factors for each orientation, determined by the discrepancy between each parent's personal expectations and the postnatal reality s/he meets*

other disturbances.

SELF STUDY HOMEWORK: re fathers see:
http://www.sussex.ac.uk/Units/CCE/socialwork_researchreports2009/TalkingDadsRe searchReport2009.pdf

> **Self-study/Group Discussion**: *'Why are the first few weeks of caring for a new-born so intensely disturbing for most caregivers?'* [answers on flipchart or in Journal]

Unconscious Identifications and **'Contagious Arousal'**:

Contagious arousal seems to explain why. Thrust into close contact with raw feelings of the pre-symbolic baby, and exposed to the redolence of *primary substances* (amniotic fluid, lochia, breast-milk, urine, feces, 'cradle cap', posset, etc), the new parent experiences a reawakening of procedural memories from their own infancy. And indeed, recent research reported in the New Scientist establishes that the brain's olfactory centres are intimately linked to its limbic system, which is involved in emotion, fear and memory.

For every parent, but more so for teens, the ongoing intimate, emotional exchange with a non-verbal baby, revitalises unprocessed feelings. *Contagious arousal* refers to reactivation of somato-sensory experience and fantasy representations (of one's own baby-self seen through the eyes of archaic caregivers) as well as implicit memories of being mothered, for better and for worse. Contagious arousal through the baby's feelings and primary substances activates a network of unconscious representations reflecting repeated emotional experience of a myriad subjective sensations, and sub-symbolic schemas of affects, actions, arousal and motivation which now come together to form *an internal paradigm of babyhood and being looked after* (Raphael-Leff, 2001) such as underpins caregiving orientations.

Adolescent are still very close to their own childhoods. Their determined attempts to free themselves of childish feelings and the primary attachment to their own carers renders them particularly at risk to revival of uncontained emotion. Suffering from stress, exhaustion, sleep deprivation and vulnerability many teenage parents find the struggle with regressive feelings and developmental issues quite overwhelming, as the baby constantly retriggers the very feelings they are trying to relinquish.

> *Just when parents need to be most grown-up, parenting revives infantile feelings*

Furthermore, today's age of time consuming, baby-excluding, electronic communication and devices means that the teenager's own emotional needs, social networking style, and concept of time and space is very different from that of the baby - which has changed little since the Stone Age!

What can we do about this? **HOMEWORK: watch** Secret Powers of Time, P.Zimbardo **http://www.youtube.com/user/theRSAorg#p/u/1/A3oIiH7BLmg**

Perinatal Distress

People whose infantile experience has been largely positive or is now idealised, may relish this reactivation of early feelings, delighting in the baby's dependence on them as a reminder of the care they imagine they themselves received from an archaic carer. This emotional experience of identification leads a Facilitator to a state of *'primary maternal preoccupation'* (Winnicott, 1956). Resilient people whose upbringing was less than good-enough may nevertheless achieve a state of internal security, by processing their feelings about their own deprivation. They become Reciprocators, aware that experience is always mixed and never perfect.

Others who have not done so before, may begin to actively utilise the reactivation during parenting of their own despondency and infantile feelings to rework and resolve less than optimal early experiences, and in the course of looking after their own child, forgive their parents their 'trespasses'. For yet others, this contagious arousal may feel like a very threatening experience which they then try to control by maintaining an emotional distance from the infant, through co-carers, routines and regulation.

Those who lack a confidante, or lost their own mothers before puberty are particularly at risk of depression (Brown & Harris, 1986) as are very young teenaged mothers. Some parents (of whatever age) feel extremely anxious in the early weeks and months, unable to bear the negative aspects of contagious arousal. They need support and frequent respite from the overwhelming state of *'primary maternal persecution'* that threatens to envelop them (Raphael-Leff, 2003). Indeed, through their own projections, at times the baby can seem like a prime persecutor and may be at risk of their retaliatory actions if they cannot get a 'breather' of time spent away.

Some new parents retreat into obsessionality - splitting 'good' and 'bad' aspects of their feelings and self-representations. They try to keep these apart, controlling them through compulsive rituals (such as hand-washing, excessive tidiness, or counting things). The 'bad' may be avoided by locating it outside, in external dangers (cats, the neighbours, the health visitor, food contamination, etc) and developing mild phobias or paranoid anxieties. Unfortunately, contagious arousal is such that defences fail, with uncontrollable breakthrough ideas involving the baby as the target or source of danger. These are not uncommon, but many mothers are not too alarmed as they distinguish between thought and action. Teen mothers may feel unable to protect themselves from this overwhelming state of high arousal in the early weeks. Their disturbances range from an identificatory fusion/confusion with the idealised infant, to extreme withdrawal, disassociation or detachment from a denigrated or feared persecutory infant, representing repudiated aspects of the

---

Precursors are found antenatally (*'Placental Paradigm'*) – hence the need for realistic plans and therapeutic help during pregnancy, before it impacts on the relationship with the baby.

young carer's own baby-self, or states of intense range and frustration at having to be on call twenty-four hours a day and night, to look after an exploitative, demanding infant. *Teenagers who have experienced violence, abuse, or trauma during their childhoods are especially at risk.* Anna Freud regarded traumatic stress as a shattering and devastating event that alters the course of future development. Cross-culturally, research find associations between childhood sexual abuse, coercion, rape and intimate partner violence with teenage conception rates (Coy et al, 2010).

Untimely pregnancy is one of many outcomes of early abuse.

Post Traumatic Stress may be intensified by the powerful state of heightened arousal during early parenthood, which threatens to re-evoke traumatic feelings from the past when they were left feeling as helpless and frightened as the baby is now.

Dissociation may seem the best way to defend against the risk of flashbacks. It does enable many people to function efficiently. However, dissociated the carer then feels removed from the baby and unable to respond intuitively and reflectively. In addition experiencing an inner emptiness due to being so out of touch with her/his own emotional core.

> When periodic respite is insufficient and counter-transference alerts you to danger, *a mother-baby unit* may support the healthy aspects of the fraught relationship.

> Note: *Perinatal psycho-therapeutic help* is needed <u>before</u> teen mothers succumb to a spectrum of depressive, anxious, obsessional or persecutory and phobic disturbances that affect the relationship with the infant. Speedy referrals!

Conclusions

- Exposure to the baby's anxieties and to primary substances impacts on the young carer through 'contagious arousal' of their early own dependency needs.
- If a young mother or father feels haunted by unlaid 'ghosts' from their past these painful traumatic experiences disrupt the ongoing parent-infant relationship and tend to be enacted in the new context with the baby.
- As health visitors know, parental insecurities and unresolved conflicts often manifest in the baby's disturbance: acute separation anxiety, feeding and/or weaning difficulties, sleep disruption, excessive crying and in extreme cases 'failure to thrive'.
- If the baby unconsciously represents part of the parent's own self or some aspect of their archaic carers this is revealed through parental overidentification with the baby, or repudiation of the infant's 'weaknesses'. These idealised or negative projections and attributions are absorbed by the infant into his/her self-image.

Key Concepts:
'Transitional object'. Secure and Insecure Anxious; Avoidant, Disorganised attachment patterns ; IWM 'internal working model'; Facilitator/ Regulator/ Reciprocator Parental Orientations; 'Contagious Arousal'; Primary Maternal Preoccupation/Persecution.

Major Themes:
Reactivation during pregnancy and the early postnatal weeks of unresolved issues from one's own infancy and childhood, as well as later traumatic life events.

Module III:
BABIES IN TEEN FAMILIES

6. Skills-Based Seminar:

Babies and Reflective Function in Teen Parents

Learning Objectives

> - Enhanced understanding of the child's representational world.
> - Basic Mentalization techniques.
> - Skills for enhancing containment, attunement, emotional regulation and contingent responsiveness.

'Mirror' neurones

From birth the baby is biologically 'wired' to be *a 'social partner'* - eliciting and seeking affection, attachment and a sense of belonging. We have all observed how avidly even a very young alert baby interacts with the environment – constantly looking, listening, touching, observing and learning. Amazingly, not only does the infant *communicate* her/his own feelings of pain, joy, puzzlement and frustration but s/he is exquisitely attuned to the feelings of others. An infant picks up unconscious feelings in the adult even when these are consciously denied.

Innate mechanisms enable her/him to register the live experience of others and to empathise with them. In a crèche, neonates respond by crying on hearing another infant's cry. Studies show that when we watch someone perform an action the same part of the brain is affected by as if we were doing it. This is due to 'mirror neurones' which also enable a newborn to imitate simple actions (e.g. tongue protrusion). Similarly, a spoon-feeding mother opens her mouth to get the baby to do the same. By recognising their similarities, attributing mental states to the infant and sharing her own, she helps the child recognise his/her own feelings, and that others too, have similar feeling states. We too unconsciously copy rhythms and mimic postures.

> *Through 'mirror neurones' the baby's mind can mirror the minds of others*

Resonance also underpins our own 'counter-transference' feelings when we feel what the client is feeling. This resonance is the basis of many familiar states – contagious laughter and yawning, tears welling up with compassion, goose bumps of anxiety and empathy for the suffering of others. Indeed, each one of us is subtly influenced by others in an inescapably intertwined way, and resonance is the basis of our selfhood. Mirror Neurones:http://www.youtube.com/user/theRSAorg#p/search/0/l7AWnfFRc7g Then find: The Empathic Civilization. [*With this and all other assignments, write your thoughts and response in your Learning Journal for your own record. See p.201]*

Empathy

consideration for the feelings of others arises through a baby's emotional responsive-ness to, and identification with, the 'stance' of the other, thus a developing capacity to temporarily shift his/her own perspective (Hobson, 2002). Once again, the corollary of the baby's growing sensitivity to *other people's differing views of the same reality,* and to the meaning they ascribe to objects, events and also to oneself, is enhanced awareness of self – the infant's dawning *self-consciousness* arises from the other's 'gaze' – becoming aware of being observed through someone else's eyes. This in turn allows for an altered form of *reflective,* rather than emotional psychic intimacy (which we could formulate as a thinking process that is the internalised dialogue between the subjective observing 'I' and the socially constituted 'me', in Mead's terminology). He was one of the first philosophers to recognise that *'the individual mind can exist only in relation to other minds with shared meanings'* (Miller, 1982:5) [p.151 in Readings]

> *Message: Oscillation between self-conscious awareness/self-reflection is a lifelong process. This training aims to provides participants with a taste of that experience.*

Containment:

The baby's acute sensitivity to both their own subjective feelings and to what others are feeling, at times can be overwhelming. Before being able to manage his/her own emotions and to understand those of others, the infant is dependent on a particular set of carers and their capacity to contain her/his anxiety and reduce confusion.

Our earliest experiences are bodily based, recorded somatically in states of arousal and quiescence. For these subsymbolic experiences to become represented in the mental realm, they must be received, processed, and transformed by a carer who can act as a *'container'* for the infant's raw, unmanageable feelings. By transforming nameless distress and confusion into tolerable, *thinkable* experiences the unbearable anxiety becomes bearable. As the child gradually 'internalises' the carer's capacity to process raw feelings, s/he evolves a 'space' to think thoughts, and can begin to process his/her own feelings (Bion, 1967). That child then possesses this function of 'thinking' and can call up an internal image of a trusted loving carer that provides security at times of separation, or perceived danger.

However, when the carer is too preoccupied with his/her own feelings to be aware of the infant's, or too afraid of intense emotion to process the child's anxieties, the baby may have to prematurely take on the function of *self-containment*. Worse still, in some cases when the carer lacks support, or is too depressed to be receptive to help, the infant may feel overwhelmed by imbibing the adult's anxieties, when called upon to act as a 'container' for the parent. A child whose feelings could not be received and understood is likely to feel flooded and confused. Consequently, relief comes from expelling those troubling feelings, projecting them outside or else cutting off from them, destroying his/her own capacity to perceive, communicate or reflect.

Parental attributions

> *Infant mental health is a function of shared emotions and intentions within the family system as a whole.*

If carers do not believe the baby *has* feelings, s/he is deprived of the building blocks for understanding the meaning of his/her emotional reactions. Sometimes, a baby who was anticipated as the one who would magically change their lives experiences the teen parent's disappointment in getting an ordinary baby. Taking this disenchantment into her/his self image s/he comes to feel unworthy of love or even, deserving of rejection. As noted above, relief comes from expelling unbearable feelings, by projecting them. When emotional 'ghosts' from the parent's past intrude, these are projected into the baby, who unconsciously represents part of the self or a figure from the past (Fraiberg, et al 1975). Old traumatic experiences are enacted with the infant enlisted into a scenario from long before s/he was born, through parental projections and attributions. Reflective functioning can prevent cross-generational transfer of trauma if the carer can process painful experience and lay their ghosts to rest. Because so much of this happens very early in preverbal life, some emotional experiences are retained in visceral and muscular symptoms which may persist into adulthood – a bodily process we call *'psychosomatic'*, as it bypasses thought while expressing psychic pain through the body, unable to put it into words. These feelings cannot be 'mentalized' so they are 'repeated' in physical symptoms or 'projected' into others (and sometimes, picked up and experienced by us as counter-transference).

Containment is related to affect regulation

Containment, like mirroring requires the parent to believe that the baby <u>has</u> a mind. In the normal course of events, given emotional 'holding', babies develop a sense of security, basking in their parents' responsive enjoyment. The carer's reflective mirroring of the infant's feelings not only leads to understanding, but to *internalisation* of the adult's ability to witness, contain, name and make sense of anxieties. We may say that a growing capacity for self-observation enables the child to become a 'witness' to his/her own evolving psychic life, providing a capacity for self-awareness, containment and processing of his/her own impulses and feelings, which is reworked again in adolescence. Some teen parents miss out on this revision, as alarmed by the revival of their own painful feelings during caregiving, they *project rather than process*.

'Containment' by practitioners

By receiving and processing the young client's communications, a practitioner can help mitigate the tension of anxiety by providing sensitive feedback. By making the unbearable become thinkable the practitioner fosters her clients' belief that anxieties *can* be contained. The teenager who feels listened to and understood is then better equipped to respond to the baby's urgent feelings.

Self-study/Group: Role play: [2 minutes] <u>A practitioner communicating with a teen mother</u>, who rather than offering safety, clearly frightens her 8 month old baby. [The person acting the 'mother' sets the background scenario]

Professional containment is predicated on reliability and trust. An empathic non-judgmental approach taking place within a defined 'home' – a secure transactional space for safe engagement. By providing a boundaried 'frame' in which confidential disclosures can be made the practitioner signals that feelings are important, that they have a *meaning* which can be explored. Intentions become more understandable once the underlying forces that motivate them can be recognised (even though these are not always conscious and accessible).

Skills: <u>Helping parents contain anxiety – their own and the baby's:</u>
Showing how the baby struggles to make sense of confused feelings helps carers to tune in to what s/he needs now. Seeing this reduces the carer's anxiety
- By imagining what the baby is experiencing, worries can be formulated
- Sympathetic feedback to the infant helps keep anxiety within tolerable bounds so it is not so overwhelming.
- This insight helps the carer to address both positive and negative emotions so they become more manageable.

If the teen parent can internalise her worker's capacity to process feelings ('mentalization'), like those growing up in good-enough circumstances, the young client can begin 'metabolising' (digesting) anxieties, her/his own and eventually, those of the child. Both the practitioners' ability to think about feelings and her/his *relaxed curiosity* act as a model for young parents, enabling them to learn something new - by letting go of control, and listening attentively to what they themselves and/or the child are trying to express.

Mutual recognition

As they try to formulate in their own minds what is happening in the baby's parents often talk to the young baby as if s/he could understand quite complex ideas: *"Oh, I'm sorry! Are you feeling annoyed that that SMS distracted me from our game?"* And indeed, although the infant does not understand the sophisticated words or logic s/he is soothed by this — picking up on the tone, facial expression and a sense of being cared for, responded to and thought about.

When the carer sees the baby *as a person with a mind and feelings*, the baby's expressions, gestures, stiffening, clinging, wriggling, crying and so on are all interpreted as part of an attempt to communicate. If a parent can sustain a reflective stance, s/he can receive these feelings and respond in a way that makes them meaningful to the infant. As noted, most reflect back their understanding of the baby's mental state in a slightly overstated way, to indicate that it is the baby's concerns that are being re-conveyed, not the parent's.

Through repeated experiences of such feedback, and solitary and joint play, the baby 'practices' facets of relationships, gradually developing the capacity to differentiate his own feelings from the other's, to modulate and eventually, to express them in words *["me tired!"]*. This self-reflection is paralleled by gradually coming to recognise the existence feelings in others *[Mummy's cross when I wake her because she's tired]*. Thus, in time, a child comes to appreciate herself as a thinking/feeling and embodied person among others, a member of a particular family within a wider societal context.

Self and Interactive Regulation

We have seen how emotional and sensual experiences with primary caregivers shape the little baby's emerging self. Their 'containment' modulates and 'down-regulates' painful affect, especially if they themselves are not too aroused by the infant's distress. In the second six months of the first year a baby who has been consistently helped can begin to recognise some of his/her own feelings and emotions.

'Self-regulation' (activation/dampening of arousal) is now more possible by finding ways of entertaining oneself and self-soothing, to keep bodily states under control (through musing, thumb sucking; playing with a chosen comforting object).

These *'transitional objects'* as Winnicott called security blankets or special possessions, make separations tolerable by existing under the baby's control and symbolising the interchange with the carer. In some ways these are magical objects, allowing the infant to sustain an illusion of being merged with the m/other and at the same time, bearing a gradual disillusionment and awareness that the carer is separate.

As the baby begins to crawl, a whole new set of experiences emerges. Mobility offers a sense of agency – an ability to explore hitherto inaccessible places, to follow mother around – or to escape from her of necessary. The extra activity changes sleep patterns, with longer stints at night, and predictable naps by day. Solids are now part of the diet, and the baby experiments with new tastes and consistencies.

Concurrently, *'interactive regulation'* continues to evolve – with reciprocal coordination of inner and relational processes in both infant and carer. Differentiation of 'me' from 'not-me' (as Donald Winnicott and Marion Milner put it) allows for the evolution of give and take play through which the baby discovers and in effect, creates, bit by bit, both self and external reality.

Reciprocal influence
Parents often become stuck in a groove. Helping them to recognise their infant's *changing needs* and growing repertoire of ways in which these are expressed, enables the baby to be seen more objectively, as a curious, vulnerable and engaging little person with acute feelings and a burning desire to communicate these. In addition to strengthening sensitive interaction, igniting the young parent's curiosity and guiding her/him towards age-appropriate responses also helps the *child* to establish a more robust connection to internal states.

Twosomes and Threesomes
Babies are far from passive recipients. Micro-analysis reveals attempts of self-regulation, as well as attempts to influence the carer's level of activity. For example, one very early form of self-regulation involves the baby briefly averting his/her gaze, to process what is happening and to recover his/her equilibrium, thereby also keeping the other temporarily at bay. However, a young carer may feel rejected by the baby's 'withdrawal'. When that movement of looking away happens, if a mother or father is unable to stand the baby's momentary diversion s/he may also withdraw, in hurt silence, or call the infant's name, poke, pull or intrude into his/her visual space. This *intensifies* stimulation at the very point that the baby needs to *decrease* it.

Seeking intense engagement teen parents may over-ride the baby's signals for emotional regulation. They may tease, tickle or persist in activities that result in mutually escalating 'over-arousal' until the interaction bursts out of control (see Beebe, et al, 1999). If carers do not help a stressed baby to recover, it may lead to chronic states of intense arousal setting a distorted biochemical baseline (high levels of cortisol), and possibly neuronal loss. How can we help?

> Psychoanalytically informed Parent-Infant therapy is required for deep changes. But practitioners who offer the young person a form of receptive listening, can have a transformative effect, enabling the teen parent to become more attuned to the baby. HOMEWORK: Read Selma Fraiberg and/or Dilys Daws (see pp. 157-8 in References).

Practitioners who observe how a baby's capacity to hold him/herself 'together' breaks down when carers ignore subtle cues of dampening arousal, can explain how this hinders the baby's process of self-soothing. By encouraging young parents to observe how mental states are expressed across a variety of non-verbal modalities, a worker can help them recognise their own child's unique temperament and reasons for doing things, thereby fostering better reflective functioning. Although so much of interaction occurs entirely out of awareness, just becoming aware that moment by moment each partner in a dialogue influences the other can change the way of thinking, and help improve the process of joint coordination of their rhythmic patterns.

This helps the carer to 'reframe' their representations of the baby as complex and sensitive rather than greedy, cranky, stupid or aloof. As experiences of mutual gratification proliferate, it strengthens positive aspects of the bond between them. Similarly, repairing ruptures also confirms that feelings of love survive passing feelings of irritation or frustration, and that knowing it is OK to make mistakes and learn from them builds resilience.

Whereas much research has focused on mother-infant dyads, micro-analysis of filmed encounters provides new evidence that even the very young infant has a capacity for *early triadic relationships* (Fivaz-Depeursinge, 2008). Indeed, we may say that the desire for an exclusive relationship with mother is merely one among several wishes of the young baby, who also enjoys threesomes. It is also clear that relationships with other babies and children takes place, and that rivalry and competition over parental resources is not the main 'construct-driver' of a sibling relationships. Numerous studies now demonstrate the importance of more than one simultaneous attachment relationship, and that one's degree of security depends on the quality of each. Different carers (even in the same family) provide a child with different attachment experiences, and more secure attachments act as a buffer against less secure ones.

Skills: <u>Developmental Guidance</u> has gained recognition since proposed by Anna Freud many years ago. Practitioners can enhance the parent-infant interaction by helping the young carer to recognise the baby's mind by -

- Demonstrating *early capacities* - preference for human faces; recognition of mother's voice, face, smell; non-verbal messages; protective gaze avoidance…
- Noting *innate sociability*: reaching out with all the senses, sound and visual tracking; seeking eye contact; vocalisations reinforced by a responsive answer.
- Showing *nonverbal dimensions of communication*, conveyed through gaze, facial expression, gesture, vocal tone, posture, touch, and movement rhythms.
- Explaining that as a dialogue involves <u>two subjectivities</u> in interaction, the baby's efforts are affected by incongruent or non-attuned response to signals.
- Helping the young parent to note the *sequences* in coordinating interaction (conversational pause and turn-taking; noting signs of having enough and different levels of receptivity (ranging from highly alert inactivity, to musing, or 'fussy', drowsy and less attentive states of consciousness or anxiety) each of which invite different responses. Need for 'repair' when things go wrong.

Interim Conclusions:
- People in close proximity mirror each other's rhythms and postures and sympathetically resonate with their unconsciously perceived feelings.
- Mirror neurones thus enable an implicit form of knowing.
- The nonverbal give and take reciprocally influences both partners in a dialogue
- Contributions in co-constructing the exchange are not symmetrical - the carer
- must provide 'containment' until the other is able to do so for him/herself.

- The baby's experience is aggregated into a form of implicit, procedural knowledge – a representational system of their interaction together.
- These processes produce a unique pattern of relating to each other.
- When relationships are secure, resilience takes the form of flexibility which can be safely applied to other close relationships.
- Chronic incompatibilities and non-contingent response necessitate adaptive defences.
- Coerced babies respond with anger rather than empathy to other children's crying.

Teenage Parents and Their Babies

Suffering from the hardships of sleep deprivation, isolation, boredom and overwhelming responsibilities, teenage parents often find it impossible to sustain their own psychological resources. They buckle under the demands of meeting the baby's developmental needs as well as dealing with their own. Like most adolescents, teen mothers (and fathers) are preoccupied with their personal stuff — which weakens their capacity for child-focused mentalization. Far from offering *'contingent mirroring'*, a frustrated teenager may feel compelled to take out their annoyance on the vulnerable infant. Intuitive attunement to the baby is especially difficult when a parent feels trapped with him/her, powerless to change things and attacked by (perceived hostility in the everyday world.

Attending to non-verbal cues may come more easily if the teenage parent recognises that the baby is a 'going concern' – growing, changing and constantly enlarging his/her passive vocabulary and range of understanding. And that eventually, toward the end of the first year, s/he will begin to be able to convey feelings in more understandable ways. This growth, however, is dependent on the carer talking to the baby now, explaining what has happened or is happening right now, and preparing the child for what is about to happen.

Reflective Function in Adolescents:
Reflective function involves a mother and/or father's capacity to think of the baby's needs *as separate* from her/his own. To do this the carer must step back from his/her own emotional experience during moments of stress or conflict in order to reflect upon the child's feelings and intentions (Slade et al, 2002).

Adolescents are still Individuating. Their

> *Reflective function means keeping the baby's mind in mind*

Maturational processes are disrupted by becoming parents. Although teens are avidly steeped in the meaning of their own 'feelings', in their self-centred preoccupation they may feel less interested in the way other people's minds function, becoming non-empathic. Interestingly, when put to the test, there is no difference in the way teenagers, both mothers and *non*-mothers, have similar physiological response when listening to audio-taped babies crying with either hunger or pain. But the teen mums report more feelings of sympathy, and seem more alert to the recorded baby's cries. However, when these young mothers are compared with adult mothers a different scene emerges: physiologically the older mothers have increased heart rate and cortisol in response on hearing the crying baby, whereas the younger mothers do not. Video micro-analysis also showed differences in the patterns of play with their children – compared to older mothers, young mums spent less time interacting, and more time looking away. Researchers attribute the lower physiological arousal to adolescent neural immaturity during the period that the medial prefrontal cortex, the brain region important for planning and executive functioning, is still developing over the teenage years (Giardino, et al 2008). Knowing teens, we may wonder how much the play findings are affected by laboratory conditions. Is it likely that less interaction and more looking away have something to do with teenagers' self-consciousness when aware of being filmed? Are they beset by self-representational conflicts between a 'cool' nonchalant self-image as opposed to being deemed a 'soppy' over-involved, sentimental parent? Do we know how they play when unobserved? This is an important question! We must wonder what happens 'behind the scenes'.

We do know that many an adolescent parent feels hard done by and stressed by the discrepancy between previous unrealistic plans and idealised fantasies and the exhausting postnatal reality: the emotional shock of unexpected hardships, dream deprivation and caring for a needy, demanding infant who is so incongruent with the ideal dream-baby. S/he feels sick and tired of the constant round of sleep disruption, unpleasant chores of nappy changing and night feeding, clearing toys, stickiness and finger food mess (especially hard for a teen parent with an eating disorder).

Then there is the matter of beliefs. Surveys have shown that many young parents do not believe that a baby as young as six months *could* experience sadness or fear, or sense parental moods. Yet most feel that an infant can control his/her emotions although research shows that this only occurs between three to five years!

As we noted, the child's *mentalization* – the ability to understand his/her own behaviour and that of others in terms of 'mental states' (underpinning thoughts, feelings, motivations) – is a function of the carer's *'reflective function'*. That is, the mother and/or father's capacity to think about feelings and to apply this to the baby.

> *The parent's ability to reflect upon, and reflect the baby's feelings, makes an important contribution to the infant's capacity to organize his/her emotions, to control affects and to build up a constant representation of the carer*

But when carer's feelings are too highly aroused, mentalizing is no longer possible. Their defence mechanisms of flight, fight or dissociation (freeze) are activated, meaning that the immediate response is to forget the other's subjectivity and to escape from emotional contact, to attack or to become paralysed in the situation (see Malberg, Expanded notes for a more detailed account). This affects the infant who has to mobilise defences in response.

Faced with total responsibility, many teenage mothers and fathers find it difficult to recognise or even consider the child's feelings, especially when the baby's, and later the toddler's, developmental processes both parallel and clash with their own. At times of competition a 'battle of wills' ensues as the parent assumes that the child is refusing to cooperate or doing something spiteful just to 'get at' her/him.

This may lead a young carer to increase her/his own controlling behaviour, which in turn leads the baby to perceive the carer as hostile and unsupportive, provoking anxiety. Such malevolent projections are then internalized by the baby and become part of his/her own self-image *["I must be a monster if she hates me so much"]*.
In addition, the baby too develops defensive strategies to deal with the carer's negative response.

Parental disillusionment is even more acute if the baby is born prematurely, is irritable, floppy or fussy following a complicated birth, or born with visible defects (e.g. cleft lip) as guilt complicates the relationship, particularly when these relate to tetrogens (cocaine, alcohol, tobacco, solvents, mercury, etc) imbibed prenatally.

Skill Building: Practitioners can foster reflective functioning in teenage parents by -
- being the 'voice' of the baby *["Daddy – I love playing with you but I get scared if you throw me too high!"]*
- helping the carer to think about the child's viewpoint:
     – asking parent/s to give you 'a running commentary' on the baby's thoughts
     – asking for their view of normal developmental patterns;
     – asking for best/worst case scenarios, etc.
- questioning: e.g. *"What do you think your baby might have been thinking when s/he became so scared/upset/angry?"*
- encouraging self-reflection: *"What were you thinking when that situation arose?" "How did it make you feel?" "Would you have wanted this scenario to work out differently? In what ways?"*
- fostering insight: *"In what way do you think your child"s reaction was different or similar to yours?" "Does this make you think of anything similar you might have experienced in the past?"*
- promoting more complex systemic understanding: *"What do you think your child might have thought you felt about it? How might this have made him/her feel?"* [adapted from Fearon, et al, 2006].

Disturbances

When an infant has to self-regulate without the support of containment or mutual regulation s/he comes to expect that carers will not help with the management of arousal states. *Lack of support* is a major source of disturbance in the infant during the first year, resulting in frequent and enduring high levels of negative affect and low levels of positive affect. The infant remains distressed for longer, with excessive crying, feeding difficulties and sleeping problems, which in turn may aggravate the situation further by engendering parental hostility. Eventually, a growing child may become *impassive*, no longer expecting to be helped. This is at the core of avoidant insecurity patterns. Carers who are inconsistent in their responses breed anxiously attached babies and those unable to monitor and modify their *own* negative feelings also have difficulty modulating the infant's levels of affect when these are too high. In fact, the interaction with a stressed adult actually *creates* stress in the infant, leaving him/her with an intrusion of chaotic feelings, undifferentiated and embedded in his primitive states of mind. This is at the core of disorganised insecure attachments.

Chronic parental stresses manifests as behavioural and personality disorders in the child

---

Defences

In mothers and fathers habitual defences derive from threats in their own childhoods. They are activated in situations when they cannot tolerate seeing their own feelings reflected in the baby. This tendency to disavow similar feelings in themselves make them unreliable 'mirrors' for their infants as they disapprovingly project their own into the child .

When *mis-attunement* is a chronic situation, the baby cannot learn to develop a smooth transition between emotional states, living in a state of *hyper-arousal* with deficits in self-regulation. Defences, such as hyper-vigilance or dissociation are brought in as strategies to avoid unmanageable affects and ward off unpredictable intrusions. Insensitively raised babies have difficulty in organising and modulating their emotional states. However, by processing their traumatic childhoods, many people grow up to overcome this, developing fine-tuned emotional understanding.

Recent research suggests that *'stimulus overload'* (where carers allow experience to exceed the baby's threshold barrier), or chronic deprivation and unpredictable, disrupted care necessitate *continual over-activity of the infant's own emotional systems.* Findings show that a child may then become habituated to stress overload.

Long-lasting high levels of arousal in infancy have been linked to ADHA, over-vigilance, anxiety and panic disorders, depression, eating disorders, addictions and borderline personalities in later life. Conversely, under perpetual bombardment, innate *'alarm systems'* that usually activate appropriate responses to danger may defensively shut down, or be managed by obsessional-compulsive defences, including harm-avoidant preoccupations and rituals intended to control all unpredictable eventualities. Interestingly, even non-psychodynamic theoreticians now agree that high levels of early stress may be accompanied by chronic feelings (such as sadness and alienation), possibly leading to persistent traits of shyness, guilt, shame or depression (O'Connor et al, 2000).

Skill Building: Basic Mentalization Techniques
- Ask yourself: *I wonder how I make the other person feel?*
- Reflect: How does the client's perception of you impact on the encounter?
- How does your perception of the client impact?
- Capitalise on the client's and her/his baby's curiosity
- Offer clients a vocabulary to think about their feelings
- Admit mistakes and laugh at yourself.
- Pitch things at the appropriate level (don't try to be too clever).
- Give your client an opportunity to think about her/his own mind (recognising this may feel scary, especially for teens who may not have done so before).
- Once you can help the young parent to express her/his own feelings, s/he can be enabled to think about the baby's.

HOMEWORK
One Plus One The transition to parenthood: The 'magic moment' - becoming parents – a vulnerable time for partners:
http://www.oneplusone.org.uk/Publications/InformationSheets/TheTransitionToParenthood.pdf

---

Self-study: Self reflection applies to the practitioner as well. Ask yourself the same sort of questions as you would your client: *"What was I thinking when that situation arose? How did it make me feel? Would I have wanted it to pan out differently? In what way? Does it remind me of anything I experienced previously?"*

> **READING** for next module: Angela Joyce – one to two year olds: junior toddlers pp 71-95; 2-3 year olds: senior toddlers pp.96-120, in *Human Development* http://books.google.co.uk/books?id=y2q9s644_3wC&pg=PA96&lpg=PA96&dq= Human+Development+Angela+Joyce&source=bl&ots=K6WaEVuYDA&sig=I50 BeWdTiLqMnStuaDLuap1TSSA&hl=en&ei=76lCTOqSLp0gTA9NmoDw&sa=X &oi=book_result&ct=result&resnum=2&ved=0CCEQ6AEwAQ#v=onepage&q=H uman%20Development%20Angela%20Joyce&f=false [Some pages are missing in this internet text. Readers may prefer to obtain a copy of the book].

Conclusions:

Patterns of interaction between the baby and caregivers form the basis of the child's *representational world* of self and others:

- The child's inner world becomes 'peopled' through exchanges with others.
- Representations of the self as *an effective agent* arise out of the carer's responsiveness, which allows the baby to feel s/he is influential
- Representations of others as helpful, soothing, playful, or pressurising, frustrating, etc derive from repeated social-emotional experiences with carers which coalesce into a 'working model' of expectations (Bowlby, 1969; Sandler & Sandler, 1998).
- The child's capacity for mentalization is a function of his/her parent/s' *'reflective function'* and capacity to think of that child's needs as separate from her/his own.

Key Concepts:

Attunement; Communication - rupture and repair. Attachment. Affect Regulation. Contingent responsiveness; 'Marked' mirroring. Defences.

Major Themes:

Infant-carer dyad's co-construction of meaning. The emotional security of the relational climate is dependent on the carer's reflective function, attunement, emotional regulation and contingent responsiveness. These are internalised by the infant to be drawn upon at times of stress.

Module IV:
TODDLERS & TEEN MOTHERS AND FATHERS

Aims:
- To increase your awareness of the developmental needs of toddlers, and ways in which these coincide and clash with the teen parent/s' developmental processes.
- To encourage involvement of fathers and other family members in primary care, play and support.

By the end of the fourth module you will have
- improved your capacity to observe toddler–parent interactions and to identify difficulties that may arise in teen-toddler relationships
- developed awareness of counter-transference feelings in interaction with toddlers and their parents, and confidence in detecting signs of referable emotional disturbance.

---

7. <u>Interactive Workshop</u>:

Teens, Toddlers & Imaginative Play

Learning Objectives

The model of 'separation-individuation' enhances understanding of motivations underlying three phases in toddler development – *'Practising'*, *'Rapprochement'* and *'Consolidation'*. Explored is the role of play as a bridge between teen and toddler, as a means of processing anxiety, sexuality and aggression; fostering creativity and rehearsing social roles in both.

Extending Boundaries

When we take a broad overview of maturational processes in toddlerhood we can map their progress from infantile dependency to greater emotional and physical self-reliance, with more responsibility for body management, and a growing capacity for symbolic thought and imaginative play. However, as we know, children vary in their milestones. Some walk or talk early, others late - due to a multitude of both constitutional and environmental factors which develop separately and interact with each other. So there are often discrepancies of attainment across age-related 'developmental lines' (A. Freud, 1965).

Sometime around or after the first birthday, the upright infant undergoes a momentous change of perspective on all she/he surveys. A 'love affair with the world' now begins (Greenacre, 1957).

Standing offers the child a different perspective, new modes of mobility, and a hands-free experience for tool using and investigation.

The perambulating child personally expands the boundaries of her/his world - finding new places, new activities, new objects and new capacities to explore.

Increasingly s/he also extends invitations to share in the excitement, by using more gestures (waving, beckoning, pointing) and a new range of rudimentary words to articulate desires, expecting mutual play. Activities too become more sophisticated as the child copies and improvises more complex actions (learning to turn on the TV or DVD player; playing with keys and washing machine controls; uprooting flowers 'pruning' bushes, feeding dollies, talking on the phone, typing on keyboards...

Another change is happening – recognition of the other as subject. The junior toddler can now follow the carer's gaze rather than looking at the finger when s/he points to something. This indicates a growing appreciation that others have a different physical perspective, and a dawning awareness that others have differing emotional perspectives, too (Hobson, 2002). This creates some insecurity and the toddler interacts more avidly, bringing offerings, showing special things, seeking undivided attention, affirmation and encouragement.

> *Alongside this revolutionary change in perceiving the subjectivity of others, the child who up to now has felt her/himself to be the centre of the world gradually begins to realise that s/he is merely part of it.*

In parallel, the parent's mental image of the child changes dramatically as the little crawling infant suddenly *doubles* his/her height by pulling up on something and stands tall and strong. The initial enjoyment of the toddler's excitement around new motor-skills may begin to pall with his/her unruly capacity to escape and to venture into forbidden areas.). For the parent, the constant vigilance is exhausting, and those heart-stopping moments of real danger with an impulsive toddler, render even the most patient carer snappy. Many parents, especially teenagers, are mortified to find themselves behaving with their toddler as their own parents did, and they swore they would not! Moreover, their inconsistencies and ambivalent identification with their own parents are absorbed by the toddler.

Attachment – Separation – Individuation

Throughout our lives two central forces can be said to organize our striving towards fulfilling ourselves — *a desire for closeness,* attachment and connection on the one hand, and for *separation* - or rather, recognition of separateness, and unique selfhood on the other. The tension between these poles of attachment and 'individuation' is heightened during toddlerhood, and again in adolescence (and at other crucial crossroads of our lives, such as marriage, parenthood, immigration, menopause, when earlier solutions to the interchange with our social environment have to be revisited). Through such renewed reworking, our adaptable *'identity'* is subtly transformed – composed of ever more complex, fluid yet enduring flexibly organized, multiple self-and-other representations within our minds.

What I wish to highlight here is that both toddler and adolescent parent are simultaneously engaged in this process of separation-individuation.

a. The 'practising' toddler – 11-15 months:

Margaret Mahler and her colleagues noted that as the 'junior' toddler expands her/his capacities, imitation facilitates both a sense of similarity to others and separateness from them. S/he becomes increasingly capable of understanding subtleties of interpersonal signals. The young toddler's new sense of influence over the environment is extremely pleasurable, especially when it is shared and reflected by an appreciative loving carer.

Babble becomes differentiated into increasingly recognisable words, and new words are practiced, taking as much delight in making sounds as in making spit-bubbles at a younger age. Parents who have struggled to understand the baby, may find this stage much easier now that the toddler can articulate needs. However, the child's thoughts are so much more complex than his/her active vocabulary that frustration of often sets in, unless the knowing carer can supply the missing words, or interpret the shorthand for uninitiated for others. Observations suggest that a curious toddler now spends up to six hours a day on play activities, learning and 'practising' new skills (Mahler, et al, 1975). Simultaneously, while exercising these new powers and freedom of action, the child has a burning desire for immediate gratification - to have everything – and right NOW!

The dramatic change from crawling to standing, then toddling, climbing, jumping and even running constitute major milestones within the family. However, the young toddler's unmitigated exuberance also provokes anxiety in carers as the toddling child cannot yet fully anticipate the consequences of his/her actions. Researchers estimate that previously permissive parents now issue a prohibition to the 11-17 month old approximately every nine minutes! (Schore,1994). The urge for unrestricted exploration begins to vie with anxiety about angering the parent.

b. 'Rapprochement' phase 16-24 months:
Proud of newfound physical capacities, the delighted toddler is always on the lookout for adventure. As the initial unsteadiness rapidly gives way to more confident walking, the young toddler takes pleasure in her/his bodily sensations and capacities – forever experimenting, and taking spills and accidents in his/her stride. However, jubilant explorations often lead to forbidden activities and places.

Having felt joyously all-powerful, the eighteen month old toddler is now confronted with both environmental constraints and his or her own limitations. Combined clinging and intentionally aggressive behaviours towards the caregiver increase as the toddler defends two seemingly irreconcilable fronts – a need for *agency* and *for closeness* - anxious about capitulating into passive surrender yet afraid of losing the carer's love (A. Freud, 1952). The new capacity to walk, and indeed to *walk away*, heightens concerns about getting lost and losing. Now able to venture quite far, to maintain confidence the toddler needs frequent emotional 'refuelling' (Mahler et al., 1975).

> **Observation: Refuelling** *What did you observe? Why is this child less confident from the others? Was the 'refuelling' sufficient?* Watch the same clip again

To meet the world confidently, a child needs both easy access to the carer and encouragement to experiment further (Lieberman 1993). Inevitably, anxieties are increased when the primary caregiver leaves home for work, or is left, as the child attends day care or a child-minder. These anxieties manifest in sleep disturbance and bad dreams by night, and contradictions by day - clinging and darting away, hitting out and wanting to be comforted, demanding to be carried or fed like a baby. However, it is important to distinguish between ordinary conflicts of toddlerhood and more severe disturbances. When a good experience has been internalised, it provides the toddler with a 'core' of security that can be drawn upon in the carer's absence. Indeed, availability of such a 'secure base' determines the 'radius' of the child's freedom to explore the world. It is directly related to the *quality* of his/her attachment (Bowlby, 1988).

From around twenty months the clash between the toddler's wish for unlimited exploration and the parental wish to impose safety restrictions or socially acceptable habits now escalates to a fifteen fold increase in the carer's use of verbal admonitions *["Don't do that!! I said NO!"]*. If curiosity predominates over injunctions the toddler persists, keen to investigate novelty, differences and similarities. Feeling persecuted by the child's never-ending questions and need to know and controlled by the child's 'disobedience', invasion of the parental bed and wish to climb up and walk along every low wall or visit every front garden on the way home - a busy parent may interpret these as wilful ransacking, dawdling or intrusion, rather than inquisitiveness. Struggling with contradictory internal impulses and restrictive external realities, the toddler becomes emotionally volatile, outraged by encroachments that challenge an illusion of magical control (Stoker, 2005; Zaphiriou Woods & Pretorius, 2010).

c. Consolidation
As in all things differentiated, the young child's growing recognition of separateness brings greater appreciation of *difference* - that other people's minds and emotions, feelings and needs of are often different from her/his own. Comparisons can hurt and different perspectives expose one's deficits. Shame now develops as a significant reaction to being observed and found lacking. The need to learn and increase competence vies with the desire for instant achievement, and tolerating failure continues to be difficult for the growing child when gravity and other reality restrictions intercede. Frustration is directed at parents, siblings or other toddlers who thwart her/his wishes. Then, others seem not companions but *competitors*. Aggression is heightened by counter-aggressive retaliatory attacks which do not help the child voice anger and channel it acceptably.

'Terrible Twos'- and 'Terrible Teens'
The 'terrible two' era breaks onto the scene, with awesome tantrums and intensely painful feelings of offence and frustration on both sides of the teen-toddler frontier. Intentional aggressive behaviours towards the caregiver are increasingly evident as the toddler defends both fronts of separateness and attachment, afraid of capitulating into passive surrender (A. Freud, 1952; Mahler et al., 1975).

Unbridled experimentation with physical objects also extends to body play. Toddlers are discovering the power of biting, hitting and temper tantrums. Researching sexual difference, they take delight in nakedness, locating, feeling and finding names for their genitals and pleasurable exploration of orifices - behaviours which vulnerable parents may find challenging. If the teen has unresolved issues around sex and aggression confrontations are likely to be particularly fierce.

The great activity of toddlerhood also heightens awareness of bodily functions – tiredness and energy; wounds and healing; hunger and satiation; digestive peristalsis; physical experiences of pleasure and pain and a deep interest in controlling or relinquishing bodily substances - burps, farts, pee and poop. Unpredictable incontinence, refusal to bathe and tactile interest in faeces increases parental mistrust of the child's inability to control bodily sphincters, posing essential questions about body management. These often result in intense confrontations between carer and child. The toddler makes a frantic bid for *ownership* – resisting any encroachments: s/he rejects enforced toilet training, insists on choosing books, clothes and food; resists help and throws a mighty wobbly when his/her style is cramped. These reactions, in turn, often goad the young caregiver into wanting to *"show who's boss"* – and a battle of wills ensues.

If the young child feels outraged by any limitations, the young carer, too, craves unlimited freedom. And, the continuing obligation for parental self-sacrifice clashes with ordinary adolescent needs for carefree play-time. While younger toddlers manifest their distress in eating and sleeping disturbances and crying, older toddlers tend towards extended displays of negativism and defiant disobedience. The *'terrible twos'* are accompanied by mood-swings, impulsive actions and awesome temper tantrums – paralleled only by the terrible inner turmoil of screaming door-slamming teenagers. Thus the 'terrible era' rages on both sides of the teen-toddler frontier, as feelings of uncontainable anger, confusion, hurt and frustration predominate.

Some toddler behaviours (like eating bogeys or taking pleasure in wetting and soiling; smelling and playing with turds), and open masturbation, may arouse disgust and uncontained fury in defence-dominated puritanical teens. Repugnant manners are especially disturbing to an adolescent parent in the throes of suppressing his/her own 'primitive' aspects. Following aggressive outbursts, including cruel teasing, physical harshness or actual violence, the young parent may feel deep shame at being unable to control of his or her own feelings while demanding that the toddler do so. Under pressure, an exasperated teen parent may find it hard to 'mentalize' and consider connections between his/her own disproportionate rage and the child's 'naughty' behaviour. In turn, emotionally abused toddlers tend to respond to inconsistent handling and retaliation by hiding persistently, hurting themselves, or even running away. But the teen parent may not see the child's accident proneness as a need for comfort, or link antisocial activities to a defensive means of expressing distress.

Young mothers or fathers who relish the child's growing capacity for separation and independence may feel bewildered by her/his bouts of clinging, or when the young toddler who demands to do it all 'bym'self' suddenly capitulates, climbing into the adult's lap, and vociferously demanding seemingly unnecessary help. Others, mainly Facilitators, feel they've had a 'reprieve', getting the baby back. It makes it easier for the parent when these apparent regressions can be understood as the toddler's attempts at *'rapprochement'* - increasing concern and remorse for her/his attacks. Seemingly irrational panic over a torn bit of paper or refusal of a broken biscuit reflects the child's remorseful anxiety.

Reparation

Before a young child is able to maintain a stable positive representation of the m/other in her absence, s/he experiences intense feelings of love and hate, splitting the idealised carer from the hated one. However, as in all fairy stories – the witch and the good fairy are but different facets of a single figure. In toddlerhood, gradual recognition that the split loved/hated good/bad caregiver is one and the same person has two effects. The child's mixed feelings become more integrated but also accompanied by regrets about his/her attacks and fear of losing the carer's affection (Winnicott, 1971; Klein, 1952). The shame, guilt and anxiety involved in this realisation can feel devastating. Caregiver tolerance helps develop the child's compassion and appreciation that others have their own emotional needs and hence, subjective reasons for their different responses.

The growing ability to see things from different viewpoints enhances the toddler's empathy but also, recognition of other's liability to judge. However, until there is a firmly established sense of self and considerable capacity for self-observation, the younger toddler cannot easily distinguish parental disapproval of a specific action from a more general disapproval of him/herself, experienced as *rejection*.

But needing some time alone, and resentful of being stuck at home, the adolescent carer may be intensely irritated by 'incessant' demands for attention. Similarly, the toddler's rowdiness, picky eating, sleep disturbances, regressive incontinence and anxious clinging all enrage the teen parent who had glimpsed freedom. When a young mother's wish to escape is thwarted she brushes aside the child preventing her departure by screaming furiously and clutching at her legs. Seeking her reassurance s/he clings ever-harder as the teen desperately tries to get away, tersely overlooking the child's urgent need to restore a sense of security.

> *Security is learning to manage sadness, anger and anxieties in a safe context with responsive carers who 'survive' without collapsing, retaliating or attacking*

Practitioners can show these apparent setbacks for what they are. Not 'naughtiness' but anxiety - the toddler's increasing concern about his/her lovability, remorse for attacks on the carer and desperate attempts to repair. Similarly, a young father who feels stymied by the toddler's seemingly irrational panic over a torn bit of paper or adamant refusal of a broken cookie would respond differently if he grasped the child's anxiety about irreversible damage and abandonment.

Practitioner's explanations can render these infuriating behaviours understandable and better tolerated by the young carer, especially if s/he knows it is a passing developmental phase. The toddler's highly charged bid for autonomy enrages the young parent because s/he too craves independence. It also undermines a fragile sense of authority. Shamed in public by the uncontrollable toddler and feeling embarrassingly out-manoeuvred and disobeyed, the teenager may resort to scathing sarcasm or physical violence to stop the rampaging toddler. Although abruptly halting the tantrum, it endangers the young parent's self-respect, neither providing understanding nor teaching appropriate anger management. Confusion prevails as parental blind spots further affect the child's capacity for self-regulation.

When the teen parent's defences fail during these fraught encounters, their own troubled emotional experiences are revived and unconsciously transmitted to be absorbed by the perplexed child. Parental ascriptions proliferate at this time. Normal acquisitiveness may be treated as greed; sexual curiosity regarded as perverted, or anger misinterpreted as sadism. Mothers with abusive partners may attribute the child's 'age-appropriate rambunctiousness' as malevolent or out-of-control aggression, originating in the violent father (Lieberman, 1999).

Adolescence as a 'Second chance'

This period is difficult for any parent, but adolescent parents are simultaneously reworking of many of these same issues themselves. Their own unresolved history, unformed personality, and difficult external circumstances make them more vulnerable to 'contagious arousal' and the turbulent feelings and fantasies their toddler evokes in them.

Note: Practitioners can alert carers to the child's anxiety and the necessity to explain. Feeling acknowledged, explanations help the child to understand dangers, and to internalise a world based on *reason rather than parental power*.

Clashes, Conflicts and Co-operation

As the third year progresses young parents enjoy the child's growing command of communicative language and greater ability to tolerate separations, failure and frustration. Simultaneously, for this very reason, they feel even more provoked by occasional 'crankiness', 'negativism' and blatant refusals to collaborate. The challenge of responding to the three year olds' contradictory declarations of adoration and intense hatred is disconcerting to a teen whose motivation for such early parenthood was a craving for love.

The area of ambivalence is particularly difficult for teen parents struggling with their own mixed feelings. An immature mother or father may find it impossible to survive the child's verbal attacks without collapsing into guilt, convinced s/he has failed. Conversely, s/he may become angry, vindictive and retaliatory. Like the toddler, the teen is still intensely engaged with heightened aggression and eroticism, and notions of age and gender inequalities. The need for protective care is a life-long experience, and even while providing care for the child, teenage parents themselves yearn for security and emotional refuelling from their own attachment figures.

As s/he increasingly identifies with carers (of both sexes) the toddler is better able to hold on to them internally, which can help to cope with separation. However, if the internalised figure is felt to be critical or domineering inside, the child may need constant reassurance, and benign acceptance to modify the cruel controls the child has set up within (A. Freud, 1981).

Individuation

During this period of late toddlerhood, language rapidly becomes more sophisticated, expanding in vocabulary size, richness and complexity, in tandem with increasing awareness of the emotional intricacy of self and others. The growing child who previously used his or her name as signifier, now says 'I' and 'me', as rudimentary symbolic thought gives way to logical structures, with a growing capacity for humour and imaginative play. Around age four, integration of different modes of functioning occurs when the child begins to perceive thoughts and feelings as *representations*, and is more capable of reflecting upon these (Fonagy & Target, 1996:470). Soaring beyond restrictions through imaginative play the child learns to negotiate both the illusion of his/her omnipotence and its realistic limitations (Raphael-Leff, 2010a)..

A sense of unique individuality builds up through numerous play and everyday activities, reinforcing an increasingly multifaceted identity and complex view of the important people in his/her life. Pride in new capacities and skills, especially those learned from peers and siblings drives a wish to exercise these, even at most inconvenient times. However, the dynamics are such that when the odds feel stacked against him/her, the young child escalates his/her demands to be consulted. An unsupported single mother who is the sole target of testing defiance, may not have the time, patience or emotional resources to remain accepting while acknowledging the toddler's frustration and even aggression, without hitting back verbally or physically. Body ownership is consolidated over the fourth year, with completion of toilet training, and mastery of skills such as skipping, hopping, galloping and bike-riding.

In Anna Freud's view: 'The separation-individuation phase of the second year of life is negotiated successfully only in cases where there is perfect synchronization between three factors: motor development which provides the means for the infant's physical departure from the mother and for his rejoining her; the ego's awakening wish for exploration and adventure; the mother's readiness to grant the child a measure of independence. If any of these influences comes in too early, or lags behind the others, development is interfered with and the infant, instead of advancing, misses out on an important step' (1981:116).

Setting limits

Young children need a safe framework within which they can accurately gage their own limits, and develop their capacities. Of necessity, parents must impose constraints – to minimise risk and restrain the growing child's defensive omnipotence and desire for boundless exploration. Ideally these combine affectionate playfulness with firm boundaries. However, this is not easy for a teenager who personally feels unable to apply restraint. Lack of a boundary can take many forms. A toddler whose parent/s cannot say 'no!' will feel triumphant but unrealistically powerful and bereft of adult protectors. Toddlers with inconsistent carers cannot be convinced of their loving acceptance, and must continuously put it to the test. They anxiously seek reassurance through clinging, compliance or mollification, try forcing the adult's hand by bullying, bribing or blackmailing, or alternatively, resorting to escalating acts of defiance, darting away and hoping to be rescued.

Attempts to instil a sense of social niceties backfire when the teen yells at the child to 'ask nicely' rather than demand. Many a young parent still needs firm limit-setting coupled with warmth and support from her/his own parents. Finding it difficult to provide age appropriate boundaries the teen may inconsistently overstate control or abandon regulation altogether, thereby increasing the child's sense of omnipotence, confused withdrawal or defiant rebellion. Furthermore, adolescent emotional lability gets in the way of establishing social restrictions and safe boundaries. Their own impulsive need for immediate gratification obstructs attempts to teach the child to wait. Indeed, a savvy toddler may reverse roles, reprimanding the parent for shouting, smoking, littering or drinking too much.

Young parents who themselves know no limits and cannot contain their own emotions, often stage counter-tantrums. Incomprehensible rage in an otherwise benign person is terrifying. With no third person to transform frightening anxieties into manageable emotions, the child's imagination runs riot or must be shut down. But nightmares include powerful dragons and witchlike parents who engender fear of unchecked passions or murderousness.

The *'why phase'* signifies the young child's determination to identify patterns and learn how the shared world works. Instruction around *behavioural control* becomes ever more significant to the senior toddler who is trying to learn social regulations. When told what to do, still resisting, even the child who fiercely negates suggestions will now try to emulate the carer. If the urgency of prohibitions was previously ignored, the growing child now both defiantly refuses them, yet in a personal attempt to control his/her own behaviour, when confronted by an enticing stimulus privately reiterates the parental 'no!', waggling a finger to resist temptation. In this transition to a more abstract sense of right and wrong, deterrents are still expressed physically.

Observation: Senior toddler folding with his hands behind his back, while sitting near a chocolate cake. *Note the sly kick the younger toddler gets for eating cake.*

But, where previously a toddler used 'social referencing' – checking the carer's face to see whether something was safe, acceptable or repulsive – s/he now asks questions. In some families rules are fair and clarified. What is permitted or forbidden is spelled out and even explained. Children are praised for keeping them. In other families, the rationale remains unfathomable as 'goal-posts' shift inconsistently, and the child is reprimanded for transgressing..

Concerned to understand and comply with social systems, the older toddler further expands boundaries by imitating peers. Parents who are aware of the child's growing capacity for reason and self-regulation, shift their expectations from demanding instant compliance to *negotiation*. They appeal to common sense about not doing acrobatics on a chair, cutting his/her own hair or poking toothpicks through the butter or agree on a compromise when their views clash.

Observation: teen mother comforting child after a tantrum

Accruing experiences of insensitive negotiation of areas of conflict and inappropriate limit-setting contribute to the child's inner estimation of him/herself as 'bad'. This exacerbates anxiety about loss of the parent's love, leading either to a 'devil may care' attitude of delinquency or conversely, to installation of a harsh internal judge and constant self-criticism

But when loving encouragement predominates, increased competences help the child towards satisfaction in his/her newfound physical, mental and social capacities and more realistic self-esteem. Senior toddlers learn to monitor their own behaviour and eventually, to take on responsibility for affect regulation, exerting control over modes of expression their carers deem inappropriate. As principles are abstracted and taken in, an internal conscience is consolidated. Obedience is no longer dependent on the carer's *presence*.

Dyads and Triangles

Teenaged mothers are often isolated and single, deprived of the company of school-attending peers, and their carefree leisure activities. The child may become her central mainstay. In her struggle to differentiate a little girl may be disempowered when her own fantasies about causing damage by separation and individuation dovetail with those of her same-sex mother, who feels abandoned and wishes her to stay close by for comfort. Their intricate conflict of interests is especially intense when a young mother, as yet uncertain about her own separate identity feels unsure of the difference between self-assertiveness and aggression. A fashion conscious teen mother may balk at her son or daughter's inappropriate choice of clothes, but toddler-dynamics are such that as the odds stack up, demands to be consulted escalate into a screaming match. Similarly, a lone mother who lacks confidence in her own entitlement to achieve in her own right, may invest her own ambitious wishes, and feminine desires in her son. There is cumulative evidence of the need for two carers (of whatever sex) in the ever smaller nuclear family. Lacking a partner with whom to 'debrief', a vulnerable single mother who is the sole target of defiant testing may not have the time, patience or emotional resources to acknowledge the toddler's frustration without hitting back verbally or physically.

Children also need to know their origins. In some cases, the child's father may not be on the horizon. Detrimental effects of father-absence are widely documented. Recent studies focus on specific positive contributions of fathers as a bold presence encouraging exploration beyond safe boundaries. Precisely because they tend to use less baby-talk, their more complex language can increase verbal facility in the growing child, and their endorsement of competitiveness fosters a desire to 'win'. However, it is not his sex or genetic connection to the child that is effective, but existence of a (male or female) *third* who can 'triangulate' an intense mother-child twosome.

Toddlers display avid curiosity about difference between the sexes how baby's are made, where they themselves 'come from'. Freud assumed that although the toddler in a nuclear family has feelings of love and hate towards both parents, during this 'Oedipal phase' s/he craves sole possession of one parent and elimination of the other, as rival. S/he must be helped to acknowledge the distinction in potency between adults and children, and to recognise that s/he cannot be the parent's sexual partner.

Experience of *a triangular 'space'* enables the child to acquire a different perspective - as imaginary 'witness' rather than a participant in the parents' union (Britton, 1998). Coming to terms with exclusion from the parents sexual relationship ultimately motivates the child to seek a mate of his/her own, outside the family of origin. In single-parent families where a child has no knowledge of another, the intimate twosome requires support and intervention of another person, who has a separate adult relationship with the carer.

Toddler-Teen Parallels

The dynamics of the toddler's passionate desire for self-assertion coupled with powerful internal struggles are not unlike those of the young adolescent upholding the right to be separate, different and independent. Both are involved with playing out *contradictory impulses of love, hate and sexuality* and age-appropriate anxieties around body-ownership, loss of love, separation and merging.

Clearly, when the toddler's carer IS a teenager the similarity of their emotional experience creates a bond of mutual excitement. Yet clashing goals provoke reactions of fury or despair when their respective wills are thwarted. *Teens and toddlers are set to challenge and antagonise each other.* If infants manifest their distress in eating and sleeping disturbances, crying and even head banging, toddlers tend towards extended temper tantrums, displays of negativism and defiant disobedience.

The *'terrible twos'* are accompanied by mood-swings and awesome temper tantrums – paralleled only by those of door-slamming 'terrible' teenagers. These are all very disturbing to the adolescent who in the throes of similar feelings may be unable to stay in control of his/her own feelings leading to aggressive outbursts, cruel teasing, physical harshness or actual violence. In response to such emotional retaliation, abused toddlers may engage in persistent hiding or running away. But exasperated parents may find it hard to recognise the connection between their own and the child's behaviour – or see the motivation behind behaviours, such as accident proneness as a need for comfort, or antisocial activities as a defensive means of expressing distress.

When a young parent has difficulty in balancing the infant's needs and their own it results in an inability to sustain the balance in the interactive inter-subjective experience between them – so that either the adult's subjective reality is acknowledged, or conversely, only that of the child (extreme Regulators and Facilitators respectively). The former type of interaction fosters later forms of *role-reversal* and *parentification* by the child during the preschool years (Main, Kaplan, & Cassidy, 1985), when the child's ability to think about her/his own subjective experience lags behind the capacity and need to reflect about emotional states in the other. Conversely, children who have the experience of the world rotating around their own needs alone, lack the interactive experience of *sharing* feelings and considering the emotional states of others.

Of necessity, parents must impose constraints – to restrict the growing child's boundless exploration and to minimise risk. This involves explanations, using praise, incentives and rewards and tactics such as withdrawing privileges and using timeout to reflect on the consequences of their misbehaviour. However, setting boundaries for the child may be difficult for a teenager who is unable to do so for him/herself. Similarly, given their own urgent feelings, it can be problematical to try and instil a sense of social niceties – the need to negotiate rather than demand, and to learn to wait rather than insist on immediate gratification, and to share rather than hog limited resources.
The young child may feel outraged by any limitations. But in turn, her/his highly charged bids for autonomy enrage the carer who feels that his/her own fragile sense of authority is being undermined. This is especially exasperating when the young carer's unresolved issues around control make it difficult to see the child's point of view. Feeling embarrassingly out-manoeuvred, disobeyed, duped or emotionally exploited by the rampaging toddler, the teenager may resort to scathing sarcasm or physical violence to control the child. While this can bring the tantrum to an abrupt end, it does not meet the child's need for respect and understanding – nor does it teach appropriate ways of managing anger. Confusion often prevails for both.

Mentalizing with toddlers:
Ideally, parental mentalization includes dual *self-reflective* and *interpersonal* components (Fonagy et al., 2003) which enable both carer and child to distinguish inner from outer reality, pretend crying or teasing from 'real' suffering or defiance. The ability to make these subtle distinctions is especially important when parents feel tested to their limits by intensely negative emotion, such as that displayed by a toddler rampaging in the supermarket.
If *'I hate you!'* is treated as a declaration of war rather than a cry of frustration, and one aspect rather than the whole of the toddler's tangle of mixed feelings, the parents'

hostile reaction may actually give them cause to be hated. Furthermore, carers who are unable to disentangle their own feelings from the child's, unconsciously project their repudiated impulses into the toddler who becomes the carrier of false ascriptions, internalising unwanted attributions.

As noted that mothers or fathers who are deficient in reflective function may become easily dys-regulated. When disorganised by the child's distress or anger what they reflect back fails to distinguish between their own feelings and those of the child. A carer who cannot step back to reflect on the reasons for the child's negative feelings, may become overwhelmed, and engage in various enactments during which s/he takes on a hostile and intrusive (frightening) or a fearful (frightened) and withdrawn role which is bewildering to the emotional child.

In sum
The toddler's intense feelings arouse equally intense responses in adolescent parents who are themselves still engaged with concerns of separateness, limitations and control. It may be very difficult for the young mother or father to maintain their cool in the face of their toddler's ambivalence and controlling behaviour, which in turn raises the toddler's anxieties about his/her own destructive powers.

However, the carer's affection, and readiness to explain their concerns and repair the relationship following these inevitable clashes reinforces the toddler's belief in being lovable and understood. Gradually, through ongoing exchanges, the little child begins to recognise that the mother or father has their own reasons for not wanting him/her to do acrobatics on the chair, or cut their hair, establishing restrictions and safe boundaries. The frequency of contact is less important for the child's well-being than the *quality of the emotional relationship* - closeness, attunement, understanding and authoritative (rather than authoritarian parenting).

Note to Practitioners:
Given that both toddler and adolescent parent/s are preoccupied with issues of love and hate, defiance and autonomy, closeness and separateness, the parent is likely to need help to differentiate their respective feelings, in order to become emotionally available, and reflective. Practitioners can encourage toddler and parent to discover each other through play, curiosity and humour by providing a 'safe base' which helps the carer to provide one in turn – thereby both strengthening the attachment relationship and promoting separation and individuation.

Interim Conclusions:
- In toddlerhood as in babyhood, development occurs not as a uniform pace and progression across capacities but operates across a variety social, emotional, motoric and intellectual spheres. At times, progress in one modality may inhibit achievements in another.
- 'Individuation' is achieved through experimentation, trial separations, expansion of experience and gradual internalisation of limits that enable a more realistic view of one's own capacities and limitations.
- Teenage parents may find it challenging to help the toddler negotiate developmental tasks which parallel their own ongoing issues of separateness, autonomy and identity

- Practitioners can help them to negotiate the challenging contradictions of toddler defiance yet need for reassurance.
- A sense of security is affirmed when a trustworthy carer can respond empathically to the child's contradictory needs, without mockery, rage or retaliation.
- The toddler then establishes an internal image of a 'good-enough' mother or father and self-esteem which, given appropriate 'emotional fuelling', allows for forays at greater distance and for longer durations away from the carer, and development of internal restraints.

Imaginative Play

The importance of play cannot be overstated. Not only is it an exciting activity that enhances parent-child bonding but play fosters a variety of crucial functions for developing the mind. It offers a vital means of emotional expression, social engagement and imaginative expansion of boundaries – providing routes for the child both to test out realities and to fulfil desires.

> **Observation** – a girl and boy toddlers playing with shredded paper. *Note the different styles of junior and senior play* (age-appropriate? gender influenced?)

Playfulness is not uniquely human but an inherent function of the mammalian brain. Social play is crucial in developing vital skills, forming alliances and integration into the group structure, learning the social communicatory-matrix. Creative play also fosters innovative uses of available resources. Studies attribute the pleasurable incentive of play to dopamine arousal. A leading neuroscientist specifies that play has *a developmental function* for the young brain –arousal of 'play circuits' promotes growth by exercising and extending the range of behavioural options 'under the executive control of inborn emotional systems' (Panksepp, 1998:p.295).

Interestingly, unlike humans, in other primates the appeal of play seems time limited, irreversibly disappearing by adulthood. Also, when we observe animals playing, it is in response to direct sensory stimuli. Human play can utilise the *imagination* to leap beyond restrictions of immediate somatic experience and material reality.

> *Imagination - the capability to form a mental representation of what is absent*

Play can integrate past, present, and future, linking observation, memory, and practice; thought, fun, and fantasy; illusion, dream, make-believe, and magical beliefs. Imaginative play allows a child to become *inventive*. The nature of playfulness is influenced by playmates – originally the carers. Parental orientations and the degree of tolerance for 'silliness', fantasy and mess all contribute to the play-style. Facilitator and Reciprocator mothers and fathers who induct the baby into the role of 'communicative partner' from the start (by responding to all nonverbal initiatives as spontaneous communications), while Regulator parents tend to delay, focusing on regulating desires and aggressive impulses and socialising the 'presocial' infant (Raphael-Leff, 1986; 2009). Some parents rely on flashy toys, children's TV or educational 'Little Einstein' DVDs to satisfy the child's need for entertainment; some rely on behavioral drugs like Ritalin to provide containment, and fast food to nourish their bodies. But play, that has neither aim, nor screen (or limiting 'glass ceiling'), offers rich nourishment for the *mind* – the shared interactive process of imaginative limitlessness, however brief it's duration in actuality.

The changing nature of play

Play usually has no other conscious purpose than sheer exuberance and fun. But it has many functions. By cultivating a channel to both wish-fulfilment and working-through of early anxieties, play provides the child with a means for *mastery* of ongoing developmental tasks. Themes repeat at various stages with new emphases as age-related interests and skills develop.

For babies, it is mutual play that dramatizes relationships, clarifying shared affects and notating bodily functions. Mutual exploration of objects, assisted gestures (waving) and hand-movements ('pat-a-cake') give way to ever-more-robust body-action games involving tickling, suspense, surprise ('round and round the garden'), and learning of body parts ('this little piggy,' 'head and shoulders, knees and toes, knees and toes'). Increasingly, games involve elements of separation and constancy (lost and found 'peek-a-boo,' drop and recover, 'where's teddy?' hide-and-seek). In time, narrative is added , with cumulative self-other awareness.

By the end of the first year, infants are adept at instigating play—remembering and reviving reciprocal fun and inviting others to replicate it (Trevarthen & Aiken, 2001). With the active control of upright posture, walking, and eventually running, the young toddler initiates interactive 'rapprochement' games, more consciously engaging with issues of separateness-yet-dependency in the anxious squeal of flight and exhilarating reunion. Chase/escape/engulfment sequences abound ("You can't catch me!" and "I'm coming to get you!"). Discovery prevails, with burgeoning language enhancing awareness of subtleties of meaning. Sensual enjoyment is increasingly expressed through bodily achievements (self-feeding, swings and slides, complex water play) and anal-type games of messiness and/or progressive power over sphincters and objects (finger painting, gloopy sand castles, and mud play), with salient words ("poo-poo, wee-wee!"), which continue to cast their magic spell for some years.

During toddlerhood, through play the curious little girl or boy can engage with what Freud (1908 p.135) termed the 'oldest and most burning question that confronts immature humanity': *Where do babies come from?* The emergent symbolism of play and speech is partly influenced and organized by the toddler's reaction to observations of genital differences, and growing awareness of social patterns of distinction between the sexes in their own culture. Play allows the child to imaginatively explore various aspects of 'gender' – the components of which include a sense of male or female *embodiment;* social expectations and *representations* of femininity and masculinity, and manifestations of erotic *desire* (Raphael-Leff, 2007a, 2010a). For the young child, these are accompanied by anxieties and personal preoccupations about bodily and behavioural complementarities and differences between the sexes.

Functions of Play
- Very early play provides an imaginative rediscovery of the continued existence of people and objects that 'disappear';
- Through symbolisation the child can call up an internal image of a carer, to provide safety at times of separation, or perceived danger (Bowlby, 1969).

- While allowing exploration of the external world, play also expands internal boundaries promoting emotional 'literacy' ingenuity and creative growth (see Raphael-Leff, 2010a).
- By synthesizing memories into mental images, play facilitates creation of a subjective 'inner world' of internalised and imaginary experience (Greenacre, 1959).
- Seen as a precursor for adult 'work' (A. Freud, 1981b), play also facilitates future-oriented anticipatory planning and contributes to self-reflectiveness.
- Play is a special mode of psychic functioning which allows a little child to demarcate the physical, perceivable world from the mental, fantasied one (Mayes & Cohen, 1992).
- It offers a means of testing hypotheses, and appreciating realistic restrictions (Dennet,1996)
- It provides a safe way of negotiating issues of lack, loss, dread and frustration, as well as fundamental anxieties about separation, separateness, origins, and sex (S. Freud, 1908b).
- Imaginative play can *compensate* for painful limitations and frustrations of reality. It promotes and restores self esteem by simulating preferred interactions (S. Freud, 1908a).
- For the oedipal toddler, play facilitates increased awareness of self-limitations, and consciousness of the difference psychic and external reality, thought and action - with integration of the 'psychic equivalent' and 'pretend' modes into a 'reflective mode' of play (Target & Fonagy, 1996).
- Through role reversals, make believe and dress rehearsals play urges a child toward *mentalization* and increasingly complex relationships with others, by having to envision what they may be feeling or thinking. This requires understanding that others do not share one's thoughts (Fonagy & Target, 1996).
- Finally play facilitates greater awareness of one's own mind as *private* increasing the capacities for both secrecy and lying—judging how much to share; creating social alliances and discriminatingly establishing intimate connections (Meares, 1993).

Teen Parents and Play

Adolescent parents enjoy fun and are likely to be playful. However, those who have missed out on play in their childhoods or currently feel deprived of their own play-time may resent providing a happy experience for their child. Joyful mutuality can suddenly turn sour, with the carer taking possession of the best toys, or enviously spoiling the child's game.

The teen might adopt a *managerial attitude* controlling the child's game. Removing toys from the toddler's reach, or indeed, excluding him/her from the game, may stem from the teenager's own desire to play with the toys or fear of what it might arouse. It can be difficult for practitioners observing this type of behaviour to abstain from becoming 'managerial' themselves. Lack of true engagement manifests in *repetitive* or *intrusive play*, or in *over-stimulation* – constantly flagging up a new toy which prevents the child enjoying or becoming 'too' involved in playing with one specific object.

Mutual play can form an essential bridge between toddler and teen parent. The importance of play cannot be overestimated. It is a fun situation which facilitates mutual understanding, but may also be seen as a 'precursor for adult work' (A. Freud, 1981) and a prime means of developing new skills of communication and social functioning. As the distinction between objective and subjective reality becomes clearer, 'pretend' modes of play replace the uneasiness of 'psychic equivalence', when the child still assumed the reality of his/her fantasy, and its omnipotent projection into the world. Through numerous role-play activities the toddler not only builds up a sense of his/her unique individuality, but reinforces an increasingly multifaceted identity and more complex empathic understanding of the important people in his/her life.

Playing together has inestimable benefits in developing understanding and empathy between toddler and teen. Play offers both participants a safe arena for reformulating their anxiety provoking experiences. By playing out a variety of roles, including each other's [*"You be the baby and I'm the mummy"*], power relations are temporarily reversed and new compassion can be generated between parent and child, enabling them to better see each other's viewpoint and appreciate their difficulties.

Through enjoyable playtime together, toddler and teen can each explore what the other feels and thinks, can master their own anxieties and use fantasy to compensate for their painful frustrations. A carer who is unable to play or who feels threatened by the emotions it arouses may dissociate or need to control the risky side of play. S/he may take steer the topic away from dangerous subjects or over-direct imaginary scenarios to his/her own script. A troubled parent may dissociate or become remote in the course of their play or else too intrusive, as s/he projects disowned feelings into the play space. This distorts the play experience by breaking the safe 'frame' of pretence - creating anxiety and confusion between fantasy play and reality.

Skill Building: Watch, Wait and Wonder
- Practitioners can invite a teenage client to sit on the floor with her infant or toddler for 5-10 minutes, and simply watch and follow his/her lead responsively, without taking over or guiding the play activity in any way.
- In parallel, the practitioner's role is to 'watch, wait, and wonder' about the interactions between mother and child without intervening by directing the mother or commenting. Waiting provides space for the infant to play out relational and developmental issues and helps the mother to watch and observe – and to 'wonder' at the complexity of the infant's experience.
- The latter may be explored later in discussion between the mother and the practitioner, inviting her to describe her feelings, including anxieties about following the child's' lead.

The Changing Nature of Play

Optimally play consists of finely attuned coordinated exchanges of mutual delight, in which the infant's communicative expressions and excited or subdued feelings are sensitively recognised and closely matched by an attentive playful companion (Trevarthen, 1989). From life's start, play features – the somersaulting fetus appears to play in the womb, the infant playing with the maternal face and body during breastfeeding, finger games and more energetic games with mother, father, siblings, and others, all of which require responsive collaboration. From earliest imitative exchanges to simple social engagement, repetitions and discriminations, then mutual exploration of objects to assisted gestures ('wave goodbye!') and hand-movements ('pat-a-cake') and ever-more-robust body-action games involving tickling, *suspense,* surprise ('round and round the garden'), and learning of body parts ('this little piggy'; 'head and shoulders, knees and toes'). Increasingly, games involve elements of *separation and constancy* —lost and found 'peek-a-boo', drop and recover, hide-and-seek ('where's teddy?'), and increasingly vigorous physical activities ('ride a cock-horse')… By the end of the first year, infants are adept at instigating unstructured play, remembering and reviving amusing moments of reciprocal fun and inviting others to replicate it (Trevarthen & Aiken, 2001).

With mastery over upright posture, walking, and eventually running, the young toddler initiates interactive 'rapprochement'-type games, more consciously engaging with issues of *separateness-yet-dependency* in the anxious squeal of flight and exhilarating reunion. Scary-beloved chase/escape/engulfment sequences abound - "You can't catch me!" and "I'm coming to get you!" *Sensual enjoyment* is increasingly expressed through bodily achievements (self-feeding, swings and slides, complex water play) and anal-type games of inserting and extracting, progressive power over sphincters and objects (the controlled messiness of finger painting, gloopy sand castles, and mud play), with salient words ("bum-bum; poo-poo; wee-wee!"), which continue to cast their magic spell for some years.

Through 'pretend' play the child practices, explores and gradually integrates earlier modes of understanding into a more reflective mode of play that experiences and recognises emotional motives underpinning feeling states that set off action ["Let's pretend that I kicked him because I was cross that he called me 'stupid' "…].

Before age three, the child has difficulty maintaining the conviction that ideas or perceptions are *representations* rather than accurate replicas of the way reality really is. His/her mode of play oscillates between *'psychic equivalence'* (belief in the reality of his/her fantasy and its projection into the world) and awareness of *'pretence'* (putting a banana to the ear). As the growing child's play shifts to an increasingly *'reflective mode'* s/he perceives his/her own thoughts and feelings as representational (Target & Fonagy, 1996).

> **Observation**: Toddler & Mother playing with shredded paper. Discuss possible reasons for her shut-down and its effect on the child. *Is her reaction dissociation or a game? What is his reaction to the younger toddler?* Watch it again.

Imaginative play can now take off as the child can engage with flights of fancy into the 'impossible' with a clear distinction between pretend and reality (Raphael-Leff, 2010a). Importantly, through active engagement of memory, past and present experience are linked as imaginative play integrates observation, illusion, fantasy and thinking — all of which contribute to a rich inner world and greater complexity of the capacity to generate pleasurable games, activities and new ideas.

An infant who is played with from the start, has had numerous stimulating opportunities to imaginatively expand the boundaries of his/her world. But, the capacity to distinguish 'pretence' depends on the child's clear sense of the carer's capacity to do so.

> For <u>troubled cares</u> - *unstructured play is risky. It can unleash frightening ideas.* Dissociation may arise as a defence against concrete enactments.
> * For the child – a carer's distorted response breaks the 'frame' creating confusion between fantasy play and reality
> * When parents are heavily involved in projection of their own disowned feelings into mutual play, the child may defend by bland repetitive play and/or impoverishment of fantasy.
> * Violent or abusive parents play out their sadism 'toying' with the child, who in turn projects it into toys. These then become hostile persecutors rather than comforters. Play brings no pleasure. Such children feel compelled to torment, destroy or even 'kill their teddy bears' (Sinason, 2001).

<u>The Capacity to Play</u>

'Playing is always liable to become frightening' unless it takes place within a protective area, such as that initially shared with a trustworthy, sensitive m/other (Winnicott, 1971, p.58). As noted, uninhibited play requires an external or internal *'secure base'*, with age-appropriate *'refuelling'* from carers when needed. Solitary play can allow for emotional processing. It also serves to defend the psyche against overstimulation (or, its corollary, sensory deprivation) when carers are misattuned.

However, even in solitude, playful exploration occurs not in isolation but in the context of accruing actual and imagined dialogues with internalised 'collaborative partners' whether adults, siblings or peers whose internal presence can encourage or inhibit aspects of spontaneity, curiosity and desire. In this receptive state, the child is open, vulnerable to perturbations. Anxious or traumatised children may display repetitive, monotonous play to defend themselves against unmanageable arousal.

Toddler Groups

Play groups in which toddlers participate with their parent/s serve several important functions: providing young companions for the child and friendly support for carers who may be bewildered by their toddler's intense conflicting reactions and new needs. When groups are organised with the child's emotional needs in mind (such as Toddler Groups influenced by the Anna Freud Centre tradition), they maintain a consistent atmosphere which changes little from week to week, providing a safe interim step between home and eventual nursery. Staff play a significant role for all their clients:
* They encourage parents to share their toddlers' play, and communicate with them at an age-appropriate level.
* They help toddlers to use play to express their excited feelings in an enjoyable and safe way, and to master anxieties about aggression and loss and separation.
* They facilitate interaction between parents so they might learn from each other.
* They try to support parents in managing the child's aggression and setting limits.
* They make mixed feelings more tolerable for the parent, and help the child to learn to delay action, to communicate his experience in words, and to distinguish between fantasy and reality.
* They may speak directly *to* the child about what s/he is feeling or *for* the child or his/her emotional state to the parent. This may be the most effective way of raising parents' awareness of their toddler's state of mind and enlisting a

contingent response from them.

- By verbalising the toddlers' feelings and supplying words to identify and legitimise her/his experience, workers also help the child to feel less overwhelmed, out of control and alone.

For instance, from an observation in a toddler group:
Seeing a little girl flinch when her mother roared loudly holding the toy tiger too close to her face the toddler group leader said *"You are frightening me, mummy. Please put the animal away"*. Noticing another toddler slide up cautiously behind his mother after he had been upset, the leader said on his behalf *"I think he needs a cuddle"* (Zaphiriou Woods, 2011).

Young mothers and their toddlers come together in various settings in Children's Centres and elsewhere. Small nuclear family units reduce the number and variety of contacts a child establishes. Currently it is estimated that 17% of children from lone mother families have fewer than two hours a week contact time with a man; 36% have fewer than six hours. Male early years workers can perform a vital role in ensuring many of these young children have quality contact time with men.

Practitioners can offer a welcoming 'transitional space' in which alternative ways of thinking and being together might happen. The important ingredient is a receptive and reflective group leader (and possibly an assistant if the group is large) to be responsible for the day to day running of the groups (including setting up, providing the mid-session snack, and overseeing tidying up). By being seen to think and work together for the good of the group, they provide a model of thoughtful co-operative partnership that the parents and toddlers may internalise. Inevitably, however, they also attract powerful (grand)parental transferences, which may be intensely ambivalent and hard to manage, and will need to be discussed when they meet after the group to share their observations and experiences. (For more details on the Anna Freud Centre parent-toddler model see Zaphiriou Woods & Pretorius, 2010).

Summary: Achievements through Play

Play tends to be devalued but it is the prime medium of learning.

- Play helps the child express feelings and make sense of the world s/he inhabits.
- Through play difficult situations can be mastered. The child can communicate anxieties and extend her/himself by imaginatively testing out new roles.
- Gradually, as the toddler plays more directly with peers, play extends emotional links between the child and others, further encouraging separation-individuation.
- Play helps instil acceptable codes of conduct, with increasing internalisation of social procedures, allowing for modified expression of sexuality and aggressiveness. These reinforce a sense of social belonging [*'this is how we do it'*].
- Play is thus a formative experience, but one dependent on the play companion.
- By first learning to play alone in the presence of a trusted m/other, the child then recreates a privileged space full of potentialities for imaginative play, symbol formation, and spontaneous experimental activity.
- This transitional state between 'me' and 'not me', between internal and external worlds is one in which defences are relaxed, creativity flourishes and cultural experiences can be appreciated (Winnicott, 1971).

Conclusions:
Imaginative play builds on interactions with internalised 'collaborative partners'. Teen parents so close to their own childhoods, may use play with the toddler a means of completing their own developmental growth; others find it challenging, threatening to arouse unresolved issues. Play also reveals interactive distress. Anxious or traumatised children who have not internalised a safe home display repetitive, monotonous play to defend against unbearable arousal, or chaotic enactments in an attempt to make sense of their predicament.

Key Concepts:
Adolescent parenting. 'Separation-Individuation; Identification; Practising; Emotional 'refuelling'; Social 'referencing'; Rapprochement; Ambivalence; Anality; Negativism; Equivalence, 'Equivalence', 'Pretend' and 'Reflective' modes of Play.

Major Themes:
Toddler-Teen conflicts and clashes resonate with their parallel dynamics of self-assertion and defiance coupled with a powerful internal struggle against dependency needs, and contradictory impulses of love, hate and sexuality. Boundary setting.

Module IV:
TODDLERS & TEEN MOTHERS AND FATHERS

8. Skill-Building Seminar:

Contemporary Parenthood, Fathers
& Emotional Disturbance in Teen Parents

Learning Objectives

- To appreciate the importance of fathers in facilitating development, fostering stability and decision-making capacities in toddlers
- Developing skills to address young fathers' needs, and problem of absence
- Dealing with intimate partner violence
- Screening questions, signs and symptoms of parental disturbance

Contemporary Parenthood – Fathers:

Over the past decades parental roles have changed considerably. Fathers were designated as breadwinners, and sometimes, supports for the 'nursing couple'. As such they were revered but largely invisible to professionals, who usually made contact with the mother during his working hours. Today, with educational parity and better female job prospects, parenting roles have become much less polarized and rigidly defined, especially among the youth. As young mothers enter the workforce, someone has to 'hold the baby' while she works. Furthermore, in today's economic climate, in certain sectors of the population, women who settle for less pay may less redundant than men.

At this time of gender convergence, studies show that if a father takes on the primary care role in the mother's absence, he can offer just as nurturing a relationship with the infant, and the growing child.

In previous eras research focused almost entirely on mothers, stressing the *differences* between fathers and mothers. Mothers were described as more empathic, seen to provide more soothing, singing, and emotional support while fathers were described as physically playful (roughhousing) and more intellectually stimulating. However, in general, fathers were seen to put less value on activities that facilitate early learning – such as reading, speaking, and pretend play – concerning themselves more with conveying information, chastisement, and dealing with the challenges of temper tantrums, sleep disruption and food fads. But, we know that apart from such complementing roles, correspondences exist and as the model of Participators, Reciprocators and Renouncer fathers shows, like mothers, fathers are each involved in parenting accordance with their personal attributes and capacities.

Similarity between the Sexes:

Numerous studies now show that fathers can be as nurturing and sensitive with their babies as mothers. They hug, caress, play, comfort, read to children and teach them to comb their hair, ride bikes, fly kites, play chess, wash dishes. The differences in parental styles previously assumed to be sex-related are found to be largely a function of *primary vs. secondary care*. When fathers are primary carers, mothers who work full-time elsewhere tend to be the ones who physically stimulate and play rough compared to their soothing, stay-at-home mates, who try to preserve the baby's equilibrium. This demonstrates that as well as personal sensitivity, attunement is a function of the amount of *time* spent with a particular baby: Intimate familiarity with the baby facilitates recognition of signals, and ongoing regular contact helps the carer learn to respond to more subtle cues.

The sexes differ in their reproductive capacities. Women can be pregnant and give birth. But with the invention of feeding bottles and milk-formula, lactating women are no longer the sole source of infant feeding. In theory all baby-care tasks now can be jointly shared – rather than the father as a lesser parent 'helping' the mother. The emotional climate is clement as long as a couple's parenting expectations harmonise and do not conflict or compete like, for instance, a Facilitator and hands-on Participator who vie to be the exclusive full-time carer; or a Regulator whose partner insists she stay home and mother full-time.

A 2010 survey conducted by the Fatherhood Institute polled UK 1,000 mums and dads and found that with only a few exceptions both aspired to *an equal sharing of parenting roles* – which the current UK *parental leave system* militates against. One study of 18 OECD Western countries calculated that increasing paid maternity leave by 10 weeks would decrease infant mortality by 4%! (Tanaka, 2005 cited by Graham Music, 2011). On the other hand, in many Scandinavian societies the maternity and paternal leave of 10-18 months at full pay can be shared (with a specific minimum 'daddy-quota'), and as women receive equal pay, and more real co-parenting is enjoyed, usually after weaning as an extraordinary high rate of breastfeeding is achieved (98% of Norwegian women leave maternity wards breastfeeding and 90% of mothers are breastfeeding at 3-4 months and 75% still breastfeeding at 6 months). In addition, the State provides free high quality childcare from 18 months enabling mothers to return to paid work.

In the UK, new paternity leave rules have come into effect meaning that parents will be legally entitled to share time off work during their baby's first year, up to six months off work each. But paternity leave is not interchangeable with maternity, as more than 40 years after the Equal Pay Act women working full-time are still paid on average almost a sixth less than men. Britain has one of the worse *gender gaps* in Europe and working mothers spend the bulk of their income on childcare. The Eurobarometer estimate is that the UK gender pay-gap will only vanish in 2067! A further gap is that of class inequality.

Furthermore, a UNICEF report on child well-being, put the UK at the bottom of the league table, arguing that the pressure of the working environment and rampant materialism combine to damage the well-being of UK children, who want time and attention but are given goods, branded items or money. This as opposed to Sweden (2nd) whose social policy and culture safeguards family time, or Spain (5th) where fathers do work long hours, but women stay home, and the extended family is present and supportive.
See http://www.chimat.org.uk/resource/view.aspx?RID=113728&src=KU

Men who wish to be full-time fathers are somewhat stigmatised in the UK, USA, Australia and New Zealand. Health practitioners tend to underplay men's emotions, still tacitly adhering to old Patriarchal values asserting that 'boys don't cry'. Mothers are still tacitly regarded as the 'expressive' primary caregivers, with fathers expected to control their emotions and fulfil an 'instrumental' role - setting boundaries, providing discipline, giving their name and financial benefits to their offspring.

Even those practitioners who laud paternal participation in joint antenatal classes and encourage co-parenting may feel judgmental of the way a *teen* father does so. They impose stereotype driven expectations that he give up beer and his mates, be 'strong', well-behaved and able to sustain the partnership with his baby's mother, without any help from anyone. New projects now specifically target teen fathers recognising the enormity of external demands and developmental pressures on them. But developing these services raises challenges for organisations according to the Supporting Young Fathers' Network. Staff may lack expertise in working with young people, or lack skills and confidence in working specifically with males. Young father workers may be marginalised, and surveys find significant gaps in service provision for the youngest school-age fathers, with few projects and agencies catering specifically for under 16 year old fathers who are most in need. Practitioners face barriers in locating them, the fathers themselves lack support mechanisms when identified, and circumstances with the mother and her family, educational difficulties, and negative attitudes of individual professionals complicate matters further. Where it does exist, support work for (older) young fathers is wide-ranging often involving a variety of delivery methods including one-to-one, group work, drop-ins and fixed-term programmes, peer support, and more mixed approaches that may combine elements of each, offering a range of services from practical advice relating to housing, benefits, education, employment, and legal issues in addition to emotional support and fatherhood work.[http://www.youngpeopleinfocus.org.uk/, http://www.youngminds.org.uk/parents, http://www.da-youngfathersproject.co.uk/, www.mensproject.org]

Importantly, interventions must be designed to engage young fathers, to encourage emotional responsibility by sensitising fathers to the effects of their involvement on the child's well-being, encouraging parenting skills, and where possible financial contribution.

The Paternal Function

In the past, the sex-based division of labour meant that primary nurturing was always supplied by a woman, for both boys and girls.

This ubiquitous asymmetrical arrangement of *female mothering* had repercussions which led to correspondingly separate social ideals of male and female development: Boys were groomed to be worldly workers and girls to be mothers. This also meant that in late toddlerhood in order to be 'masculine', a boy had to dis-identify from everything he had imbibed in the first few years, disavowing tenderness, nurture, and anything which smacked of the 'feminine'. Masculine meant different from the female mother. On the other had, daughters found it harder to separate off from the same-sexed mother, relying on the father to 'rescue' them. This gave rise to an idealisation of men ('knights in shining armour'). As Nancy Chodorow claimed, it also provided the driving force mothering in females, who desired to reproduce the triadic base, compared to the male dyadic (mother-son) structure which in adulthood was mirrored by wife-husband and did not require a child to complete it (1978). Could paternal nurturing change this in the next generation?

Adolescence as a 'Second chance'

The 'paternal function' was originally considered to be acting as a 'third'. Providing an external incentive for the growing child to give up his/her initial demands for unconditional mothering. In Jaques Lacan's original (1956) formulation, it was not the *person* of the real father who breaks into the dyadic world of symbiotic 'fusion' to liberate the infant, but his 'name' – the father as representative of a symbolic system organised in language. In a patriarchal society, the father also represents the Law, a symbolic delegate of the exciting outside world beyond the control by the child...

Feminists have tried to equalise the imbalance, with increasing numbers of women now partaking of what had been a man's world. Missing in these formulations is recognition of *differences* not between the sexes, but among women (Facilitators and Regulators, for instance) and among Participator and Renouncer fathers. And recognition that even in traditional divisions of parenting, mothers too have always performed the 'paternal' function of introducing otherness, thinking, limits, language and a different perspective to that of the baby. Yes, it is much easier when there is an *actual third* to whom the mother relates, who can help set boundaries to assuage the baby's separation from the maternal birth-giving body, and foster the growing child's sense of separateness, subjectivity and agency. The third needn't be a father, or even a man. Research into children of lesbian couples find that it is the *quality* of the parental relationship that is crucial rather than the sex of the parents. But how to achieve that quality?

Among teens, the stronger the relationship the greater the likelihood of paternal involvement. As noted, men living with their pregnant partners produce more prolactin which increases nurturing, and lowered testosterone after the birth. But, as Penelope Leach found in 2009 only 3% (!) of all fathers are primary caregivers of babies in the early months, rising to 7% at one year. However, many do participate in child care. When in the 1970s fathers were allowed into labour wards, paternal bonding (or 'engrossment') became apparent. Today, two generations later, we must realise that the main difference is the specificity of having grown inside and emerged out of the mother's body. When children of both sexes are brought up with 'hands on' fathers they can identify with the *nurturing qualities of both parents* (as well as other of their capacities), rather than girls and boys having to relinquish those of the opposite sex – which in turn, increase the likelihood of paternal nurture..

Young Fathers

Some midwives do expect fathers to be involved. In some quarters there is now a tacit anticipation that they will come to scans, attend antenatal classes and help with panting in labour, becoming a competent dad right from the birth. In a very young couple these expectations may be a tall order, especially if the pregnancy was unintended. Many teen conceptions are unplanned, occurring in the context of casual 'dating', sexual experimentation or even non-consensual sex. The pregnancy may bring not celebration but increasing conflict and a deteriorating relationship between the expectant partners, and their disapproving friends and/or families of origin.

Joint parenting may not be realisable at all where very young parents are concerned, particularly if their own relationship was not solid to begin with. Even 'tight' BFF (best friends forever) cohabiting mothers and teenage fathers face multiple socioeconomic challenges, including poor housing, disrupted schooling, and enforced revision of future plans. At a time of high youth unemployment and belt-tightening strategies, they are further disadvantaged by the dearth of jobs, inflationary prices and increased costs of raising a baby. Paternal

> *Parental roles must change with the needs of the growing child.*

contact can continue even if he no longer loves Mum. And contact changes over time. Like many mothers, young fathers who were bewildered or 'bored' by babyhood, may come into their own when the infant begins to toddle and talk. At this stage of 'practising' encouragement in exploratory forays coupled with limit setting, and later help in negotiating the rules of sharing and antagonism in peer relations is the order of the day. Captivated by the newly mobile child's enthusiasm, fathers who are not living with the child's mother may now feel inclined to become more involved in playful activities such as taking the child out to the playground or swimming pool. While those involved on a daily basis are aware of the discrepancy between the child's physical and cognitive capacities once-a-week dads may egg the toddler on beyond the limits of safety. Parenting intervention programmes can do much to encourage warm and enjoyable involvement and to enhance awareness of the importance of a caring father in the life of a growing child, even to the point of increasing the child's future popularity at school.

Spending time with his novelty-seeking toddler may excite the novelty-seeking teen father, but also offers him a 'second chance' to re-negotiate a safe way of chasing thrills. A young father who is still in the throes of his own individuation can re-engage with his own attachment needs, mitigating some of the stresses and strains of his own early life by engaging warmly with his child. In winning the toddler's love and admiration by being helpful and loving, a father can further his own growth, developing confidence not only in his competence, but his tender manliness.

Through interactive play with his child, a young father not only encourages the child's physical and social skills, but thinking and problem-solving abilities in himself too. Above all, he is modelling someone who *cares*. His boisterousness and encouragement to take risks may contrast with a primary caregiver's tendency to regulate and decrease excitement. But, importantly, he can retain his enthusiasm while ensuring that his energetic play style does not endanger the child.

As the child grows, even a mother who previously curbed the father's involvement for a variety of reasons may now wish him to help her mitigate the pressures of the toddler's separation-individuation. For examples of active paternal involvement, see:
• http://www.young-fathers.org.uk/images/pdf/youngfather_booklet.pdf
• http://www.youngfathers.org.uk/index.php?option=com_content&view=article&id=62&Itemid=48

> **Role Play***: [5 minutes, 4 volunteers]*:Task: a tantrum throwing toddler an 'escapist' father, a concerned mother and a mediating practitioner *(audience supplies scenario. Leader collects comments with discussion of alternative options. Asks players (still in role) about their feelings during this exchange).*

Paternal care

Surveys show that many new fathers who do have jobs are dissatisfied with their *work/family balance* and would prefer to spend more time with the baby. Aware of the chance to raise their child's 'social capital' by providing good experiences, sharing their street cred and social skills and networks, and their particular knowledge of the world, some dads make considerable efforts to find a way to spend time regularly with the child, usually at the expense of some of their leisure activities. But in the current socioeconomic situation, with higher unemployment among younger men and the lower female wage discrepancy favouring them as workers, some teenage fathers have become *unwilling primary carers*.

A caregiving young father may feel encumbered by the baby in the sling or buggy, unable to drop into the pub or participate in the rowdier activities of his mates. A teenager may ride this as a temporary condition but another may feel aggrieved and humiliated, feeling that since the baby arrived his own situation has steadily worsened – his emotional concerns are neglected by his once attentive partner, their sex-life is affected, and she may seem more preoccupied with the child than with himself. If the father's self esteem is fragile the partnership may not last, jeopardising the relationship with the child. Studies indicate that adolescent fathers are particularly likely to be absent fathers

> *Only 50% of young fathers have ever lived with their child anytime after the birth.*

Absent fathers

Statistics show that non-resident biological fathers are at risk of losing contact with the child. 20-39% do not see their kids for at least one year and another 20%–40% see their children less than once per week. Moreover, in surveys, they often do not even acknowledge having a child! But - fatherhood can take many forms.

Small group: Discuss how to encourage a non-cohabiting father to have contact. Given considerable strain and uncertainty about the future, consider visits, paternal nurturing, long distance communication, financial support, gifts, text messages, telephone or skype calls, etc. **Self-study:** jot down your views in your Journal.

We know that there are many practical factors which prevent young couples living together – most notably, lack of suitable housing and financial disincentives. There may be parental opposition to the relationship, or the couple may have split up, or never have been an 'item' in the first place. It is important to distinguish between a non-custodial father who wishes to remain involved with his baby, and may have to make an extra commitment to do so against considerable odds. [see http://www.dads-space.com/JustinsStory for the story of a father's battle to maintain contact with his children when separated from their mother/s]. As opposed to one who *chooses* not to be involved.

Under-involved fathers

Surveys suggest that these fathers are themselves more likely to have been brought up in stressful environments with absent fathers, and/or insensitive, harsh, or unpredictable carers. Boys who go on to become teen parents tend to have lived in poor neighbour-hoods, in large, low-socioeconomic status families – and with lone-mothers who have low educational aspirations. Paternal absence is associated with low grades, low school attendance, drop-out and early childbearing.

Many lack a role model for paternal activity, and also for a healthy partner relationship. Without help, young fathers find it hard to sustain a warm interactive relationship with the child/ren, and the women in their lives. It is a circular argument. We know that conduct disorders and antisocial behaviour problems in adolescence (sometimes stemming from maltreatment in childhood) also include risky sexual behaviour, which leads to impregnation.

One study found that absent fathers were specifically characterised by *insecure attachments*, with a low threshold for the experience of negative emotions such as fear, anxiety, and anger; and more symptoms of anxiety resulting in alcohol and marijuana dependency. Their work regularity suffered from months disabled by mental health or drug problems, due to which they therefore engaged in more illegal and abusive behaviour and had accumulated more criminal convictions (Jaffee et al, 2001). This social and psychological profile of poor adult adjustment among men who choose to be absent fathers has been confirmed by independent reports. Like all quantitative research, it makes generalisations to which there can be exceptions. Nonetheless, in their very absence, fathers have long lasting effects!

Negative effects of father absence: research findings indicate that:

Clearly, many non-genetically related fathers provide excellent paternal care. However, investing in some one else's offspring may

A child living without a biological father is more likely to
- live in poverty and deprivation
- have ADHD, conduct disorder, trouble in school and problems getting along with others
- have higher risk of health problems
- be at risk of suffering physical, emotional, or sexual abuse, or to run away from home

call forth primitive rivalry and there is an elevated sevenfold likelihood of mistreatment of step-children. In many cases, the so-called *'Cindarella effect'* consists of decreased care, protection, and interactive play. Live-in step-fathers may show increased antagonistic interaction involving arguments, spanking or downright neglect, abuse and violence.

'Father hunger' during adolescence has serious effects:

Teenagers living without fathers are more likely
- to become teenage parents
- to experience problems with sexual health
- to offend, smoke, drink alcohol, to take drugs, play truant,
- to be excluded or leave school at 16 with conduct problems

Numerous studies show that fatherlessness is related to lower qualifications among teens, unemployment or lower income, or life on benefits. Young men who grew up without fathers are more likely to experience homelessness, to be caught offending and to go to jail, and suffer from long term emotional, psychological and health problems. They tend to enter partnerships earlier and to dissolve these and are more likely to have children outside marriage or outside any partnership (see http://www.civitas.org.uk/pubs/experiments.php)

Mentalization: what makes paternal absence so detrimental?

While research shows detrimental socio-economic effects on boys growing up with absent fathers, recent finding are that *girls without fathers* reach sexual maturity earlier! They start get their first period on average a year before their peers, seek male attention and engage in sexual activity, often with older men, seemingly to find fatherly protection and care. Some of these become teenage mothers. However, clearly, the important factor is *lack of an ongoing connection with one's father* rather than him not living in the home. As noted, a non-residential father can keep up a warm and loving relationship with his child/ren, even on a daily basis. Conversely a live-in father may be emotionally unavailable or even abusive, and two-parent domesticity is not always advantageous. However, single parenthood does have socioeconomic and emotional repercussions.

Lone parenting

In general, findings are that even amongst older career women, lone mothers tend to have fewer financial resources than had they been in a couple. More importantly, an unsupported single parent (of whatever sex) with no partner or confidante to share both joys and

Lone mothers face twice the risk of depression as do cohabiting mothers

stress is more likely to suffer from exhaustion, depression, anxiety and other adversity-related psychological and health problems. Conversely, couple-dom has its downsides and living with a mentally unstable partner raises the higher likelihood of being/becoming disturbed oneself (see p.112).

It is impossible to generalise as there are many reasons for single parenting: it may be a deliberate choice, including women who undergo artificial insemination from a sperm donor. It may be due to a father unwilling to be named, or one deemed unsuitable by the mother or her parents; a relationship severed by death, prison or other circumstances, etc. The few in-depth qualitative studies of children who grow up without fathers suggests that decisive factors in the child's mental health are truthful discussion and information about paternal origins. Children who are abandoned by their

Crucial elements: the presence of the father in the mother's mind, and what, how and when the child is told about him.

fathers feel unloveable and less able to sustain self-esteem. They are more likely to be depressed and to attempt suicide. Some carry the burden of supporting the jilted mother; others feel that she too has betrayed them, by finding another partner.

American statistics confirm the UK findings collated by dadsworld.com
- 63% of youth suicide is from fatherless homes. *BANM, 1997*
- 90% of all runaways and homeless children are from fatherless homes. 32 times the USA national average
- 80% of rapists with anger problems come from fatherless homes – x 14 national average. *Justice & Behavior*
- 85% of children with behavioural problems – x 20 national average. *Center for Disease Control*
- 71% of all high school dropouts - x 9 national average from fatherless homes. *National Principal's Assoc. Report*
- 75% of all adolescent patients in chemical abuse centers - x10 national average. *Rainbow's for all God's Children*
- 85% of all youths in prison are from fatherless homes x20 national average *Source: U.S. Dept. of Justice*
- Daughters of single mothers without a father involved are 53% more likely to marry as teenagers, and are 711% more likely to have children as teenagers; 164% more likely to have a pre-marital birth and 92% more likely to get divorced themselves.

Currently, separation from the mother means that unless she grants it, the biological father will not be entitled to *'Parental Responsibility'*. A young dad may feel apprehensive about the demands of the Child Support Agency will make if he agrees to be named on the birth certificate. But if he is *not* registered yet would like to remain involved, he may find himself in a disputed situation, lacking visitation rights or the power to make decisions about important areas of the child's daily life and future, including health interventions or educational choices.

> Note to practitioners: It is important to convey this information during the pregnancy. In conflicted situations, it is possible to make an arrangement for continued contact through mediation by family members or a professional agency, which can work out agreements in the best interests of the child about the nature of the relationship, parenting rights and access issues.

Interim Conclusions:
- Both sexes are capable of empathy and nurture.
- Attunement is not a function of the parent's sex, but of the amount of time spent, and quality of interaction of each carer with the baby.
- Parenting provisions must change with the growing child.
- Antenatal practitioners are in a prime position to alert the family to the importance for the child, of continuing contact with the father or another supportive figure.
- Postnatal practitioners who are receptive to the hardships of non-resident fathers who wish to be involved can encourage them to maintain a partnership in parenting even if they no longer have a relationship with the child's mother.
- With help and awareness of the importance of two carers, the child's young mother and father can work together towards providing what is best for their child under their own particular life-circumstances, at this point in time.

Emotional Disturbances
in Teen Mothers & Fathers, and their Children

Parenting is by no means all fun and games. Nonetheless, the nature, content and quality of interactive play reveals a great deal about a person's emotional state, and defences against anxieties. We tend to think of emotional disturbance taking the form of depression or violence, but it can affect the simplest of play scenes. Some parents suffer from internal turbulence or devastating apathy which render them unable to be playful. They cannot not rise to the occasion, drinking a pretend cup of tea with gusto and gratitude. Nor collaborate with the child's need for funny exchange without imposing their own anxieties.

As we have seen, a traumatised withdrawn parent may feel inhibited from playing with his/her child for fear of it stirring up uncontainable feelings. Sometimes play is sporadic, and sadly, for some less disturbed young carers, the *child* is the plaything – a dolly to be dressed, played with and put back into the box, out of mind!

Clearly, a young carer's inability to engage with the baby's *mind* will impact on the child's emotional, social, intellectual and even physical development. When the primary person in life is not just unattuned but *fails to relate,* the basic elements of subjective selfhood remain incomplete – empathy, security, learning. fantasy and reciprocal play (Raphael-Leff, 2001). But as we have learned, a secondary carer who is empathic may buffer the impact of the first. In a parental couple, encouraging a better relationship between them is one of the most important factors ensuring a child's sense of security (see Cowan & Cowan, 2002).

A disturbed parent may be less responsive, or inconsistently and ineffectually so. A *personality disordered parent* is deeply hurtful, even dangerous. They imbue joint play with their toxic fantasy life, imposing horror stories on the child. For the little girl or boy who imbibes these destructive forces, play itself becomes dangerous. As in physical abuse, any form of unstructured play threatens to unleash frightening ideas or memories to a child overburdened by terrifying internal scenarios. In cases where the child's trust in external protection is violated by incestuous, violent or traumatic happenings and the worst imagined scenarios materialise into a morbid reality, and not only the child's body but mind — the very relation to reality is severely jeopardised. People abused as children are over-represented among severely ill adult mental patients.

Signs, Symptoms and Defences

One view of adolescent pathology is that it is *a breakdown in the process of integrating the physically mature body as part of the representation of the self* – that is a break in the developmental process whose primary or specific function is to establish the young person's sexual identity (Laufer & Laufer, 1984). This is a concise way of thinking about a whole host of mental ills that can and do arise during adolescence. However, in addition to the 'sexual' body, there is the 'strong' body – capable of aggressive destructiveness to self and other. This is very pertinent to teen parents whose developmental processes are disrupted by parenthood, and who are responsible for a vulnerable child. In addition the high velocity roller-coaster of intense emotionality in teenagers has a direct effect on the infant.

> *In general, symptoms and defences of children brought up in small nuclear units tend to reflect their adaptive responses to the relational climate of their shared emotional world, including the harmony or mis-match of child and parental rhythms and temperament.*

Any child caught in the throes of a parent's disturbance is at risk. But the parent too, is the product of a baby-carer exchange. Findings from attachment research shows that the defensive manoeuvres of children and their carers intersect, and patterns are transgenerational. Whereas previously, defence mechanisms were regarded as protective devises formed by an individual, today, like symptoms, they are regarded as manifestations of *interpersonal processes.* For instance, the conflicted behaviour shown by toddlers with disorganised attachments is linked to fearful, hostile or frightening responses of their caregivers (Lyons-Ruth, 1999) even when these do not directly apply to themselves. These are carers who are unable to reflect about the impact of their own volatility on the child. In turn, the child's frightened or hostile reaction triggers further emotional counter-reactions which add to the emotional morass.

Inevitably, a carer's shaming or rejecting reactions are absorbed by the child, who then bans the expression of some of his/her own mental states. The interiorised prohibition is, instilled as an internal barrier, which then selectively excludes facets of inner experience, now disavowed by the child! This internal ban leads to cognitive and psycho-social developmental deficits in the child, and poor mentalization which is then enacted cross-generationally. Growing up, these unprocessed emotional states can erupt in their raw state with the child in their care. Unsymbolised experience underpins many childhood disorders including depression, attention-deficit/hyperactivity, anxiety, obsessional, conduct and eating disorders.

> *Today, one in ten young people are affected by serious diagnosable emotional disturbances that severely disrupt their daily functioning in the home, school, or community.   Young parents bring these to their parenting.*

Child Protection Issues:

Babies, toddlers and adolescents are at greater risk for developing mental health problems when their early experience failed to provide a *'facilitating environment'* that fosters resilience and realistic self-esteem. Childhood factors precipitating disturbance include early physical or emotional abuse, trauma, loss of a loved one, frequent relocation, discrimination, poverty and/or exposure to violence, parental alcohol addiction or drug use. Emotional disturbances range from mild to severe.

In 'multi-problem' families, typically involving substance abuse, domestic violence, and emotional abuse and neglect of children, intergenerational transmission of disturbance creates an ongoing cycle of chronic stress and adversity as children grow up to repeat their carer's failures when raising their own child.

Most practitioners have been trained to identify warning signs and symptoms of emotional or physical abuse or neglect in children. They know that abused children usually present as scared – unhappy, nervous, withdrawn and isolated or sometimes angry, rude and manically unable to settle. Sexual abuse can sometimes be detected in genital injuries, precocious sexual knowledge (in words, drawings or play) or sexualised behaviour with other children, and/or flirtatious eroticisation of relationships with adults, even strangers. Violence may leave its marks.

But in cases of emotional abuse, often all we can rely upon are countertransferential feelings. In chaotic situations, our own defendedness as well as the client's secrecy and wiliness complicate detection. The perpetrator has a vested interest in concealing abuse and children usually are threatened not to disclose, or are kept under strict surveillance. An innocent carer may be unaware, or in a state of denial. Practitioners may be loathe to consider that 'nice' people might be guilty of abuse, or conversely, that a child may thrive in what appears to us a horrific mess.

Effect on practitioners:

In the ordinary course of events, practitioners are so overloaded with routine tasks and heavy caseloads that it is difficult recognise subtle maltreatment, much less to contemplate sparing extra time, effort and emotional wrangling in clarifying our perceptions. However, our aim is to ensure the each child can be safe and happy by identifying and supporting and strengthening healthy aspects as well as detecting weaknesses of individual carers.

> *Our main task is to reflect how parental history affects the ongoing parent-child relationship, and to assess the child's emotional experience of their home.*

In suspected cases of abuse, neglect, or abandonment or when a young mother proves unable to take care of the child despite home supports, we have the difficult task of coming together with a variety of different practitioners who must find a way of working and thinking together as an integrated system to find the best solution for that individual child, whether this involves foster care, or some part of the family of origin. Multi-disciplinary and multi-agency services designed to safeguard and promote the welfare of children may feel intimidating and the evaluation process is fraught with stress, anxiety and complex feelings as crisis measures may be taken to remove the child from his/her home on a temporary or permanent basis.

In our deliberations we must be aware that although we seek to be as objective as possible the decision-making process is implicitly affected by *subjective interpretation* of the facts — the emotional responses and identifications of all the practitioners involved — hence the importance of self-reflection.

Disturbance in early parenthood

In the general population almost half of all new mothers and some quarter of all resident fathers experience some form of emotional disturbance in the first years following birth of a child. Much of this postnatal distress is linked to *discrepancies between antenatal expectations and the postnatal reality* – for instance Facilitators who are unable to devote themselves to the child as planned, or Regulators who are doomed to do so (Raphael-Leff, 1985; Sharp & Bramwell, 2004). In addition, mothers of different orientations have different anxieties and are susceptible to different types of depression and at different times (Raphael-Leff, 1985b; van Bussel, et al, 2009).

> **Distress in societies in transition** is exacerbated by:
> * Geographical mobility with rapid urbanisation
> * Inner-city pressures, discrimination, social isolation
> * Dispersed extended family; loss of support systems
> * Loss of traditions and community networks
> * Stratified age groups – lack of contact with babies
> * Increased life-events and street crime
> * Socio-economic stresses/unemployment/adversity
> * Breakdown of sexual/romantic partnerships due to unrealistic expectations

Postnatal disturbance is more severe in vulnerable or young parents who also feel ineffectual, trapped with the baby, ignored, humiliated or infantilised by professionals, and offered little financial or practical support. *Vulnerability factors* include previous depression or a family history of disturbance.

Children of postnatally depressed mothers have a three-fold risk of emotional disorders, and detrimental effects of PND persist long after maternal distress abates (Murray, 1997). As noted in the first modules, patterns that are set early tend to persist. Studies suggest that babies of postnatally depressed mothers seem to develop a hyper-sensitive stress response, with a greater risk of becoming depressed in adulthood than those who did not live

> *Teenage mothers are three times more at risk of postnatal depression than older mothers.*

with a depressed parent. And there are deficits. Children of angry parent/s continue to have difficulties soothing themselves and others; controlling their anger or understanding emotional states. Emotional disturbance is related to seclusion and lack of support.

> **Discussion:** *How can practitioners help?* Both antenatally and in the early months postnatally, they are in a prime position to offer both practical support and compassion. Clients may be on their best behaviour, hiding their painful or 'shameful' feelings. But in many cases, gaining their young client's trust, practitioners can encourage expression of emotional experience. Observation of the parent-infant pair and counter-transferential 'alarm-bells' must guide referral for specialised professional attention.

As we have seen, the quality of early care also establishes the way we *perceive* stress affecting our resilience, and how we deal with stress later in life, especially when *providing* care for others. During the early period of relative helplessness, infants are helplessly reliant on their carers to regulate their affects, to soothe them when over-aroused, and restore a sense of well-being when stressed. People who have had responsive parents learn to 'self-regulate', developing what we call *resilience to stress*. In us all, the complex chain of biochemical reactions to stress remain a response to emergency situations. But people who grew up with carers who chronically conveyed hostility or resentment of the child's needs, or those who ignored distress, leaving him or her in a state of high arousal for longer than is bearable — have *an over-sensitive stress response.* When aroused they do not habituate. This is likened to a thermostat being 'set' too high very early in life (Gerhardt, 2004).

In adolescence relatively minor stress may trigger anxiety disorders, manifesting in excessive worrying, which in teen parents may be directed at the child's health or well being); incapacitating phobias (which sometimes relate to the child), and depressive disorders characterised by states of hopelessness with suicidal thoughts, or helplessness and apathy that seriously disrupt baby-care. In fact, the young child may be parentified, and expected to care for the ailing parent.

We noted that many teenage parents experience social isolation due to loss of their school friends and divergence between their own lifestyle and that of their previous peer-group. The disadvantages of being young and inexperienced in a world of adult parents are exacerbated by *insecurity* and *low self-esteem.* Current and/or a history of childhood *abuse or trauma* contribute to a greater sense of powerlessness, and inability to cope with everyday demands, especially the emotional and economic pressures of parenting. Stress is further increased by family conflict, physical complications following the birth, life events and/or problems with the infant. And low weight babies, lack of breastfeeding and erratic households worsen the prognosis.

> **Skills:** practitioners can mitigate stress by creating a community of teenage support groups, mentors and friendships with other young parents, and encouragement to utilise some of the available provisions and variety of services.

Effects of paretal disturbance on children:
Postnatal distress is experienced by almost half of *all* new mothers and a quarter of (live-in) fathers. Surveys show that much parental disturbance goes undiagnosed, and even many older mothers and fathers *do not recognise that they are ill,* and keep their feelings from family, professionals and friends.

Disturbance does not usually have a single cause. Distress is the result of a combination of factors. As we learned, in early parenthood 'contagious arousal' retriggers unresolved emotional issues from the past, and as teenagers are in the throes of reactivated emotions anyway, teen parents are most susceptible to this, as it constitutes a double dose. But why do so many past issues remain unresolved? As we noted, childhood is now seriously curtailed, becoming sexualised in pre-adolescence. This leave less time to process our childhood issues. But moreover, I suggest that the small size of today's nuclear families both generate intense emotions, and no longer allow us to work through our own infantile conflicts. Previously, in large families, this was done following the birth of each new sibling. But today, many parents have never even seen a newborn before handed their own, and many of those early feelings erupt. Finally, unlike requiring a license to drive a car, they are given the baby to take home with full round-the-clock responsibility for his/her well-being with little or no preparation and dwindling support. No wonder the situation is fraught!

It is heightened by socioeconomic deprivation, lack of emotional resources and practical support, and above all, social isolation – although some of that is due to the distressed person's withdrawal, shame and anxieties about interacting with others.

> Perinatal disturbance is precipitated by
> * worry and anxiety about *responsibilities* of taking care of a baby, or
> * disappointment following *a difficult delivery,* and a fragile baby affected by birth complications, or low weight;
> * Discrepancy between antenatal (idealised) expectations and postnatal reality.
> * *stressful life events*, such as losing a job, moving house, family conflict or the break up of a relationship; the death of a relative,
> * a poor family relationship, or violent partner.

Disturbance in New Mothers:
In addition to broken nights, dream deprivation and exhaustion, a biological mother also contends with recovery from labour and possible birth damage, hormonal fluctuations, painful engorgement or mastitis and frightening orgasmic feelings is she is breastfeeding. Not surprisingly, perinatal breakdown among new mothers is very common.
A comparative study of fifteen

> Postnatal depression [PND] is rarely experienced on its own.

centres in eleven countries showed that some form of morbid unhappiness after childbirth comparable to postnatal depression is widely recognised.
This distress is associated with crying babies, difficulties with feeding and concerns about the health of the baby in the context of isolation, lack of emotional and practical social support, poor relationships with partners, family conflict and tiredness (Oates et al, 2004). Milder emotional and behavioural changes affect 50-80% of all new mothers in the UK in the first week after the birth (the 'blues'), and around 10-13% of

recently delivered women are said to develop a severe depressive illness, although I shall argue that the overarching concept of 'depression' conflates a variety of postnatal disorders.

But teen mothers have a threefold rate of postnatal disturbance.
Many mothers continue to feel intense feelings of bewilderment, a sense of incompetence, loneliness and even despair over the first postnatal year. This is aggravated in young mothers who are less emotionally mature, and often have not built up resilience or consolidated the social resources needed to balance their own needs with those of the baby.

Intrusive thoughts of deliberate harm
In a study of 100 middle class women and their partners, in, the first month following the birth almost all parents had worries about accidental harm befalling the baby, including sudden infant death syndrome. About half also had unwanted intrusive thoughts about deliberately harming the baby, often beginning in pregnancy. Reported thought content included suffocation, shaking, stabbing, drowning or losing the infant; throwing the baby off the balcony or having unacceptable sexual thoughts. High parenting stress and low social support predicted the occurrence of thoughts of intentional harm. These ideas felt strange or aberrant, and distressed the mothers more than fathers. By three months half of them reported engaging in harsh parenting, but the only overlap with the intrusive ideas was 'screaming at the infant' (Fairweather & Woody, 2008).

While studies such as this provide evidence of the normative ambivalence of early parenting – it is important to note that the majority do not act on these ideas. However, crucially, we know that some babies are at risk from intentional acts of parental violence, and it can be very difficult to identify these.

> **Group Discussion**: *What are the difficulties in identifying signs of a child at risk?*

Disturbance in Fathers:
A meta-analysis of 43 studies was conducted by the Eastern Virginia Medical School team involving 28,000 parents from 16 different countries including the UK and the US. Findings showed that new fathers generally seemed happiest in the early weeks after the birth of their baby, with depression kicking in after three to six months by which time between 10-25% had developed post-natal depression (Paulson & Bazemore, 2010). This is more than twice the rate of men in the general population (4.8 percent). One wonders whether timing is related to the brevity of paternity leave. Another study based on a literature search from 1980 to 2002, identified twenty research studies showing that

> *Maternal depression is identified as the strongest predictor of paternal depression during the postpartum period (Goodman, 2004).*

during the first postpartum year, the incidence of paternal depression ranged up to 25·5% in community samples, but from 24% to 50% among men whose partners were experiencing postpartum depression!.

> **Group Debate:** *Why are live-in partners more affected?*
> Almost half of those who live with an ill person suffer depression or some other disturbance in their own right. This is either due to the strain of living with an ill partner, or due to 'assortative mating' (choice of a similarly susceptible partner).

The strong correlation of paternal postpartum depression with maternal postpartum depression has important implications for family health and well-being suggesting that co-habiting partners of an ill mother or father should also be screened, and that prevention and intervention efforts for depression in parents must *focus on the couple and family* rather than the individual. There is now evidence that paternal depression during the postnatal period can have a specific and persisting detrimental effect on their children's early behavioural and emotional development.

A very large study showed an increased risk of conduct problems in boys in fathers who were disturbed during their babyhood (Ramdachani, et al 2005). [These effects remained even after controlling for maternal postnatal depression and later paternal depression]. What is depression? And how do we detect it?

Depression

People suffering from depression usually find it difficult to process their own feelings without being overwhelmed by them. The day-to-day stress often interferes with a parent's *reflective functioning*. However, we must not generalise as some mothers are still able to relate sensitively to the infant despite their depression, when this is not child-linked. Others cannot even drag themselves out of bed to look after the infant. They may feel horrendously guilty about letting the baby down, or that the baby must be avoided as s/he is inextricably linked to their illness. This tends towards persecutory feeling rather than depressive ones. Some parents feel afraid to interact with the baby for fear of contaminating him/her with their own 'bad' intrusive thoughts and fantasies. Others fear the baby might contaminate them! Yet others focus intensely on the infant, curtailing his/her world as they feel too anxious of all that may befall them if they leave the house and/or too ashamed to keep in touch with friends.

Because of the risk of taking antidepressants while breastfeeding NICE-recommended treatments for postnatal disorders are *'talking cures'*. Moderate illnesses improve rapidly within the first weeks of individual therapy. Parent-Infant therapy might be advocated in addition, to resolve complications in their relation which have arisen as a result of the mother being indisposed. Psychodynamically oriented therapies or perinatal counselling offer a chance for self-reflection within an intimate therapeutic relationship or a confidential group of like-minded people in which new mothers or fathers can explore the root causes of their feelings.

Skills: *Symptoms of Depression:*
- Pervasive low mood, prolonged sadness (inability to get up and dressed; feeling irritable with unexplained tearfulness)
- anxiety without an external cause; panic attacks or feeling trapped
- difficulty concentrating, lack of motivation
- lack of interest in self and the new baby
- feeling lonely, guilty, rejected, or inadequate
- feeling emotionally overwhelmed; unable to cope,
- tiredness, yet difficulty sleeping, or early waking unrelated to the baby
- physical signs of tension, such as headaches, stomach pains, lack of appetite, and a reduced sex drive. [However, some of the last are also common experiences after any childbirth].

Psychoanalytically informed psychotherapy groups offer a safe setting for exploration of interactions with other group participants and with the leader/s. By paying attention to primitive anxieties and defences, members learn about themselves by sharing a group experience and learning to understand and integrate some conflicting aspects of themselves.

Some GPs advocate interpersonal therapy, or Cognitive Behavioural Therapy (CBT) as a means of solving problems relating unhelpful thinking patters, dys-functional emotions and harmful behaviors. In very severe cases of disturbance, such as puerperal psychosis, symptoms can include hallucinations, delusions and suicidal thoughts.

Because of the preponderance of irrational behaviour, in these cases there may be a danger to the baby or herself. Tranquillisers or anti-psychotic medication are usually prescribed by a psychiatrist, preferably with a short stay in a mother-baby unit as a possible treatment option.

Suicide:
While few mothers kill themselves, the UK Confidential Enquiry into Maternal Deaths (CEMD) reports that psychiatric disorders contribute to 12% of all maternal deaths (10% of which are due to suicide). This must be seen in the context of decreased rates of maternal mortality due to birth complications in the UK.
As noted, teenage impulsivity and dramatic gesture increase the risk of unintended suicide. NICE notes that psychotherapeutic talking treatments for antenatal and postnatal depression tends to be effective. However, women who do not receive help may remain depressed, sometimes for many years, with negative effects not only for the mother's reflective function and the baby's developing sense of self, but also for other family members who have to step into the gap to care for both. About a third of women have a recurrence of postnatal depression after a subsequent birth, and not surprisingly, it tends to affect women whose own mothers had PND.

Note to Practitioners: Although 'Postnatal Depression' is the common diagnosis, *co-morbidity often occurs*, including anxiety and mood disorders. Depression can coexist with persecutory disturbance (phobias, paranoia, projections), or various other forms of distress, such as OCD with unpleasant intrusive thoughts.

Anxiety

How stress and uncertainty are perceived is related to one's early life experience. Incapacitating anxiety may be a constant accompaniment of pregnancy, and/or is activated after the birth.
The nature of apprehension varies from mother to mother – she may feel panicked or agitated.

Skills: Symptoms of Anxiety:
- feeling worried all the time
- feeling tired and unable to concentrate
- feeling irritable
- sleeping badly
- feeling depressed
- experiencing palpitations, sweating, dry mouth
- muscle tension, trembling, numbness, tingling
- shallow, fast breathing, dizziness, faintness
- indigestion, nausea, stomach cramps, diarrhoea

Her anxiety may focus on the baby or involve concerns about her own safety, or that of significant others. nxiety can manifest in sudden, acute panic attacks during pregnancy with sensations of choking or fear of dying. It may take the of a form of nagging, chronic anxiety which has long term effects on the fetus as well as impacting on the baby postnatally. It may only arise postnatally. In predisposed women an over-sensitive stress response means that the high arousal of anxiety is quickly activated and slow to subside. If her anxiety centres on a specific feature such as bodily damage in labour, she may seek reassurance in technology or control the pain and uncertainty, even requesting a caesarean section to avoid a vaginal birth, and to minimise the terrifying helplessness and her involvement in the potentially 'humiliating' process of labour.

Postnatally, anxieties may become so persecuting that the threatened teenager tries to control the risk of succumbing the them through *dissociation:* cutting off from her emotions which unfortunately leaves her feeling empty and out of touch with herself.

> **Note:** *depression, persecution, anxiety and childhood abuse are all associated with high levels of smoking, unhealthy eating, alcohol consumption, 'recreational' or medicinal drugs and other risk-taking escapist behaviours (including self-harm, suicidal attempts and externalizing enactments).*

Persecutory Disturbances

Depression has been the focus of many studies. However, disturbances also include *persecutory feelings* about the baby, phobias, obsessions and intrusive thoughts of harming the baby feature, which may feature as part of antenatal or postnatal depression. When these cluster, and especially if focused on the baby, they warrant recognition in their own right as *persecutory states.* This is an important distinction.

> *Parents suffering from persecutory disturbance [PNP] tend to be hostile, intrusive and suspicious (in relation to the child, whereas PND depression sufferers are withdrawn, guilt ridden, and anxious as parents (see Raphael-Leff, 1986; 2001).*

This differentiation between postnatal persecutory disturbances [PNP] and post-natal depression [PND] makes sense of research findings of two types of mothers whose children have 'disorganised' attachment, described as predominantly hostile/ intrusive frightening mothers as opposed to 'fearful' (see Lyons-Ruth & Jacobvitz 2008).

Needless to say, the nature of a young woman's perinatal emotional dis-

> *The timing of disturbance reflects the weakest links in the carer's own upbringing, now revisited with her child.*

turbance reflects the *meaning* she ascribes to her own feelings, and the defence mechanisms she uses to escape awareness of these, or to relieve her distress.

Some issues will push her hypersensitive 'buttons'. For instance, her threshold for picky eating and food refusal will be determined by her own unresolved issues around food. These will intensify during weaning and introduction of solids; whereas for others, issues of autonomy and control will be retriggered in heightened form when the child becomes involved in toilet training. Subsymbolic disturbances from a time of very early pre-verbal regulation in her own infancy will manifest in psychosomatic experiences, affecting interactive bonding with her baby in ways that she cannot understand or put words to. This also related to OCD (below).

Skill Building: diagnostic questions for postnatal distress.

It is important for practitioners to make timely and rapid referrals when necessary. Although these are presented here as separate entities, it is now recognised that there is a great deal of overlap between various disorders. Some health visitors and midwives are trained in administering the EPDS. Others may ask THREE crucial questions:

1. *'During the past month, have you often been bothered by feeling down, depressed, or hopeless?'* [PND]
2. *'During the past month, have you often felt anxious?* [Anxiety]
3. *'Has your baby done things just to annoy you?'* [PNP]

If the answer to 2 of 3 of these questions is 'yes', then postnatal disturbance is likely and the GP should be alerted.

Obsessional Compulsive Disorder

OCD is an anxiety disorder accompanied by unwanted and repeated thoughts, feelings, ideas, sensations (obsessions), or behaviours that make people feel driven to do something (compulsions). These only provide temporary relief and not performing them can cause great anxiety. The aim of obsessional defences is to try and split 'good' and 'bad' aspects of themselves and others, and to keep them apart through compulsive rituals and avoidances such as counting, checking, hoarding, cleaning, etc. [*"If I don't step on a crack in the pavement nothing will happen to X"* or *"If I wash my hands seven times, no harm will come to Y"*]. Likewise, feared aspects of the self may be experienced as so disturbing they cannot be faced, so they are expelled and projected outwards, to be located in external dangers, which are then avoided by practices such as unwanted intrusive thoughts [*"I must throw the baby out of the window"*] can feel very dangerous as the person who is afraid they could lead to action, or believes that *thinking is doing*. Although these ideas may appear paranoid or even and potentially psychotic OCD sufferers generally recognize their obsessions and compulsions as irrational, and may become further distressed by this realization.

Pregnancy and the early postnatal period are times of great susceptibility for someone with a predisposition to obsessional personality traits. With all the uncertainties and intense emotional arousal antenatally and with early parenting, defences and rituals become less effective, and breakthrough thoughts might arrive, seemingly 'out of the blue', with ideas of harming the baby.

Phobias and Paranoia

Phobias may arise following a distressing or traumatic event. They involve extreme fear of a neutral situation or anxiety about something that is not actually dangerous. Common phobias include:

- **agoraphobia** – fear of public places where escape seems difficult (like crowds, queues, buses, trains or bridges). Some teenage sufferers may feel unable to leave home unless accompanied by someone.
- **social phobia** – anxiety about being with other people; unable to talk to acquaintances for fear of embarrassment or judgment.
- **specific phobias** – such as a fear of spiders, needles, heights or flying.
- **Tokophobia** (parturiphobia) – fear of pregnancy, labour and birth

As noted earlier, virtually every expectant mother has concerns about accidents, and one in two mothers have intrusive ideas about harming the baby. This are can be distressing, but is especially so a perfectionist who wants to be an ideal mother (or father). In this particular group, thoughts are accompanied by extreme anxiety about actualising these ideas, therefore provoking defensive rituals.

Paranoia is a delusional sense of persecution. The threat is usually defined, and sometimes involves elaborate beliefs about others conspiring against one. Unlike OCD, there is little insight into this as irrational thought process. And unlike phobias, in which the outcome can be unspecified, paranoia involves deliberate malevolence.

I have not referred here to psychotic illness such as schizophrenia, bi-polar disorder, mania, or autism as these are rare and unlike depression, anxiety and OCD, do not usually begin in adolescence.

SELF-STUDY HOMEWORK: a useful [16 minute] film of children talking about the effects on them of a mentally disturbed parent. The Royal College of Psychiatrist's Website
http://www.rcpsych.ac.uk/mentalhealthinfo/youngpeople/caringforaparent.aspx
Also see: http://www.rcpsych.ac.uk/Files/stigma_video.mpg
And http://www.parentchannel.tv/video/stress-and-depression-14-19?gclid=CK3r-5ehpKMCFQ1t4wodpnuy6Q

Intimate Partner Abuse:

In transitional societies such as Britain where couples live separately from the protection of an extended family, abusive behaviour often increases within the sexual partnership during the perinatal period. There are many deep causes why a young expectant father may feel aggrieved at this time:

- de-masculating effects of a low earning capacity coupled with extra financial pressures.
- the humiliated sense of infantilisation in a non-cohabiting young couple, each still living with their own parents.
- detrimental effects of binge drinking, substance abuse, belligerent mates, poor social skills, etc.
- the pregnant girlfriend's introspective preoccupation or refusal to make love.
- a sense of being overlooked at this time when all the attention is lavished on her
- anxiety about exclusion and losing his favoured position with birth of this baby, as happened with birth of a younger sibling
- murderous envy of the procreative maternal body

Skills: Referral for partner violence

Perinatal violence must not be tolerated. It heralds child abuse in which the parent identifies the child as a persecutory part of his/her self to be bludgeoned into submission. If there is any suspicion of intimate partner violence it is incumbent on the practitioner to probe tactfully and make referrals to specialists.

If the violent partner is present during the interview, the practitioner can try and elicit his recognition of the need for help with affect regulation and anger management. While this provides 'first aid', the reasons for violence are deep and intractable and usually necessitate ongoing specialised psychotherapy

Feeling demoted, the young man may seem compelled to act belligerently, in an attempt to re-establish his macho masculinity by throwing his weight around. This begins by humiliating the partner, escalating to emotional 'put-downs', hard-hitting swearing and verbal attacks, intrusiveness, possessive jealousy and control over her phone, email and social activities, or may involve financial exploitation, or deprivation, physical threats to her body or possessions, actual destructiveness or violence and sexual mistreatment.

While it is true that young women can also be violent, they are injured more badly than men. Male perpetrators tend to hit or beat their partners while females tend to slap, throw objects, or use verbal or psychological aggression. As in all abuse, the recipient is *dehumanised,* and the man 'forgets' that his pregnant partner has her own thoughts and feelings, too. If she has low self-esteem and unconscious guilt she will feel unable to resist, believing she deserves to be punished, and while the abuse is abhorrent, the pivotal factor for the couple may be the bitter-sweet confusing moments of 'repair' – when the aggression stops and the perpetrator explains that 'you made me do it', emphasising how the rage is driven by love and care.

If the couple are motivated to understand their entangled predicament, intervention of a sympathetic practitioner may lead to referral for *couple counselling.* This is important to prevent escalation if violence has not occurred, and where there seems to be enough of a healthy base to hope for a parental partnership between them even if the sexual relation ship is over.

Alternatively, the woman may be helped to appreciate the validity of her self-respecting anger. And need, as a mother to cultivate self-assertion, and her capacity to become an active, decision-making adult, protective of her own needs and those of her baby.

Skill Building: Dealing with aggressive abuse.

This delicate topic can be mentalised by discussing with the teen (and partner?):

- the prevalence of physical aggression in teen couples, and ways it and various forms of possessive jealousy are misinterpreted as 'love'.
- the anxieties pregnancy may arouse in a young father-to-be.
- the ways in which bullying, humiliation, shame and self-blame due to poor self-esteem can cause a young woman to collude with her partner's aggressive behaviour, perceived as a justified punishment, or even a sign of care.
- the baby's sensitivity to a negative emotional climate.

Challenge the macho gender stereotype stressing that violence is unacceptable; that like rape it is not a sign of manliness or protectiveness but a knee-jerk reaction of expressing feelings through action rather than words

---

Some useful brief films: http://www.thehideout.org.uk/over10/default.aspa
http://www.thehideout.org.uk/over10/whatisabuse/videos/default.aspa [unicef]

Note to Leader: Emphasise the need to recognise disturbances that are *beyond the scope of the practitioner's own expertise.* And the importance of continued support, after speedy referral of the pregnant woman or new mother or father for specialist treatment, for her client in her capacity as a known and trusted carer.

Post Traumatic Stress Disorder (PTSD)

PTSD is a type of anxiety disorder that may occur in the days or even years following experience of a traumatic event that involved the threat of injury or death to oneself or others. A psychological trauma may be defined as the emotional reaction to an inner or outer demand or happening that is experienced as *overwhelming.*

> *Trauma involves a degree of intensity that is too great for to be endured, which has far-reaching effects on psychic organization.*

Traumatic events are often dissociated and stored as sensory and affective fragments, which unlike narrative recollection, cannot or may not be recalled in words and meaningful ways. These involve intense visualisations and sensually perceived traumatic recall with repetitious behaviour and trauma-specific fears, and often drastically changed attitudes towards life and the future. Young people who have been exposed to extreme stressors such as experiencing abuse or witnessing violence or death, struggle in school, often isolating themselves from friends. The World psychiatric Association notes that many studies state the same finding – that young men tend to display more externalising behavioural problems with girls showing more mood or anxiety symptoms, and a tendency to dissociate. Memory of the trauma disturbs day-to-day activity, disconnecting them from daily reality of their lives, with flashbacks of the trauma seeming more real that current events.

Extreme emotional states that have not been worked through live on inside us profoundly affecting our everyday experiences, unless we detach ourselves from them. Even when a child is removed from a traumatising home, old expectations and anxieties are transferred into the new situation of foster care or residential home, and the process of developing intimate relationships with new carers is powerfully influenced by intrusive memories.

Due to the double turbulence of adolescence and parenting, and the greater accessibility of unconscious factors in pregnancy in dreams, imagery and vivid daydreams, defences often fail. To a survivor of sexual abuse, having a fetus moving about inside her may feel like an unbearable physical invasion of her bodily privacy. Similarly, a young woman who has pushed memories of a relational trauma out of her mind by dissociating, now finds herself invaded by flashbacks and distressing uncontrollable thoughts. The original traumatic event is involuntarily re-experienced in a very dramatic way during the perinatal period with physiological reactions, nightmares and repetitive intrusive images, smells and feelings.

We distinguish the powerful shock effect of a *one-off traumatic experience* from the accumulation of frustrating tensions. *Recovery* from relational trauma is related to attachment status. Resilience enables accommodation, whereas processing is affected by insecurity. We also distinguish between trauma that occurs in adulthood from its effect in childhood, while resources are forming. *Cumulative trauma*, such as that of living with a personality disordered parent, affects the growing child's sense of self-worth. The maltreated little girl or boy yearns for love, preferring contact with the carer to abandonment or rejection.

As the Hungarian psychoanalyst Sandor Ferenczi observed already in 1933, the child maintains an illusion of a good carer by internalising the abuser's 'badness', but feeling guilty and responsible for the abuse has a profound effect on self-other representations and perception of reality. In the developing child this results in permanent disturbances, and in many cases disintegration, fragmentation, and atomisation of the self through dissociation and splitting, which persist even if the child is removed from the abusive household. This may result in what today we call Dissociative Identity Disorder [DID] or 'multiple identities' (see Sinason, 2001).

<table>
<tr><td>

Skills: Identifying Symptoms of PTSD fall into three main categories:

'Reliving' the event
- Flashback episodes, where the event seems to be happening again and again
- Repeated upsetting memories of the event
- Repeated nightmares of the event
- Strong reactions in reminiscent situations

Avoidance
- Emotional 'numbing' or sense of not caring
- Feeling detached or having no fututre
- Lacking interest in normal activities
- Avoiding places, people, or thoughts that remind one of the traumatic event
  Inability to remember important aspects of it

Arousal
- Difficulty concentrating, startling easily
- Having an exaggerated response to shock
- Feeling more aware (hyper-vigilance)
- Feeling irritable or having outbursts of anger
- Having trouble falling or staying asleep
- Guilt and survivor guilt.

Physical symptoms (also typical of anxiety/stress)
- Agitation, dizziness, fainting, loud heart beats, headache   *[PubMed Health, USA]*

</td></tr>
</table>

The powerful state of heightened perinatal arousal may overwhelm some young mothers who due to unresolved traumatic events in their pasts, are more susceptible to internal turmoil and re-activation of negative self-representations. During pregnancy, a trauma-tised teenager may try to defend herself and protect her unborn baby from these terrifying states of altered consciousness by trying to maintain an emotional distance from her loved ones, her partner and/or family. Or by denying the pregnancy's impor-tance, or indeed, trying to 'forget' that it will result in a baby. A mother who regains her dissociative defences can provide competent routine care but feels disconnected from her baby's emotional states, and her own, devoid of curiosity about the baby's inner experience.

Child abuse as a perversion.

Perversion, is a syndrome in which a sense of powerlessness is converted to one of power by aggressive dehumanization of a victim into an object for one's own satisfaction. Chronic emotional deprivation and betrayal of trust in childhood can lead to perverse sadomasochistic enactments later in life. *Sexual perversions* such as pedophilia, rape, compulsive exhibitionism coincide with inducing pain in oneself or another person, and sex without relatedness.

Whereas men mainly externalise, using the penis (or a symbolic equivalent - gun, knife, stick) in carrying out perverse fantasies, in women, the whole body is used, including self-inflicted abuse (anorexia, promiscuity, drug abuse or burning), as representing attacks on m/other. An abused, isolated, neglected, and denigrated mother trapped in a state of powerlessness except for power over her child may be unable to resist the pull to use the baby who seems an extension part of her, to meet her own sexual needs and/or satisfy her aggressive impulses through fetishism, violence and Munchausen-by-proxy (Welldon, 2011).

> *Many abused children manifest low self-esteem, and defences such as denial, projection, dissociation and self-destructive behaviour, both drawn to and trying to avoid dreaded situations of re-traumatisation.*

Effects of abuse in childhood

Children whose parents are unable to protect them from danger, or indeed, are perpetrators experience horrific happenings within or outside their family, shatteringly betrayed by abuse of power and authority by the very people they trust most. This likelihood is increased with violent, drug or alcohol addicted parents. Abuse includes witnessing abuse of another, including intimate partner violence. Reactions to child-abuse are multilayered and the terrible sense of confusion and bewilderment reinforces the child's powerlessness, when the abuser is a family member. In cases of father-daughter incest the victimised child may attempt to preserve a loving image of the carer by taking the blame, which leads to self-hatred, shame and confusions between love and sexuality, neediness and pain, tenderness, cruelty and sadism.

Not surprisingly young people who have experienced traumatic experiences of childhood neglect, abandonment, violence or sexual abuse are overrepresented across a variety of foster-care facilities. In the UK there are currently 80.000 children in care each year. Most Looked After Children (LAC) have not only lost their home, but are psychically homeless – lacking a place inside a parental mind. When at 16, these vulnerable young people are forced to leave the care system, and are sent out on their own to fend for themselves, a third end up severely disadvantaged, homeless or in prison. In the absence of support in accessing services, many feel second class citizens and lose any trust they may have managed to sustain. [see National Children's Bureau findings on care leavers and pregnancy].

> *One in five of those leaving Care at sixteen will become mothers within a year!*

'Identification with the aggressor' as Anna Freud called it results in developmental distortions and deficits with self-blame changing the child's self-concept. Defence mechanisms against acknowledging the trauma further undermine the capacity for reality-testing and self-protection in abusive situations. These primitive protective defences include denial, repression, splitting, encapsulation and dissociation.

Growing up, the young person gravitates towards the familiar, preserving the original tie by seeking the form of primary sado-masochistic relationship s/he had with the abuser, including intimate partner violence. The perpetrator's implicit feelings of anxiety, helplessness, and despair are passed onto the victim. The violence is arousing and possibly eroticised. Deficits in psychic structure increase vulnerability to depression and annihilation anxiety. On a physiological level, it is now known that traumatogenic experiences can also affect immunologic functions and endocrine activities that produce psychosomatic disorders, restlessness, irritability, sleep disturbance, hyper-vigilance, and hyper-arousal in the traumatised child.

Adolescent symptoms such as somatisation, eating disorders, depression and suicidal behaviour, hyper-sexuality, gender identity issues and antisocial behaviour often represent disguised enactments or displaced repetitions of the original trauma. When generational boundaries have been transgressed, the practitioner can serve as a safe model for the adolescent to identify with, with whom confusions can be clarified within firm boundaries.

'Ghosts' and Enactments

> ' *a thing which has not been understood inevitably reappears;like an unlaid ghost, it cannot rest until the mystery has been solved and the spell broken'* (Freud,1909:122).

Ultimately, the internal confusion and compulsion to *repeat* the trauma until it is 'laid to rest' may lead a person to become a perpetrator, identifiying with both aggressor and/ victim, replicating traumatising patterns in self-destructive behaviour, and with other vulnerable powerless people, including his/her own child. The unconscious sado-masochistic attachment between parent-child rests on perception of the baby as a self-accessory, identified with the parent's own child-self, and hence both idealised and seen as a monster.

To people brought up in chronically turbulent households, anger is often associated with caring, and violence is regarded as a prime mode of relating to other human beings. Pathological cycles of repetition and repair become addictive. As noted, in cases of sexual abuse, especially when it occurred before puberty, emotional confusion prevails. Subsequent self/other representations are coloured by memories of the actual trauma of abuse mixed with fantasies about its undoing, and an ongoing preoccupation with 'if only' stories and preferred responses one might have made. The unresolved traumatic experience maintains an inner tension between dissociation and sexualisation, and unconscious pressure to *reproduce the internal scenarios externally*, so as to make sense of them, to lay the 'ghost' to rest.

> *When past traumatic experience has not been worked through, there is a danger it may be re-enacted with the baby, treated as a self-extension.*

A parent may dissociate when exposed to tender or to angry feelings which s/he feels unable to manage. Feeling threatened by any display of assertiveness by the child s/he may feel compelled to crush it or veer between feeling like an intimidated victim of abuse to becoming a frightening enraged perpetrator. Some sado-masochistic games may be disguised as 'innocent' play - tickling that escalates beyond tolerance thresholds, dangerous bouncing, looming and startling, disregarding the infant's anxious responses.

Therapeutic help
The World Psychiatric Association estimates that worldwide 10-20% of children and adolescents suffer mental disorders, but only a quarter of them receive professional help. 90% of countries have no mental health policy for children. We in the UK are incredibly priviledged to have a national health service that can offer free medical and psychiatric care, and child guidance clinics that cater specifically to children and adolescents. Young parents with children straddle both categories. Mixed individual and joint parent-child work can help to contain both the child and the parent's physiological and psychological hyper-arousal, and derailed developmental processes. Importantly, therapy also facilitates the parent's recovery of dissociated memories and

intense affect states from their own disorganised infancy or childhood that are being re-enacted with the baby in their care. By holding the young parent in mind and providing the experience of a new relationship, the emotionally available therapist offers a chance to validate their feelings, to grieve their losses and tolerate ambiguities, through which the quality of current family attachments may be improved. [For clinical examples see Fraiberg et al, 1975; Daws, 1999; Raphael-Leff, 2001, Malberg & Raphael-Leff, 2012); Baradon et al, 2005; Slade, 2006].

Some children and adults benefit from individual long-term therapy in which the therapist can respond to transference enactments by providing words, clarifying unintegrated traumatic memories and increasing coherence by labelling feelings and gradually disentangling what belongs to whom (see Appendix 6). Therapeutic groups allow for growth of insight and respect through an exchange of experiences with other people who have become unacceptable to society (see Welldon, 2011).

Antisocial Behaviours: Conduct Disorder and Delinquency

Finally, in *violent families*, or in the absence of a paternal figure, adolescents may turn to delinquency, crime or gang-related activity to satisfy the need for a macho stance or to drug use or dealing as an escape route. Gangs offers a sense of belonging by excluding/attacking others, with ready-made uniforms, masculinity test and confirmatory initiation, heroic leaders and exciting 'phallic' activities such as impregnating as many girls as possible, extreme risk-taking, rebellion and mild vandalism which may escalate into sadomasochistic homo- or hetero-sexual rape, and aggressive exploitation, gang warfare, raw violence, and even murder. When a baby's father is a gang member, in prison or if there is no mitigating third in an enmeshed mother-child dyad both female and male practitioners may have to serve as the sane 'paternal' figure. Child or family therapy, including members of the wider family network may be effective (see Malberg & Raphael-Leff, 2012 for clinical examples).

Conclusions:

Disturbances are interactive. The child's defences and responses to stress reflect their own adaptations to parental disorders which render the carer more rejecting, hostile, inconsistent, ineffectual or less responsive and poorly attuned - all of which lead to cognitive and psycho-social developmental deficits in the growing child. Resilience is a protective factor, comprising self-efficacy, security, and assets such as and resources such as supportive care systems. Conversely, risk factors are those that weaken or threaten protective systems.

Key Concepts: Intersubjective responses; Identification with the aggressor; absent fathers. Lone parenting. Depressive and Persecutory disorders. Contagious arousal; Child Protection Issues. Cumulative trauma; Child abuse as a perversion; intrusive thoughts;

Major Themes: Defences are adaptive responses. Disturbances take many forms, including co-morbidity of depression, anxiety, persecutory distress, obsessional disorders, PTSD, and unconscious enactments.

HOMEWORK for next Module: Dan Pink re motivation:
http://www.youtube.com/user/theRSAorg#p/u/0/u6XAPnuFjJc

Module 5:
FAMILIES, GROUPS & ORGANIZATIONS

Aims:
To review the crucial functions of the family in the context of contemporary psychosocial changes. To promote cross-agency and interdisciplinary team work, and understanding of group dynamics and institutional defences.

By the end of this last Module a practitioner is expected to have
- developed better observational skills and subtle psychodynamic under-standing of underlying interactive forces in individuals, small & large groups
- greater awareness of the effects of their own initiatives and counter-responsive reactions in work situations.
- acquired greater insight into personal strengths, biases and blind-spots; and insight into habitual defence patterns.

---

9. Interactive Workshop:

Family Dynamics

Learning Objectives
Debating the functions, ethos and effect of familiar issues (such as the family) is intended to stimulate curiosity and critical thinking that can generalise to other topics.

Societies in transition
Worldwide over the past decades since the 1960s, family formation and structure has been changing dramatically. Why is this so? Greater awareness is attributed to social forces (e.g. feminism, Student and Civil Right's Movements), scientific advances (e.g. the 'pill', new reproductive technologies), and disasters causing population and family decimation (AIDS, wars, migration). These changes contribute to an experiential culture which generates particular attitudes and values, in turn affecting individual choices and bringing about new adaptive social patterns, and new defences against common anxieties.

Social and individual forces are intertwined. In societies-in-transition contemporary family composition has changed rapidly and in some new ways to adapt to unprecedented circumstances. With erosion of traditional societies, the many 'allo-parent' child-raisers must be replaced with non-relatives, state provisions or purchased child-care. Multiple patterns coexist. In addition to social acceptance, wars, climate change, religious imperatives and socio-economic

Self-study & Group: Formulate contemporary family patterns *[jot answers in Learning Journal]*
- lone-parent (female or male)
- non-cohabiting and 'live-in' partners
- same-sex parents [gamete/embryo donors]
- 3-generational, or polygamous (several 'wives')
- grand-parental or child-headed families (no parents – common in AIDS decimated areas)
- composite ('blended') step-families
- unrelated small groups/communes/gangs
- adolescent parent/s

necessities instigate patterns of residence, mobility and migration which determine the nature of efficient family units.

Family Functions

Given these many transformations we can no longer take for granted old definitions of the traditional family function as *a reproductive unit,* privileging its own to ensure survival of its genes (especially given falling birth rates, assisted reproduction by surrogates and donors, and adoption/fostering). Neither can a family be regarded as a means of *property transmission of property* or even as a *co-habiting unit.*

We used to see a family's role as generating children. In contemporary families, we still assume that it is the presence of a child (of whatever origin) that turns a single parent, couple, or other carer/s into a 'family'. Of course, the question of whether there can be a family without a child is a tautology, as every generation is child of a preceding one.

> **Self-study/Group Discussion***:* What is a family? What are its features and functions? *[write in Learning Journal or Leader writes salient points on flipchart, conveying the following ideas if they do not arise spontaneously]:*

Family Features

Across the board, families seem to have several distinguishing features.
- The family as *a socialising, regulating force and agent of society* – is the interface between the social and the individual.
- A common family function is of *cultural transmission.* Those who are older and more fully socialised, nurture and pass on skills, tools and understanding to younger or less knowledgeable people. This is as true of adolescent parents as of others.
- Developing a family culture or ethos*:* the family as a psychosocial entity has the function of offering *an identity* integral to that family, and possibly, that genealogical lineage.
- In larger families, children are exposed to *multiple perspectives,* including those of other children and young people, with whom feelings are discussed intensely.
- Genetic or non-related family members may be co-opted, sharing common values, linked 'destinies', or a wish to preserve or promote improvement of the younger generation's quality of life.
- The family has a *protective function* – meeting the members' basic needs for food, shelter, sleep, safety, (sex) – and acting as a defence against external forces, perceived as hostile.
- Other features are *durability* and *continuity* – the trust that despite failures, family members belong, and can continue to negotiate proximity over time. However we know that some families fail to provide this (for instance Personality Disordered parents often 'dump' their children if something goes wrong).

Family as Playground

In some ways the safe family acts as a *playground* – an experimental context to try out different roles and imaginary states. The family meta-structure can provide the *security* that enables illusion and fantasy to flourish. The child can 'play' with different sets of identities and evolve a stable yet fluid self-structure that enables him or her to safely switch between different roles and contexts without fragmenting. Yet the process of achieving coherence within one's internal organization constitutes a life long evolutionary progression. A well-functioning family will go on providing a 'facilitating environment' (in Winnicott's term) enabling each individual to reach his/her own *highest potential*. In its daily workings the family supplies the child with *a set of relations* that are sufficiently emotionally invested to create an imaginative world around them, and *a play-space* with others, including peers, to develop linguistic and other social skills within and away from the close familial understanding. [Again – both Attachment and Separateness].

The Mindful Family

While most families still signify procreative or genetic kinship - with today's efficient (and female based) contraception (and infertility treatments), family formation usually signifies a *choice*. They elect to have a child and implicitly, choose to undertake responsibility to promote the development of younger members rather than following an obligation dictated by shared blood or inevitability. 'Baby-partners' tend to choose each other for complex unconscious reasons, which include procedural reminders of the original attachment figures. Today, family members do not necessarily carry a single family marker. Many women no longer take the name of the father of their children, nor do kids in composite families share the same surname.

Families try to generate a range of emotional experiences that each individual child will need to survive and to experience the world in a meaningful way – which varies cross-culturally, and with each family ethos

---

As we have learned, each family unit evolves its own *'relational climate'* (Raphael-Leff, 1991). Through early give and take, the family acts as the *'cradle of thought'* (Hobson, 2002) and emotional 'literacy' for the growing baby. In view of our central emphasis on primary interaction in this training, another way of seeing families is as 'containers' for impulses and anxieties, and instigators of human processes such as *mentalization*. Conversely, the very proximity and continuity may establish entrenched positions, allocating each member an immutable place or designated role in the family, which affects self and other representations. If its boundaries are too constricted, the family acts as a constraint - not a container but a prison. And when the interactive processes are misattuned or abusive, it may form the coffin, rather than cradle, of reflective thought!

Unconscious transactions

Given the close physical quarters, and the intimate corporeal care in families, boundaries around the body are fluid, as body-image stretches and contracts to incorporate representations of self with other. Through constant interaction, minds too are permeable, as *one mind enters another mind*.

Family relations carry the potential for a person to identify – internalising facets of another that transcends the physical boundedness of each. Projective and introjective identifications allow for imaginary control over and imaginary possession of the other by psychic appropriation – metaphorically 'inserting' parts of oneself into the other or 'taking' the other into the self. This emphasises the importance of the family commonly conferring belonging that promotes a sense of security and internalised self-esteem which is 'portable' to other places, situations and time. This psychological 'home' cannot be taken for granted in families who reject, eject or lose their members (children taken into care, abandoned street children, or given to institutions by overburdened parents) and families that instil a sense of 'insecurity' and/or inflict emotional damage. This is particularly so when *incestuous relations* occur within the family [whether father-child or mother-child (of either sex) or siblings]. Incest crosses generational boundaries actualising oedipal fantasies; it destroys trust, creating sibling rivalries, and preventing the capacity to think.

The Emotional Family:
The strong passions played out in the intimacy of a small familial constellation are the seedbed within which the child co-creates primary relationships and learns to understand the meaning of basic feelings such as love, hate, anger, envy, jealousy, empathy... Family relations provide the *template* on which 'internal working models' of relationships are constructed (Bowlby, 1988).

What is most pertinent is that unconsciously, each family member defines his/her own notions of an *emotional family* and who it consists of – whether this relates to biological or social parents, or expands to include chosen others, who may supply what is missing or enhance what the family provides.

This mental idea of family is all-pervasive, leading to a distinction between the theoretical (possibly idealised) version of the family-group and alternatively, the actual one of *lived experience*, co-created day-in day-out in full-blooded (and sometimes bloody) exchanges between members, and their introjected family values. These emotional families vary even within the same extended family as well as cross-culturally, in different societies.

Family as Forger of Identity
Regardless of its composition, a family is a group of people linked by a common *'founding myth'*. In addition to offering nurture, protection and support, the family is designated to carry out a general function of helping the child to process and resolve fundamental questions and anxieties, by teaching meaning, values and a particular construction of the world (according to its own belief system).

Some of these questions relate to the child's preoccupation with genetic history:
Who am I and were do I come from? How are babies made? What are my origins? Whose tummy did I come out of? As well as *'Who looked after me?'* and even, *Who would I be if I weren't me?*

These questions incorporate fantasies about the *originary union* - as one has to come from somewhere. The gradual discovery that I did not always exist nor was I self-created impels the crucial question 'how did **I** come to be?'

If an adolescent parent answers 'you were a mistake' they may not be fully aware how hurtful and demeaning this is. Even if the conception was not consciously intended – the fact that contraception was avoided, the pregnancy not terminated, the baby not given up for fostering or adoption reflects some form of acceptance, however unplanned (barring total disregard or denial of consequences).

Other problematic families are those who conscious maintain ignorance about the child's origins. This causes disruption to historicity, forcing the child to invent their place in a mythical context. Confusion about origins is found to be more disturbing than
unpalatable
facts.

| In a 'safe' family, questions can be asked even if unanswerable. |

Mothers and fathers too, affect the child's mind when they themselves are preoccupied with their own anxieties, shame and fantasies of procreation, which determine what they tell or do not tell a child – especially in situations of assisted asexual reproduction and donor gametes, rape or sexual promiscuity where it might prove impossible to trace the child's origins.

Finally the *wider social context* must be noted, including other institutions (e.g. education, health, social services etc) which take on some of the care roles or even surveillance of the family on behalf of the State. These provide a variety of perspectives and confer a broader *sense of identity* – a fluctuating sum of expectations, self-images, values and beliefs that operate in each context, with a sense of belonging to larger groups, including community, nation, even continent.

Contemporary Teen Families

Western societies are in a state of transition. Along with new freedoms there are additional pressures on parenting, which today is no longer confined to marriage, or even cohabitation. Fifty years after the contraceptive pill was first introduced, pregnancy is assumed to be a chosen state, although clearly, 'accidents' do happen. For complex reasons, especially in the USA and the UK, peer pressure towards early motherhood has increased the rate of teen pregnancy (40+ per 1,000 women under 18) – although not so in a variety of other westernised countries, such as Japan, Switzerland, the Netherlands and Sweden with equally young sexual activity, but teen birth rates of less than 7 per 1,000. In the UK, about half of all teen conceptions end in abortion. Reduction of

> **Brief discussion**: <u>What determines these different rates?</u>
> *Why has 1 in 5 British teens been pregnant by age 18?*
> *Why does the UK have the highest underage?*

the social stigma around 'unwed' mothers has meant that very few babies are now given up for adoption. The majority of young women who give birth choose to keep their babies, even in the absence of a partner. Seeking to establish a loving (and genetically related) family of their own, children who have grown up in care are disproportionally represented among teenage mothers, as are girls who did not have a father.

Education is often the first casualty of the lone young mother's double burden of both baby-care, and subsistence provision. Brevity of school educational is strongly associated with poorly paid jobs, child poverty and social disadvantage. However, many outcome studies fail to separate this socio-economic disadvantage from the effects of adolescent parenting. A common finding is that children of teen mothers have lower grades at school and poorer cognitive-linguistic abilities but it is unclear how this correlates to the high level of postnatal 'depression' in young mothers (relating to forbidden abortion, unwanted child, lack of partner, family conflicts, isolation, poverty - insufficient resources in short) or whether it relates to parental education, or is a function of dis-regulatory effects of parental immaturity - poor reflective function specifically related to pubertal physiology and biochemistry.

Conversely, protective factors such as good family and/or social support, a strong couple relationship (whether heterosexual or homosexual) are shown to enhance maternal caregiving and the future prognosis for the child. In Western societies, the level of family breakup is high. UK statistics indicate that only one third of children born to co-habiting parents continue to live with both throughout their childhood (vs. 70% of those born to married couples).

In the case of *all couples*, research confirms that relationships tend to deteriorate when sexual partners become parents (Cowan & Cowan, 2002). Having a baby changes the day-to-day patterns of engagement, both within a partnership and between the couple and their respective families. Cohabiting couples are shocked at the impact on their previous lifestyle and divisions of labour. Even longstanding couples among adult expectant parents tend to overestimate the extent to which contemporary fathers will be involved in baby-care. Mothers are often disappointed when their expectations (and the father's promises) are not met postnatally, which inevitably has negative effects on couple satisfaction. Adolescents are totally unprepared for the degree of upheaval in their sexual and social relationships after the birth, and those with romanticised notions are doubly disenchanted.

Oscillating Pairs and Family Triangles
Shifting from an intimate sexual twosome to incorporate a young third is always fraught - and in triangular relations, one person often feels left out. The infant's capacity for 'triangular communication' with both parents at the same time is more robust when 'scaffolded' by parental coalition ['two for one' alliance], and undermined by their dissention, when the infant has to regulate the 'two against one' conflict (Fivaz-Depeursinge, 2008).

Many teenage parents find that the only way they can afford to stay together is by living with one of their respective families. However this arrangement may exacerbate jealousy about the other's closeness with the baby in the one who lives apart. Urgent and heartfelt arguments may erupt regarding loyalties, and who constitutes the 'prime' unit: the sexual partners, the new family threesome, the family of origin, or the mother and baby dyad, and/or other children within the family. Much energy and thought has to be invested into finding the best ways to co-parent together despite non-cohabitation and non-resident fathers who wish to remain involved may need help to spend regular time with the child and to maintain a parenting relationship with the mother.

While more mature partners may find the internal resources to negotiate the feelings aroused by oscillating pairs and family triangles – the strain of contagious emotional arousal, disrupted sleep, constant vigilance and fitting in to other people's lifestyles may prove too much for a budding relationship between teenagers. Separations often occur against a background of unequal commitments in premature parental responsibility. The tensions for a young father between carefree adolescence as a period of finding a sense of self, and fatherhood's demand that he enable the growing child's a sense of self may feel impossible to sustain. As contact with the mother diminishes many young fathers lose touch with their offspring as well.

> MESSAGE: The importance for the child of having paternal contact or some knowledge about the father is a central theme to be discussed, as is the issue of maternal co-parenting with someone other than the father in his absence – another male partner, a female one, her own mother or parents, etc.

Family Dynamics
If the family is an overarching concept, recognisable despite its many variations – a central question is *how do we understand the human need to form it?* From a psychological and group dynamics point of view, it is even intriguing to speculate on

the impact of its specific organization on the way the child's mind develops.

> *Family interaction provides the most basic form of shared understanding.* Re
cap
itulation:

Most carers of young babies intuitively speak a form of *'motherese'* – a high pitched, repetitive, rhythmic baby-talk (Trevarthen, 1974). They spontaneously match the baby's prevailing emotional 'mood', and then tend to 'mirror' it back. What is interesting is that they do so in an exaggerated way, thereby providing *'social biofeedback'* which gradually enables the baby to recognise his or her own emotions, and to differentiate these from the carer's own feelings (which are not overstated) (Gergley & Watson, 1996).   In healthy development, the caregiver's capacity to extend a view of the child as feeling and thinking (having a mind), helps him to co-construct their shared reality, thinking about his own mental experiences. *Empathy* and consideration of the feelings of others similarly arises through the infant's emotional responsiveness to, and identification with, the 'stance' of the other, by a developing capacity to temporarily shift his/her own perspective. Through 'pretend' play the child further practices and explores experience, and gradually integrates earlier modes of understanding into a 'reflective mode' of experiencing and recognising psychic reality (Target & Fonagy, 1996).

The outcome of an infant's growing sensitivity to other people's differing views of the same reality, and to the meaning *they* ascribe to feelings, objects, events and to oneself, is *enhanced self-awareness* in all family members – alongside the growing child's dawning self-consciousness of being seen through the eyes of the other (Hobson, 2002).. This allows for an altered form of psychic intimacy and reflective function – beyond the purely emotional, instigating change in Facilitator and Regulator orienations towards Reciprocation.

Family dynamics vary for each child who takes his/her place in the family, depending on parenting arrangements; the number, ages, sex, personality and spacing of children; and the respective psychohistory of each carer in their own families of origin. Family myths and secrets, arrested images and non-conscious influences live on in attributes ascribed to each particular child, and even in the name s/he is given. Children unconsciously absorb unvoiced parental feelings, and familial trauma such as perinatal losses, which register in a child's sense of guilt or triumph over unborn babies before or after themselves. Even in the absence of these, only children may feel they have demolished all successors

Triangulation

As the child internalises primary relational patterns these constitute the internal foundation for an expanding world of relationships and social structures. In addition to the dyadic dynamics elaborated in the module on babies, the psychoanalytic formulation depicts family dynamics as triadic – an *Oedipal paradigm* of one looking in at a relationship between two others – usually construed as the father and mother's sexual union from which the child is excluded (but at times, it is one or other parent who is excluded). It is not necessarily the sex of the other partner that is important, or even the reality of his/her presence – but the parent's involvement with someone other than the child. A sibling, too, is an important element in the child's awareness of separateness. S/he too may be seen to form one point of the 'triangle' (another relationship that parent has), or as a fourth element – with potential for competition between siblings themselves, or them ganging up on the two parents. An isolated only child with a single parent may have to achieve early triangulation by good/bad splitting of the carer. The danger is one of *dyadic enmeshment.* In a mother-infant pair this may be as a consequence of the mother's negation of the existence of a third outside the mother-child twosome.

The absence of the child's father in her own mind, or her overt preference for the child over him. A further aspect of triangulation are the two who make one. Each child evolves a different intrapsychic elaboration of the originary *'primal scene'* of his/her own conception. This may or may not have a base in reality. Generative identity, the sense of oneself as a potential creator, has at its roots a male and female (or egg-sperm) coupling that engenders a third.

Nuclear units
Given the variety of contemporary families there can be few set rules about hierarchy and function, such as who in the family has the right to make decisions. Nor do western families necessarily maintain old-style segregated sex-role or generation-age differentiated power structures and task divisions. [An example of rapid change of the power structure within the family is in the disparity in Japan between previous feudal respect for the wisdom of elders, and current location of technological expertise in the young generation, leading to cross-generational conflict and disrespect].

With ever-smaller family units, unprecedented tensions and separation anxieties arise between family members in an insular household, unlike the jostling lives, and comings and goings of many surrogate mothers, fathers, siblings and relatives.

> *Notably, small nuclear units appear to generate more intense emotions and greater permeability of psychic boundaries between close dyads, than in a larger multi-generational household.*

It is important to remember that the small nuclear family only emerged with urbanisation and industrialisation. Today the changed family may follow any of the many family constellations mentioned above, or possibly even consist of a childless couple. There are few western traditional societies, which like Norway and some of the other Nordic remain relatively untouched by socio-economic geographical dispersion, or the enforced migrations of famine, disease and war. Envelopment within a large extended family, that provides continuity of traditional childrearing practices across generations. Extended parental leave at full pay and state provision free, unified, high quality childcare from eighteen months until eighteen years, and well-endowed centralised service provisions, safeguard common values, attitudes and ethics. More importantly, a positive family-work balance exists across the variety of institutions, engendering a unified coherent home-based life-style. This differs from the many contradictory choices and tugs-of-war that exist between institutions in societies in transition, such as our own. Allegiances are fractured between many, often conflicting systems, such as corporate-work, economic, educational, health, social and leisure services, each of which makes disparate demands on our time, and take priority over our families, often remove members for long periods of time, on a daily basis.

Social Narratives

In all societies, even traditional societies ones, every relationship is different, even within the same family. As we learned in relation to babies and toddlers, family relationships are co-constructed through back and forth conscious and non-conscious bi-directional influences, each specific interactive pair co-creates a particular *'relational climate'* as I called it, developing their own mutually generated patterns of expressive exchanges and interwoven rhythms of activity. In addition to social constraints, what is permitted or forbidden in each specific intersubjective ambiance initially depends on the degree to which the older companion participates in the interaction and is attuned to the full range of the child's affects.

This profoundly social interchange embeds each baby in the mother tongue, local language (which may be different), sociocultural customs and expectations, and ways of making meaning. As we have seen, the key to sensitive interaction lies in the carer's accessibility to (and self-regulation of) his/her own emotions. Recognising these facilitates acknowledgement of the *child's* feelings, including negative ones. However, co-carers may have different approaches to parenting. Their respective inter-relationships – to each other as well as to the child/ren and others – will in turn, affect their *reflective functions*, quality of mentalizing, verbal commentaries, playful interactions and non-conscious as well as intentional communications which form the foundations for the child's values, beliefs and emotional expression.

Loss of traditional patterns force individuals back on choice of their own parental orientations, generating a variety of different life-styles and childrearing patterns. Family-formation varies (single, couple, same-sex, assisted reproduction with donor gametes; mature or teenage parents; composite step-family, cross-race, mixed ethnicity/religion, etc) such that today, every family member differs on many previously homogenous variables.

<u>Conclusions</u>:

Throughout this training, the central theme has been *the interactive psychosocial nature of constitution of the self.* Emotional transactions within the small family unit are rife with identifications, impositions, fantasies and unresolved issues from earlier periods of life - both child and adult's.

- Adolescent exploration of intense emotions (i.e jealousy, rivalry, envy, hostility) which provoke emotional outbursts within the family of origin increasingly take place in the interactive arena of school, sports or music clubs and social groups.
- Intense allegiances to peer-groups facilitate a process of renegotiating self-image, sexuality, gender and generative identity outside of the immediate family.
- Like the toddler's excursions into the world of peers – the teenager relies on differentiation and identification, both the expanding environment and a small group of loyal friends to consolidate their individuation.
- This occurs through non-committal and experimentation with temporary roles and identities, within a peer-sanctioned system of evolving, strategic adaptations which enable the teen to cope with his/her changing body-schema, repressed urges, aggression and psychosexual expectations.
- Ideally, inter-relationships include members of same and opposite sex, with growing awareness of differences and similarities across and within sexes.

- Femininity and masculinity are artefacts defined by the teen's own subculture and sexual orientation emerges out of various personal fantasies and experiences of erotic desire, sexual attraction/attractiveness and/or rejection.
- Complications arise when pregnancy interrupts these ongoing maturational processes, and parenthood imposes demands over and above those of adolescence.
- A new family is founded, often to bypass the tangled emotional ties to the family of origin. However, unresolved parent-child issues are transferred and reactivated in the new unit – with a 'second chance' to resolve them.

Key Concepts: Family Functions and Ethos; the relational climate. Oedipal conflicts;

Major Themes: Primary dyadic and triadic relational patterns internalised by the child constitute the foundation for an expanding world of relationships and social structures, applied to relationships and groups outside the family.

Module 5:
FAMILIES, GROUPS & ORGANIZATIONS

10. <u>Skill Building Seminar</u>:

Teams, Groups & Organisations

Learning Objectives

> To gain better understanding of group and institutional dynamics, defence mechanisms and their applications to work situations

We all belong to a multiplicity of informal or regulated groups. These include family, friendship circles, recreational or interest clubs, educational or religious groups, etc. However much they differ in size and complexity, common features are the *interdependence* of group members, their *interrelationships* and *shared representations* of the world – the tacit beliefs, values and norms which regulate their mutual conduct. Group members cultivate connections among themselves, and feel a sense of group identification. They interact, communicate and influence one another, motivated to remain in the group as long as it seems to represent them and provides various forms of satisfaction, including a feeling of enhanced energy from joining forces with a charismatic leader.

As the originator of group-dynamics theory noted, group ways of thinking are reinforced by ongoing group processes through 'emotional contagion' which can suppress individual integrity (Lewin, 1951). This danger is greater in closed groups or residential institutions, and has implications for the care system where young people bring their own expectations, replicating these in the new setting. We know that small 'family' groupings and regular work groups are effective in mitigating some of these identificatory dynamics, helping even young children to better understand their own motivation in blindly following peers or a bullying gang leader. Furthermore, even among mature adults, defence mechanisms develop collectively in social groups under the pressure of common anxieties that afflict group members. These can cause even experienced practitioners to behave in less mature and productive ways.

Teams

Sometimes, in more formally structured groups, members are designated to work together as a team, focussing on achieving a particular goal which requires their coordinated interaction. The increased complexity of contemporary projects often presupposes *interdisciplinary* collaboration, to benefit from different perspectives, skills or forms of expertise. Team members may democratically select a leader to facilitate the exchange between the team members.

Most teams confer a sense of belonging and self-worth on members, but group goals and individual rewards often change after completion of specified tasks, bringing about a possible change of leader and membership sub-groupings.

> **Role Play**: A team of 4-6 different practitioners (disciplines specified by group) meet to <u>discuss a 'hot' issue</u> (chosen by group). *After 3-5 minutes – STOP, 'REWIND' – and explore the non-mentalizing group process occurrences. Then START AGAIN.*<u>Message</u>: This training itself reflects some of the large and small group dynamics we learn about. Most practitioners also work in teams. The Leader can call on this experience with questions: *'What makes for a topic 'hot'? 'What kind of problems can arise through inadequate communication channels?'*

Sometimes interrelated groups or teams aggregate to become *an organization* defined by a *'we' attitude* – a common purpose and specific ideology. Conversely, a larger body may establish sub-groups or teams who are delegated to accomplish a specific task, and are accountable to the large organization.

Working in teams can be rewarding, especially when group members pull together and are considerate. But when teams are required to work with severely traumatised clients with unresolved losses, and/or those at high risk, such as some teenage parents and their babies, practitioners may be preoccupied with their own anxieties about tolerating and making sense of powerfully evoked emotional states. These feelings reverberate around the team, as do defences against them.

> **Self-study/group:** How do we classify groups?
> *[Jot down thoughts in Learning Journal].*

One way of classifying groups is according to their *purpose* - work groups (including teams), creative groups (reading groups, chamber music, art projects, etc); gratification groups (social, recreation and sports); social-action groups, etc. Groups also differ in the degree of their *cohesiveness* (usually linked to smaller size). Loyalty of their members is in turn related to approval of *the specified task*, the shared beliefs, common values and implicit *goals* of the group, and *motivation* to fulfil these. Factors such as the formality of organization, rigidity of hierarchical structure and leadership style (authoritarian, democratic, 'laissez faire' delegating), and degree of voluntary participation or coercion of members also define *the emotional and relational climate of the group.*

Groups persist and flourish while others dissolve or disintegrate. Tensions can arise between and within groups due to *internal conflicts* (such as ideological shifts, conflicting aims, dissident subgroups) and/or *external forces* (altered circumstances, real or imagined threats, etc.)

Work Groups
One way in which work groups are often evaluated is through their *efficiency.* Productivity can be measured but such tabulations do not really reflect the group potential or the work process itself, which is subject to complex resistances and unconscious forces. Viewed through a psychodynamic prism, each group operates an 'emotional life' composed of assumptions, 'primitive' fantasies and states of mind which often operate in contradiction to the explicit aims of the group, and to the conscious aims of group members.

> The specific group's *'ethos' or 'culture'* is a function of the conflict between each participant's individual desires and the group 'mentality' (Bion, 1962). In most groups, including families, individual members may have to renounce or compromise some of their interests to achieve the collective aim.

Basic Assumptions
Exploring group dynamics, the psychoanalyst Bion (1962) [pronounced 'Bee-on'] found that when individuals come together to form a group – it bifurcates between two levels of emotional activity:
• A seemingly rational and cooperative work group geared to growth.

•   Another level in which three anti-growth types of basic assumptions alternate: *dependency, pairing or fight-flight.*

When the group reflects a basic assumption of **dependency** the group members ignore each other and relate only to the idealised leader, feeling a hunger for nurture, guidance and protection.

The group with a **pairing** basic assumption has a different leader unconsciously in mind – an unborn messianic saviour who will come about by a coupling of two group members, co-opted to monopolise the group.

In the **fight-flight** basic assumption group members seek a substitute leader within the group under whom to unite to fight against or escape from a perceived threat. They hope for instantaneous satisfaction in their attempt to rid the group of persecutory feelings by panic flight or uncontrolled attack. [For a proposed fourth assumption see Hopper, Expanded notes, p.194].

The more powerful the group's basic assumptions and primitive anxieties, the more trivial the conversation in the group, and action will prevail over use of language as a mode of rational thinking. Loss of the personal distinctiveness of each member, adds to their sense of depersonalization.

The group leader too, will absorb the desires, frustrations, rage and anxieties of the group, and possibly become caught up in the many projections and transference attributions by the participants, unless s/he can make sense of the *counter-transference*.

Importantly, these group dispositions and dyna-mics may be

> **Group Exercise:** Task is to come up with a name for the group
> [5 minutes] *[Break into small groups of 6-8 people. Feedback from groups about the group process.* [1 minute for each group]

found in *any* group situation although they are better observed in a work group.

Institutional Defences

If organizations and interest groups may constitute temporary arrangements, *institutions are permanent structures* of social order and cooperation within a society. They may include institutions such as: the Family; Religion; Education; Scientific institutions; Hospitals and other medical and psychiatric institutions; Military, Legal and Penal systems; Communication, Mass and News media; Factories and Financial Corporations, etc.

Although our work may be within an institution, we do not often consider the emotional forces and mechanisms employed by that institution to manage *institutional anxieties*. A study of nursing practices in the late 1950s (Menzies, 1960) applied psychoanalytic ideas to studying the unconscious dynamics of a London teaching hospital. It revealed how such institutions evolve *'social defences'* to insulate their workers against experiencing difficult feelings.

The findings of that study showed that the system in which nurses work could create a pattern of care that enabled them to distance themselves from anxiety-provoking work-situations - patients who are suffering, disfigured, in pain or terminally ill. Also from anxieties about death, and those arising from administering unpleasant procedures, coping with physical intimacy, exposure to disgusting bodily substances and/or fear of contamination.

> Organised but often unconscious institutional procedures include:
> - Horizontal lines of authority.
> - Policies that *fragment care* and *ritualise practices* (in this case, with centralisation and medicalisation of treatments).
> - Users granted minimal participation in decision-making,
> - Workers too, may be denied continuity of care, and insulated from seeing the consequences of their actions on their all too human clients

Subsequent studies have confirmed that work situations which arouse anxiety necessitate defences to enable practitioners to cope. But these create an ineffective system, or one that is geared to staff convenience and is relatively unresponsive to the needs of its clients (e.g. very early morning floor polishing on hospital wards).

Women often feel dissatisfied with the care they receive in hospitals during pregnancy, labour and the first days postnatally. This has been identified as relating to lack of continuity between staff, poor communication, rigidity and little choice or control. Many complain they do not get personal attention from known midwives; when they feel confused and frightened their anxieties are not addressed. Partly due to ways in which midwifery is organised in institutions, defensive strategies may reflect underpinning anxieties felt by the professionals themselves, about being flooded with unmanageable feelings:

> *Institutional defences aim to distance workers from others' and own fragility*

- Over and above professional detachment, midwives may be encouraged to inhibit and deny their empathic feelings.
- 'Patients' may be treated interchangeably so as to minimise individual 'demands' and personal contact.
- Antenatal care itself may be ritualised – a routinised 'production line' approach which depersonalises patients through gowns, jargon, namelessness, lack of eye-contact…
- Birth may be treated as a medical event, with an emphasis on pain reduction rather than an increased sense of agency in labour.
- Breastfeeding help may focus on 'latching' rather than the emotional experience of feeding a new little person with the juices of one's body (and from the breasts treated by the media as sexual)

> **Group discussion:**Midwives: Emotional Needs
> - Staff support group to express feelings
> - Training in psychological understanding
> - Enhanced job satisfaction in continuity of care and time for human connection
> - Broader areas of responsibility for clients (vs. tasks)
> - Debriefing after traumatic births
> - Opportunities to grieve losses (especially in NICU)
> - Open channels of communication allowing opportunities to vent grievances; a confidential complaints procedure
> - Individual and/or group counselling

> **Group discussion**: Specialist Midwives
> *What anxiety arousing situations do they experience in their work?*
> Time constraints depend on pertinence of the topic to participants.
> Leader invites ideas about what emotional threats consist of – see below:

Many other professionals experience anxieties, especially when working with emotionally needy, traumatised or poverty-stricken clients; those experiencing addictions or mental illness, or presenting threats of behaving antisocially, having violent outbursts, an/or inflicting suffering upon themselves or others.

> Emotional threats to antenatal birthing practitioners:
> *   Witnessing the primordial experience of birth.
> *   Chronic tension of uncertainty.
> *   Acute stress in emergencies.
> *   Exposure to maternal pain, physical and/or mental illness.
> *   Contact with naked physicality and primitive emotions [screams, expletives, curses - pain, fear, rage, eroticism, intimacy].
> *   Midwife's dual identifications with both baby & woman.
> *   Contact with primal substances [amniotic fluid, blood, meconium, vernix]
> *   Exposure to intense transference manifestation (acute idealisation or denigration).
> *   Birth complications/deformity of baby.
> *   Danger of maternal or neonatal damage or death.
> *   Mysteries of origination.

Other institutional defences involve:

> *   *an impersonal approach* of denying feelings in oneself or the client.
> *   operating rigid rules, routines, box-ticking and aloof 'professionalism' or hectic over-activity with no time to contemplate.
> *   Hiding, denial or distortion of unpleasant realities,
> *   deceiving workers or clients, or fobbing them off.

As we noted regarding intolerance, stripping people of their identifying characteristics and/or treating them as *interchangeable,* and maintaining *a task oriented attitude* towards featureless clients, body parts, performativity 'targets' or treatment procedures are all well-documented ways of avoiding seeing the recipient as a whole vulnerable person, as fragile and fallible as ourselves.

> Leader may ask participants for examples from their workplaces.

Staff themselves experience low morale, little job satisfaction, a high rate of frustration and 'burn out' when there is no time to reflect on their work and little space for self-motivated intiatives. But even when dissatisfied practitioners seek more gratifying forms of work, in many organisations there is *resistance to change.* When disputes arise within the organisation itself or between staff and clients, a rapid escalation to mutual blaming and recriminations may occur, as a defensive attempt to locate guilt elsewhere – rather than a genuine attempt to explore, listen to each other and resolve the problem, with potentialities for benefits to all (as we saw in the very first exercise of the 'secret history')..

Nonetheless, armed with observations, self-inquiry and greater understanding of institutional dynamics, members may bring about transformations, such as that engendered by some enterprising midwives and childbearing women in the late 20th century. In the 21st century practitioners' increased reliance on technology and electronic monitoring, and impossible case-loads detract from warm human-contact at the very time when it is most needed.

> *In conclusion, we are members of the 'caring professions'. Keeping the client's mind in our own minds is the most important aspect of our work. We can only be receptive to our clients, if we have mental space and time for reflective thinking.*

Conclusions:

Groups can vary in size and complexity – ranging from families, through teams and work groups to institutions. Shared features are *interdependence* of members and their tacit beliefs, values and norms which regulate their mutual conduct. The explicit purpose of a group may be undermined by implicit assumptions and resistances. Some institutions evolve social defences to protect group members from unbearable feelings. But these affect reflective functioning with clients. Understanding this obviates the need for these defences and reduces their tacit influence.

Key Concepts: Group Mentality. Shared representations. Basic Assumptions. *Dependence: Pairing: Fight-flight*: institutional anxieties, social defences.

Major Themes: Unprocessed feelings can disrupt rational decisions and intents, in both individuals and in groups. The capacity for mentalization and ability to stand back and think about these disruptive processes allows for reparation and change.

Endings

We are approaching the ending.

Growth during a training course is positively correlated with the degree of sorrow experienced at its end. Good endings can be a bittersweet experience – a sense of loss yet achievement, an opportunity to review and revise.

Like pregnancy, some experiences are time-limited, with the ending as a new beginning. If the conclusion is well negotiated, leaving may become a major developmental achievement in which what has been learned can be put into effect.

This training has emphasised ways in which new emotional experience is taken in to become part of the self. Reflective functions of colleagues or carers are internalised by creating an inner representation with whom one can 'dialogue'.

For our young clients, leaving our programme will be accompanied by mixed feelings – gratitude and sadness at losing a warm and caring authentic relationship in which they have been able to 'become' themselves – to play, be curious, celebrate their strengths, re-work current and previous experiences of loss (of freedom, expectations, childhood, friends). Their pride in having accomplished something valuable with you will mingle with feelings of anxiety about managing on their own, without you.

For them, leaving may be taking a firmer step forward toward adult development, having retraced their steps and renegotiated some incomplete aspects of separation-individuation. This includes transforming the tension between dependence and independence into acceptance of ordinary lifelong interdependence. Young clients may have gained a better capacity for affect regulation and tolerance of frustrations, anger and anxiety. And, an increased awareness of self-reflection as a tool for thoughtful processing of conflicts and better integration of contradictions, leads to a more coherent life story, more realistic self-esteem and expectations - all contributing to better parenting and the potential for further self-development.

Finally, for you too, this good ending provides *a 'second chance'* to take pleasure in achievements, and to help your client leave home' in a different, active and conscious way with new confidence in her/his own capacity to reflect upon feelings.

Self-Study/Group Discussion: <u>What constitutes a good parting?</u>
[Use flipchart, then add these points if they have not arisen spontaneously]
- achieving *a capacity for mentalization* – tools for thoughtful processing
- better tolerance of anxiety, insight re internal conflicts, more coherent story, integration and self-reflection (in self & client)
- *Plan* ending in advance with the client
- *Remind* client before the termination date
- *Hear* client's views of your intervention to date
- *Review 'journey'*: were their/your objectives met?
- *Discuss* disappointments, frustrations, gains - how this separation reverberates with earlier losses
- *Acknowledge* mixed feelings - of pride, abandonment, anxiety, relief, sadness
- *Mark* the event. Discuss *Follow Up/* future contact?
- *Express your gratitude* – for the mutual learning experience

---

Summary:

Over the course of this training we have explored developmental issues, discerning healthy care and factors that influence pathological development, such as: chronic misattunement of early caregivers, intergenerational transmission of unprocessed trauma, adverse psychosocial conditions and living in high risk communities.

We have asserted that the simultaneous high arousal and demands of adolescence and parenting constitute a double crisis which affects teenage parents' emotional self-regulation and capacity to mentalize. Their tendency to explode or escape when things get tough creates confusion in the child, who is unsure of the degree of his/her own influence and agency. It also has an impact upon practitioners working with teen parents, and generates disturbances in the caregiving systems around them.

It is therefore important for practitioners to process the powerful experiences stirred up by teenage clients and their children, which so often are due to projection of their internal representations and 'relational climates', including expectations of antagonistic, abandoning or abusive parental behaviour. When versions of these traumatic experiences are externalised and enacted between adolescent clients and their workers, they come to be spread around the network. transference dynamics rotate among workers, spreading blame or guilt, and projecting unbearable feelings. These dynamics may be repeated between practitioners and their managers with repercussions experienced among team members, consultants, also affecting inter-agency connections.

We can draw on the conceptual thinking about groups, teams and organisations presented here to understand the complex dynamics involved. But ideally, small confidential reflective work groups, or special meetings can provide the boundaried safety to explore and understand the powerful co-created dynamics of working with teen age parents and their offspring.

THE END

Part 2: **TRAINING PACK**

Glossary, Expanded Notes, Learning Journal, Readings, Handouts:

GLOSSARY *

Glossary of Psychoanalytic Terms and Concepts
used in workshops, seminars or readings on this course

ACTING OUT: impulsive use of dramatising action to bypass remembering
AFFECT: feelings attached to an idea
AMBIVALENCE: coexistence of love and hate towards the same person (in contradictory/split emotions as opposed to mixed feelings)
ANALITY Fr
eud's second stage of libidinal development (after the 'oral' phase) is linked to toilet training, preoccupation with expulsion/retention and the symbolic value of feces=gifts=money.
ANALYSAND: a person in analysis (patient, client)
ANXIETY: a psychosomatic signal of impending subjectively defined danger which may relate to specific concerns (i.e. separation or castration), and can vary in nature (as in depressive or paranoid anxieties). In heightened form anxiety often accompanies other disorders. Its absence may be a sign of disturbance.
ATTACHMENT THEORY: evolved from the ideas of psychoanalyst John Bowlby who proposed that as a vestige of archaic dangers, infants seek close attachment to the mother, seeking security in her presence. Anxiety is related to separation from the primary carer and from birth, proximity to the mother is maintained by five component instinctive responses: sucking, smiling, clinging, crying and following.
Confidence in the mother's availability underlies a child's emotional stability, forming a 'secure base'. To Bowlby, anger is seen as a response to separation/frustration rather than innate. And expectations are deemed to be accurate reflections of <u>actual</u> experiences as children build up an *'internal working model'* of the carer. Subsequent research established that a child might relate simultaneously to several attachment figures, with different degrees of security in each of these relationships. Unattuned, neglectful or unpredictable carers may lead to insecurity in the infant, which at 12 months can be measured through responses to brief separation and reunion under replicable laboratory conditions. [Ainsworth's 'strange situation'].
Securely attached babies tend to have at least one attuned caregiver. Insecurely attached infants are categorised as: Ambivalent, Avoidant or Disorganised respectively manifesting clingy, anxious, agitated behaviour; seemingly 'self-sufficient' and indifferent to separation; showing confused, chaotic bizarre behaviour on reunion [Sroufe].
Use of the Adult Attachment Interview [AAI] to explore expectant mothers' feelings about their own attachment figures is found to be predictive of the (unborn) baby's future attachment [Fonagy, Steele et al]

---

* Partly adapted from my Glossary in *Parent-Infant Psychodynamics – wild things, mirrors and ghosts,* J Raphael-Leff (ed), London: Whurr/ Wiley, 2003

The three types of insecurity above are linked respectively to a carer who discourages autonomy; or is dismissing/neglectful; or dissociated/anxious and preoccupied with his/her own unresolved issues [Main]. Also see Expanded notes for Module III.

ATTUNEMENT: refers to the carer's capacity to communicate an empathic understanding of the baby's emotional state in a different mode (i.e cross-modal matching of timing, form, and intensity). TUNING is a related concept designating a response congruent to the infant's state yet differing, so that it alters that state (i.e soothing) [see Stern; Emde; Beebe].

BASIC ASSUMPTIONS: Groups and social systems generally can be considered in terms of their more conscious, formal work group formations and their more unconscious, informal defensive basic assumptions formations, i.e., those patterns of relating that are co-created unconsciously by people in groups in order to protect themselves from extreme anxieties that emerge when they regress. Bion proposed three such patterns - *Dependency, Fight/flight*, and *Pairing*, each characterised by roles towards which people are drawn on the basis of their own distinctive personality characteristics. Based on the work of Foulkes and Turquet, Hopper proposed a fourth basic assumption of *Incohesion: Aggregation/ Massification* which offers protection against the fear of annihilation associated with the failed dependency of traumatic experience.

CATHEXIS: emotional energy invested in someone or an idea

COGNITIVE DISSONANCE: psychic discomfort felt when presented with opposite and competing ideas (vs. 'ego-syntonic' ideas).

COLLUSION: being drawn into complicity.

COMPULSION TO REPEAT: Freud said '… a thing which has not been understood inevitably reappears; like an unlaid ghost, it cannot rest until the mystery has been solved and the spell broken' [Freud, *Analysis of a Phobia in a Five-Year-Old Boy*, 1909,p.122].

CONDENSATION: an unconscious mode of functioning whereby several different elements coalesce, as in dream images

CONTAGIOUS AROUSAL: a process defined by Raphael-Leff by which early implicit emotions are retriggered in the parenting situation through exposure to the baby's preverbal feelings and primary substances (amniotic fluid, breast milk, lochia, urine, infantile faeces).

CONTAINMENT: Bion's concept of maternal care which necessitates emotional receptivity to the baby's anxieties and a capacity to 'metabolize' these before handing them back in 'detoxified 'form. This form of 'containment' is also used as a metaphor for professional care.

COUNTER-TRANSFERENCE: emotional responses to another which provide clues to unexpressed experiences in both. This is usually applied to the responses of a therapist to his/her patient in which the practitioner tries to sustain the countertransference feelings stirred up as opposed to discharging them, in order to subordinate them to the analytic task.

CULTURAL COMPETENCE: an ability to understand and interact effectively with people of different cultures. This entails an awareness of one's own cultural worldview and potential bias, a generally receptive attitude towards difference (age, gender, ethnicity, etc), and willingness to question one's own assumptions.

'DEAD' MOTHER: notion of a physically present mother but psychically absent leading to robotic caretaking with the infant being treated like a doll [Andre Green].

DECATHEXIS: loosening of emotional ties

DEFENCES: mechanisms used to protect oneself from realizing internal or externally derived painful experiences or threats to one's integrity. Mainly defined by Anna Freud, common defences are denial, projection, splitting magical/obsessional undoing, dissociation and regression

DENIAL: a mental state when threatening feelings and ideas attached to them are withheld from consciousness.

DEPRESSION: ranges from a healthy response to loss to a pathological form of mourning usually directed at an internal figure that is both needed and hated [see Freud's Mourning and Melancholia, 1917]

DEPRESSIVE POSITION: a concept originating in Melanie Klein's theories regarding infantile development. When a young child realises with concern that the person he loves and hates/attacks is one and the same (rather than a 'good' mother and another 'bad' mother). A desire for reparation arises

DIALOGUE (dialectic) between two or more people who may hold differing views, yet wish to pursue truth by seeking agreement with one another.[1] This is in contrast to debate where they wish to persuade prove one another wrong.

DISPLACEMENT: a process of detaching energy from one idea and its investment in another according to an unconscious associative 'chain'.

DEVELOPMENTAL LINES: an organizing principle in considering the assessment and classification of childhood disturbances established by Anna Freud (1965) to broaden developmental theory to include observational correlates highlighting differential growth of facets of the total personality. The interplay of four basic developmental lines lead from infantile dependency to emotional 'self-reliance', the ability to work, to have satisfactory love and peer relationships and secure possession of one's own body. By adding clinical descriptions to each step, the schema could be utilised to construct psychoanalytic profiles to assess variability around the norm, to classify types and degrees of disorders and to evaluate the effectiveness of therapeutic efforts.

'DYADIC CONSCIOUSNESS' - the interweaving of co-created processes between the baby and the carer that is unique to that particular relationship (Tronick, 1989; Lyons-Ruth, 1999).

'EMOTIONAL REFUELLING' is used to described how during the 'practising' period of the 'separation-individuation' process a child gains emotional sustenance from his/her mother through visual, auditory and/or direct bodily contact.

EROGENOUS (erotogenic) ZONES: areas of the body from which erotic sensations arise and/or excitations focus [Freud 1905]

FANTASY: an imaginary internal scenario which may be unconscious, or more accessible as in a day-dream. [Sometimes the former is spelled 'phantasy'].

FREE ASSOCIATION: an uncensored form of communication used in psychoanalytic treatment by which the patient allows his/her thoughts to wander and tries to express any thought that comes to mind. The aim is to lower resistance and to discover new connections.

GUILT: an indication of a capacity for concern and internalisation.

HOLDING: Winnicott's concept of reliable care, sensitive to the growing baby's changing physical and psychological needs during the period of 'absolute dependence' followed by the carer's 'graduated failure', which enables the 'relatively' dependent infant to gradually take over these functions.

IDENTIFICATION: psychic crossing of bodily boundaries between people through primary identification — fusion/confusion of self and other; projective identification — imaginary control over the other by 'inserting' parts of oneself into the other; and introjective identification, which like its physical prototype of incorporation, is a fantasy form of appropriation by 'taking' the other (or aspects of them) into the self.

IDENTITY: rather than implying a fixed and coherent entity this concept has come to signify a fluctuating sum of relatively durable yet imaginatively fluid self-representations (Raphael-Leff, 2010).

ILLUSION: an intermediate area of psychic experience in which a (false) belief reflects a desire or wish [see Winnicott].

INTRA-PSYCHIC: an interplay of internal processes within a person's psyche.

INTROJECTION is a term describing a process of taking in (a reciprocal concept to Projection). The distinction between 'introjection and 'identification' is that 'introjects' are seen as less assimilated or integrated.

INTERPERSONAL: dynamic forms of relating between two or more people.

INTER-PSYCHIC: exchanges in which through transmission and reception of unconscious communications each person unwittingly affects and is affected by the other.

INTERNALISATION: a process of inner representation of significant relations.

INTERSUBJECTIVITY: a meeting of two minds. This is fostered in infancy by caregivers who are capable of responding to their infants' emotional states as shareable but separate from their own ('affect attunement'). They treat their babies as subjects long before they develop the awareness of having a mind (around 9 months).

INTROJECTION: a fantasy process of taking in a desired or threatening quality, figure or situation to keep/control it 'inside'.

LIBIDINAL PHASES: oral (sucking & biting), anal (expulsion & retention), phallic (exhibitionistic & anxious) and genital sequences of erotogenic bodily loci and modes of being in a child's development [Freud, 1905; Abraham, 1927].

LIBIDO: from the Latin for wish or desire. In Freudian terms - 'Libido is an expression taken from the theory of the emotions. We call by that name the energy…of those instincts which have to do with all that may be comprised under the word "love"'[Freud, *Group Psychology and the Analysis of the Ego* (1921 p.90)].

MENTALIZATION: refers to the attitude and skills involved in understanding mental states in oneself as well as in others, and their connections with feelings and behaviour. This capacity may range from genuine curiosity about thoughts and feelings to thoughtfulness yet lack of empathic understanding, to apparent indifference or disregard for wishes and feelings of others [Fonagy & Target; Slade]

MIRRORING: This is a concept used differently by various psychoanalytic schools. Here the focus is on the reflective interaction in infancy seen as the foundation of inter-subjectivity [maternal 'empathic' mirroring (Kohut), rather than a literal image in the mirror (Lacan)]. Winnicott proposed that the mother's face was the baby's mirror, in which s/he sees her/himself reflected (1971). Research confirms that carers reflect the baby's feelings in an exaggerated way that enables the infant to distinguish these from their parents' own emotions [Gergely & Watson].

NARCISSISM: ranges from healthy self-love to a pathological form involving excessive emotional preoccupation with self narcissism.

NEGATIVISM in toddlerhood reflects an attempt to assert autonomy, under the threat of potential submission to passivity and regression. Negativism is usually possible only if the mother's love can be taken for granted.

OBJECT: in psychoanalytic jargon this is usually used to indicate the human object of a person's intellectual or emotional perceptions and desires (as in 'object choice' which could be a 'narcissistic' choice of someone like oneself; or 'anaclitic' choice based on differences).

OBJECT CONSTANCY: a term [adapted from Piaget by Hartmann] to describe a stage of relating during which the mother comes to have a continuous existence for the child.

OEDIPUS COMPLEX: Freud's depiction of a triangular relationship in which a child or adolescent feels powerfully positive feelings and desires towards one parent (usually of the opposite sex) and rivalry and jealous hatred of the other's claim to the loved one's affections.

OMNIPOTENCE: an overestimated unrealistic sense of one's own capacities. Renunciation of omnipotence is seen as an important developmental step in toddlerhood, and again during adolescence. Mahler attributes it to the child's realisation during the rapprochement subphase that his/her wishes and mother's do not always coincide, curtailing the 'magic of symbiosis': the child can neither maintain a 'delusion of 'grandeur' nor belief in parental omnipotence. To Winnicott, by allowing illusion, then gradually failing the infant and surviving his/her attacks, the 'good enough' mother enables the child to take over some of her caretaking capacities, thereby relinquishing omnipotence.

OVER-DETERMINATION: a multiplicity of unconscious elements and levels contributing to the significance of a symptom or idea.

PATERNAL FUNCTION In Lacan's original (1956) formulation, it is not the person of the real father who breaks into the dyadic world of symbiotic 'fusion' to liberate the infant, but the father as representative of a symbolic system organised in language. Seen also to represent the Law of a triadic system of relationships. Missing is the recognition that even in traditional divisions of parenting, mothers too perform this function, in myriad ways, as they introduce otherness, limits, observing, thinking, linking, and a different perspective to that of the baby. Idealisation of the father as an exciting delegate of the outside world continues to operate as a powerful cultural representation within psychoanalysis, too.

PHOBIA: a situation specific irrational fear (e.g. closed or open spaces, spiders, etc) which serves to tether 'free-floating' anxiety.

PRACTISING SUBPHASE (from 9 to 16-18 months), in which the crawling child, and, later, the walking toddler, feels 'in love with the world', elatedly asserting motoric freedom. This is followed by the 'rapprochement' subphase with its 'ambitendency' between desire and anxiety regarding independence [described by Mahler et al, 1975].

PRIMAL SCENE: imaginary or real scene of intercourse between the parents, the meaning of which the child re-interprets according to his/her own sexual preoccupations at each developmental phase.

PROJECTION: a fantasy means of locating threatening or unacceptable feelings or characteristics of the self in another person. What is rejected in oneself is expelled and attributed to others, thereby making it available to deal with externally.

PROJECTIVE IDENTIFICATION: an unconscious projection of one's own state of mind into someone, with the unconscious motive of communicating   and/or controlling that person or perhaps defending against awareness of painful feelings of separateness. The other then may be unconsciously experienced as containing or embodying aspects of the self (whether good or bad). This is different from

INTROJECTIVE IDENTIFICATION: where the other is felt to be taken into the self and identified with there [originating in Klein, the concept is diversely used by many different theoretical schools].

PROTO COMMUNICATION: new micro-analytic research techniques confirm that very early collaborative infant-carer exchanges achieve high levels of efficiency in turn-taking, precision of timing, pitch, intensity and rhythmicity (Trevarthen) across different modalities (Stern). Under normal circumstances there are also numerous misunderstandings and disruption which necessitate continuous reciprocal efforts   to repair mismatches in order to achieve and maintain mutual states of affective matching and synchrony in sound, touch and gestural communication (Tronick).

PSYCHIC GROWTH: Freud (1911) outlined a gradual replacement of the 'pleasure principle' in infancy with the 'reality principle'. Psychoanalytic elaborations since then describe various catalysts for psychic reorganization and change. In general, the capacity for symbolic representation, and a developmental shift from illusion to greater realism ascribed to (tolerable) absences or 'gaps' within environmental provisions of safety, reliability and empathic containment. These foster the baby's discomforting awareness of his/her own dependency, separateness and limitations. This is seen to lead the infant towards reality testing and relinquishment of omnipotence. However, unconscious motives for psychic growth differ in designation as compensatory, substitutional or reparational [see Bion, A.Freud, Klein, Mahler, Winnicott].

PUBERTY: described by Freud [1925] as the period in which erogenous zones become subordinated to the genital zone, setting up new sexual aims (different for males and females), and finding new sexual objects outside the family.

RAPPROCHEMENT: the toddler's conflictual defiant yet clinging stance during the second year, when the desire for independent autonomy clashes with lost omnipotence and awareness of separateness, dependency and limitations [Mahler, Pine, and Bergman].

REACTION FORMATION: defensively adopting the opposite position to a threatening impulse.

REFLECTIVE FUNCTION: a capacity to 'mentalize' about one's own interiority and subjectivity. Interest in the way other people's minds function [Fonagy & Target]. The mother and/or father's capacity to keep the child's *mind* in mind, and to think of that child's needs as separate from her/his own. This also involves the carer's capacity step back from his/her own affective experience in order to reflect upon the child's uniquely subjective intentions during moments of stress or conflict [Slade et al, 2002].

REFLECTIVE SELF-AWARENESS: a combined intellectual and emotional process of awareness, holding in mind both the subjective and objective aspects of self and other, during 'a meeting of minds'.

REGRESSION: a transition or reversion to earlier modes of experience, expression and relating that are less sophisticated in terms of complexity and differentiation. Social systems can also be considered in terms of structural regression, especially under certain circumstances such as traumatic experience.

REGULATION: the carer's modulation of the baby's most basic physiological aspects through affect-matching, mirroring and selective attunement which contributes to smooth transitions between states and fosters the infant's own self-regulation, interpersonal communication, and sense of self.

MUTUAL REGULATION also occurs through emotional communion and a dynamic interplay between the perceptions, affects, and proprioceptions of infant and carer, as each influences the other, creates a variety of interactive regulatory patterns [Beebe & Lachmann].

REPRESSION: a mental activity to prevent (forbidden) ideas or desires being admitted to conscious awareness. Freud discovered that these unconscious wishes could return in distorted or unrecognisable forms in symptoms, dreams, slips of the tongue or actions.

ROLE RESPONSIVENESS: receptivity to the client's unconscious use of the practitioner's psyche to activate enactment of their transference wishes and fears. Role-responsiveness (defined by Joe Sandler, 1976) is co-determined by both parties' wishes and needs, with the practitioner's 'free-floating responsiveness' complying to the role the client demands of him until s/he can recognise the situation and step back from it.

SEPARATION-INDIVIDUATION: Mahler's term for the process whereby the infant gradually separates from his/her mother (caregiver) and develops a relatively stable coherent sense of self and of others. This consists of phases such as 'symbiosis', 'differentiation', 'practising' and 'rapproachement'. Recently revised with ideas of Attachment Separation [see Lyons-Ruth].

SOCIAL REFERENCING Looking to a mentor (parent/carer) to establish whether a social or environmental situation is safe. In classical experiments (Klinnert et al., 1983; Emde et al., 1991) infants were enticed by interesting toys to cross a glass surface that looked like a cliff. After hesitating, infants crossed only if mother's face indicated that it was safe to do so.

SPLITTING: another mechanism for dealing with anxiety by dividing the threat. Both self and other (or different aspects of oneself) are experienced in unrealistically extreme terms, whether idealised [good] or denigrated [bad].

SYMBOLISATION: figurative representation of an (unconscious) feeling, conflict or wish, or translation of ideas into imagery or words (often multilayered and constantly revised).

THEORY OF MIND - a child's growing understanding that s/he and others possess 'minds'. From appreciation around one year of others' intentions (demonstrated in cooperative play), by age two there is a capacity to reflect on his/her own emotional states and by three, to distinguish between internal mental states and external behaviour, and to use theories to explore and predict people's actions and mental states, albeit sometimes inaccurately; by four there is an awareness that minds are separate, and a means of interpreting or constructing reality Five-year-olds appreciate multiple perspectives, can imagine and mentally simulate the feelings and behaviours of another person, recognising that beliefs dictate emotional reactions [Trevarthen; Hobson; Fonagy; Beebe].

THE SOCIAL UNCONSCIOUS: an essential concept for the socio-cultural school of psycho-analysis and for the disciplines of group analysis and 'group relations studies' involving the application of psychoanalysis to the study of group structures and processes. It refers to aspects of mind and personality that are constrained by socio-cultural factors and forces throughout life from conception onwards. Hopper argues that aspects of the self (the innate ego of adaptation and the emergent ego of agency) are always based on both a body-ego and a society-ego of which we are mostly unconscious, although in principle it is possible through comprehensive psychoanalysis and group analysis to become aware of these intertwined structures of the mind. A second aspect of the social unconscious refers to those constraining socio-cultural factors/forces themselves, which metaphorically reflect the unconscious collective mind of a social system, a group, family, organisation or even a society as a whole [see Hopper 2006-7].

TRANSFERENCE: unconscious wishes and impulses related to early emotional experiences which are reactivated and relived in present encounters, especially apparent in the clinical situation.

TRANSITIONAL OBJECT: Winnicott's concept of a comforting toy or object [e.g. teddy bear or security blanket] within the infant's control, which by providing some dimension of the mother's qualities, bridges 'me' and 'not-me', helping make the transition from seeing her as 'merged' to being a separate person, 'perceived rather than conceived of' (Winnicott, 1971, p. 114). In adulthood, playing, creativity and cultural experience are seen to take place within a similarly 'intermediate area'—a TRANSITIONAL SPACE.

UNCONSCIOUS: a system of repressed wishes and impulses or merely unavailable ideas and fantasy scenarios, governed by rules of its own, such as timelessness, absence of negation and doubt; hedonism and indifference to reality restrictions.

WORKING THROUGH: an emotional process whereby insights and understanding of unconscious motivations and conflicts become integrated as skills and self-awareness.

·

READINGS: Recommended & Additional

References from this Theoretical Textbook are included under their appropriate headings in this list of Readings, which you may wish to peruse now or in the future.
Training Reader:
The book below contains many of the readings that are not available online:
Parent-Infant Psychodynamics – wild things, mirrors and ghosts, J. Raphael-Leff (ed), London: Whurr 2003; Wiley, 2006; Anna Freud Centre, 2009.

As many people do not have access to a professional library, wherever possible, free online resources have been suggested. Unfortunately, some references are neither available on the internet nor on Kindle. [Most of the books mentioned here are obtainable at Karnac books online: http://www.karnacbooks.com]

Abuse
Recommended Reading:
- Ferenczi, S. (1933), Confusion of tongues between adults and the child: The language of tenderness and passion, *International Journal of Psycho-Analysis*, 30, 225-230, 1949
- Welldon, E.(2011) *Playing with Dynamite,* London: Karnac

Adolescence
Recommended Reading:
- Freud, A. (1958) Adolescence. *Psychoanalytic Study of the Child* **13**: 255-78
- Laufer, M & Laufer, E (1984*)* Adolescence and the final sexual organisation. In: *Adolescence and Developmental Breakdown: a psychoanalytic view,* chapter 1, pp 3-20. London: Karnac Books
- Rose, J.(2005) Adolescence, chapter 9 in E. Rayner, A. Joyce, J. Rose, M. Twyman & Christopher Clulow, *Human development: An introduction to the psychodynamics of growth, maturity and Ageing, 4th edition,* London: Routledge, *pp 162-178*

- Rosenblum, D. S., Daniolos, P., Kass, N. and Martin, A. (1999). Adolescents and Popular Culture: A Psychodynamic Overview. *Psychoanalytic Study of the Child* 54: 319-338
- Waddell, D (2005)*Understanding your 12-14 Year Olds,* London:Jessica Kingsley
- Waddell, M (2009) Why teenagers have babies, *Infant Observation,*12:3, 271-281
- Winnicott, D.W. (1971) Contemporary concepts of adolescent development and their implications for higher education, pp. 147-150, part of chapter 11 in *Playing and Reality,* London: Routledge

Additional reading:

- Anderson, R and Dartington, A(eds). *Facing it Out: Clinical Perspectives on* Adolescent *Disturbance.* London: Karnac Books.
- Blos, P. (1962). *On Adolescence. A Psychoanalytic Interpretation*: New York: The Free Press of Glencoe.
- Blos, P. (1965) The second individuation process of adolescence. *Psychoanalytic Study of the Child*, 22:162-186. Also in M. Perret-Catipovic & F. Ladame (eds) *Adolescence and Psychoanalysis*: the story of the history, chapter 5. London: Karnac Books, 1998 pp 77–102
- Harris, M (1976) Infantile elements and adult strivings in adolescent sexuality. *Journal of Child Psychotherapy*, 4:29-43.
- Ladame, F & Perret-Catipovic, M. (1998). Normality and pathology in adolescence. In: M. Perret-Catipovic and F. Ladame (eds) *Adolescence and Psychoanalysis*, chapter 10, p 161 – 172. London: Karnac Books.
- Laufer, M (1976) The central masturbation fantasy, the final sexual organisation and adolescence, *Psychoanalytic Study of the Child,* 31: 297-316.
- Patton, G., & Viner, R. (2007). Pubertal transitions in health. *The Lancet, 369,* 1130-1139.
- Waddell, M (2002) *Inside Lives: Psychoanalysis and the Growth of the Personality.* London: Karnac (2002).

Antenatal Disturbance

Recommended Reading:

- O'Connor, T.G., Heron, J., Glover, V (2002) antenatal anxiety predicts child
- behavioral/ emotional problems independently of postnatal depression
- *Journal American Academy of Child & Adolescent Psychiatry,* 41:1470-7
- Van den Bergh BR, Mulder EJ, Mennes M, Glover V (2005) Antenatal maternal anxiety and stress and the neurobehavioural development of the fetus and child: links and possible mechanisms. A review. *Neuroscience Biobehaviour Review* 29:237-58.

Attachment:

- Bowlby, J (1969) Attachment and loss, vol.1.*Attachment.*London:Hogarth Press.
- Bowlby, J. (1980), Attachment and Loss. Vol. 3: *Loss, Sadness and Depression.* New York: Basic Books.
- Bowlby, J. (1988), *A Secure Base.* New York: Basic Books.
- Brazelton, TB & Cramer, BG *The Earliest Relationship. Parents, infants and the Drama of Early Attachment,* Karnac Books, London 1991
- Dozier, M., Cue, K. & Barnett, L. (1993), Clinicians as caregivers: Role of attachment organization in treatment. Journal of Consulting & Clinical Psychology, 62:793-800.
- Holmes, J (1993) *John Bowlby & Attachment Theory,* London: Routledge.

Additional reading:

- Bretherton K., & Mullholland KA.(1999) Internal working models in attachment relationships: A construct revisited. In *Handbook of Attachment: Theory, Research and Clinical Applications*, ed. J. Cassidy & PR. Shaver. New York: Guilford Press, pp. 89–114.
- Main, M. Kaplan, N., & Cassidy, J. (1985) Security in infancy, childhood and adulthood: A move to the level of representation. In Growing Points of Attachment Theory and Research. Monographs of the Society for Research in Child Development, ed. I. Bretherton & E. Waters.Vol. 50. Chicago:Chicago University Press, pp. 66–104.

Babies

Recommended Reading:

- Beebe, B, Lachman F & Jaffe J (1997) Mother-infant interaction structures, presymbolic self and object representations, *Psychoanalytic Dialogue 7:133-92*
- Joyce, A. (2005). The second six months: The baby getting organized. Chapter 4 in E. Rayner, A. Joyce, J. Rose, M. Twyman & Christopher Clulow, *Human development: An introduction to the psychodynamics of growth, maturity and Ageing, 4th edition, London: Routledge, pp 23-46.*
- Music, G (2011) *Nurturing Natures: Attachment and Children's Emotional, Sociocultural and Brain Development*, London: Psychology Press
- Trevarthen, C (1974) Conversations with a two month old. *New Scientist,* May 2nd Chapter 3 in *Parent-Infant Psychodynamics – wild things, mirrors and ghosts,* J Raphael-Leff (ed), London: Anna Freud Centre, 2009, pp.25-34
- Tronick, EZ (1989), Emotions and emotional communication in infants. *American Psychologist* 44:112-119. Updated version, in *Parent-Infant Psychodynamics – wild things, mirrors and ghosts,* Raphael-Leff (ed), London: Anna Freud Centre, 2009 pp.35-53

Additional reading:

- Bick, E (1968) The experience of the skin in early object relations. *International Journal of Psycho-Analysis*, 49:484–486. Chapter 6 in *Parent-Infant Psycho-dynamics – wild things, mirrors and ghosts,* J Raphael-Leff (ed), London: Anna Freud Centre 2009, pp.70-74
- Bion, W. R. (1967). A theory of thinking. In London: Heinemann,pp. 110-119.
- Fraiberg, SH (1959) *The Magic Years.* New York: Charles Scribner's Sons.
- Schore, A.N. 1994: Affect regulation and the origin of the self. Hillsdale, NJ: Lawrence Elbaum.
- Stern, D. N (1985)*The interpersonal world of the infant.* New York: Basic Books.
- Trevarthen, C. And Aitken, K. (2001): Infant intersubjectivity: research, theory and clinical applications. Journal of Child Psychology and Psychiatry 42, 3-48.
- Zeanah, C., Keener, M., & Anders, T. (1986). Developing perceptions of temperament and their relation to mother and infant behavior. *Journal of Child Psychology and Psychiatry and Allied Disciplines*, 27:499–512.

Counter-transference:

- Heimann, P. (1950). On Counter-Transference. *International Journal of Psychoanalysis* 31: 81-84
- Little, M. (1951). Counter-Transference and the Patient's Response to It. *International Journal of Psychoanalysis* 32: 32-40

- Sandler, J. (1976). Countertransference and Role-Responsiveness. *International Review of Psychoanalysis*, 3:43-47
- Salzberger-Wittenberg, I (1970) *Psychoanalytic insights and relationships, Psycho-Analytic Insights and Relationships – A Kleinian Approach,* London: Routledge & Kegan Paul. [Chapter 18 in *Parent-Infant Psychodynamics – wild things, mirrors and ghosts,* J Raphael-Leff (ed), London: Anna Freud Centre, 2009, pp.*245*-55]
- Winnicott, DW (1949). Hate in the Counter-Transference. *International Journal of Psychoanalysis* 30:69-74. Also in *Through Pediatrics to Psycho-Analysis*. London: Hogarth, 1975 pp. 194-203.

Culture:

Recommended Reading:
- Eleftheriadou, Z. (1994). *Transcultural Counselling*. Central Books.
- Thomas, AJ & Schwarzbaum, S (2006) *Culture and Identity. Life stories for counsellors and therapists*. London: Sage

Additional reading:
- Pedersen, P.B. (1997). *Culture-Centered Counseling Interventions: Striving for Accuracy*. London:Sage.
- Raphael-Leff, J (2005) *Psychological Processes of Childbearing*, London: AFC
- Miller, D.L. (Ed) (1982). *The Individual and the Social Self: Unpublished Essays by G. H. Mead.* University of Chicago Press.

Developmental Theory

Recommended Reading:
- Fonagy, P & Target, M (2003) *Psychoanalytic Theories: Perspectives from Developmental Psychology*, London: Whurr publishers

Psychoanalytic (classical)
- Abraham, K (1924) A Short Study of the Development of the Libido, Viewed in the Light of Mental Disorders In: *Selected Papers on Psychoanalysis* London: Hogarth Press, 1927 New York: Basic Books 1953, pp. 418-501
- Mahler, MS, Pine, F & Bergman, A (1975) *The Psychological Birth of the Human Infant. Symbiosis and Individuation.* New York: Basic Books.
- Britton, R (1998) *Belief and Imagination – explorations in psychoanalysis*, NLP London: Routledege & Institute of Psychoanalysis

Research
- Gerhardt, S (2004) *'Why Love Matters: How Affection Shapes a baby's brain,* Psychology Press
- Hobson, P (2002) The Cradle of Thought – exploring the origins of thinking, London: MacMillan.

Additional reading

Representations
- Dennett, D.C (1996) *Kinds of Minds - towards an understanding of consciousness,* London: Weidenfeld & Nicholson.
- Sandler, J and Sandler, AM (1998) A theory of internal object relations. In: *Internal Object Relations Revisited,* chapter 8, pp 121–140. London:Karnac.
- Stern, DN (1995) The nature and formation of the infant's representations. Chapter 5 in: *The motherhood constellation*, London: Basic Books.

Intersubjectivity

- Beebe, B & Lachmann, F (2003). The Relational Turn in Psychoanalysis: A Dyadic Systems View from Infant Research. *Contemporary Psychoanalysis.* 39:379-409
- Benjamin, J (1990) An Outline of Intersubjectivity: The Development of Recognition *Psychoanalytic Psychology.* **7:** 33-46
- Fonagy, P & Target, M (2007) Playing with Reality IV: A theory of external reality rooted in intersubjectivity, *International Journal of Psychoanalysis.* 88:917-37
- Lyons-Ruth, K(1999)The Two-Person Unconscious. *Psychoanalytic Inquiry,* 19: 576-617
- Trevarthen, C & Aitken, K (2001) Infant intersubjectivity: research, theory and clinical application. *Journal Child Psychology and Psychiatry.* 42:3–48.
- Winnicott, D W (1953) Transitional objects and Transitional phenomena, Chapter 1 in *Playing and Reality,* London: Penguin 1971, pp.1-30
- Winnicott D W (1988) The Emotional development of the human being. In: *Human Nature*, Part II, p 33–64 London: Free Association Books.

Fathers

Recommended Reading:

Psychosocial

- Brown, JR and Dunn, J (1991) You can cry mum: the social and developmental implications of talk about internal states. *British Journal of Developmental Psychology,* 9**:** 237-256.
- Dunbar, R (1996) First words. In: *Grooming, gossiping and the evolution of language*, chapter 7, p 132-151. London: Faber and Faber.
- Phillips, A (1998) Learning not to talk. In: I. Ward (Ed.) *The Psychology of Nursery Education,* p 27–42. London: Karnac Books for the Freud Museum.
- Raphael-Leff, J (2008a) Participators, Reciprocators & Renouncers: Paternal orientations in the 21st century.*Pychoanalytic Psychotherapy* [S. Africa]16:61-85
- Trowell, J & Etchegoyen, A.(eds) (2002) *The Importance of Fathers,* London: Institute of Psycho-analysis Psychology Press

Research

- Goodman, JH (2004) Paternal postpartum depression, its relationship to maternal postpartum depression, and implications for family health, Journal of Advanced Nursing 45:26-35
- Jafee, SR, Caspi, A & Moffitt, TE (2001) Predicting Early Fatherhood and whether young fathers live with their children: prospective findings & policy reconsiderations *Journal of Child Psychology & Psychiatry* 42:803-815
- Paulson J & Bazemore S. (2010) prenatal and postpartum depression in fathers and its association with maternal depression: a meta-analysis, *JAMA* 303(19):196
- Ramchandani, P., Stein, A., Evans, J. & O'Connor TG (2005) Paternal depression in the postnatal period and child development: a prospective population study, *The Lancet* 365:2201-2205

Additional Reading (Psychoanalytic):

- Abelin, A (1971) The role of the father in the separation-individuation process, in JB McDevit and CF Settledge (eds.) *Separation-Individuation*. International UP
- Greenson, RR(1968) Dis-identifying from the mother: its special importance for the boy. *International Journal of Psycho-Analysis*, 49: 370-4.
- McDougal, J (1989) The dead father. In: D. Birksted-Breen (ed) (1993) *The

Gender conundrum. London: Routledge.

Families

- Cowan, P. & Cowan, C. (2000) When partners become parents: The big life change for couples. Mahwah, NJ: Erlbaum.
- Fivaz-Depeursinge, E.(2008), Infant's triangular communication in 'two for one' versus 'two against one' family triangles: case illustrations *Infant Mental Health Journal* 29/3:189-202
- Winnicott, D W (1967) Mirror role of Mother and Family in Child Development. Chapter 9 in *Playing and Reality* London: Penguin 1971, pp. 130-138

Gender

- de Marneffe, D. (1997). Bodies and Words: A Study of Young Children's Genital and Gender Knowledge. *Gender & Psychoanalysis.* 2:3-33
- Freud, S. (1908b). On the Sexual Theories of Children.S.E.9, pp.205–26.
- Klein, M (1932). The effects of early anxiety-situations on the sexual development of the girl, in *The Psycho-Analysis of Children,* London: Hogarth.
- Raphael-Leff (2007) 'Femininity and its unconscious 'shadows': gender and generative identity in the age of biotechnology' *British Journal of Psychotherapy* 23:497-515

Groups & Institutions

Recommended Reading

- Hopper, E. (2006-2007) Theoretical and Conceptual Notes Concerning Transference and Counter-transference Processes in Groups and by Groups, and the Social Unconscious: Part I. *Group Analysis*, 39/4:549-559; Part II *Group Analysis*, 40/1:21-34; Part III *Group Analysis*, 40/2:285-300.
- Menzies, I. (1960). A case study in the functioning of a social system as a defence against anxiety. *Human Relations*, 11:95-121.

Additional reading

- Bion, W. R. (1961) *Experiences in Groups and Other Papers.* London: Tavistock
- Hopper, E. (2003) *The Social Unconscious: Selected Papers.* London: Jessica Kingsley Publishers.
- Lewin, K. (1951). Field Theory in Social Science. Ed. D. Cartwright. New York: Harper and Row.
- Obholzer, A. and Roberts, V.Z. (eds) (1994) *The Unconscious at Work.* London: Routledge.

Maternal Orientation

- Raphael-Leff, J (1985) Facilitators and Regulators, Participators and Renouncers: mothers' and fathers' orientations towards pregnancy and parenthood. *Journal of Psychosomatic Obstetrics and Gynaecology*, 4:169-184.
- Raphael-Leff, J.(1986) Facilitators and Regulators: conscious and unconscious processes in pregnancy and early motherhood. *British Journal of Medical Psychology.,* 59:43-55.
- Scher, A. & Blumberg, O (2000) Night-waking among One-year-olds: A study of Maternal Separation Anxiety, *Child:Care, Health & Development.*26:323-334
- Scher, A. (2001) Facilitators and Regulators: maternal orientation as an antecedent of attachment security. *Journal of Reproductive & Infant Psychology,* 19:325-333
- Sharp, HM and Bramwell, R (2004) An empirical evaluation of a psychoanalytic theory of mothering orientation: implications for the antenatal prediction

of postnatal depression.*Journal of Reproductive and Infant Psychology* **22**:71-89
- Van Bussel, J.C.H, Spitz, B. & Demyttenaere, K (2008) Anxiety in pregnant and post-partum women. An exploratory study of the role of maternal orientations, *Journal of Affective Disorders,* 518:232-242.

Mentalization & Reflective Function
- Allen, J.G. (2006) Mentalizing in Practice. In Allen, J.G. & Fonagy, P. (ed) *Handbook of Mentalization-Based Treatment* pp. 3-6, London: John Wiley. Ltd. http://books.google.co.uk/books?hl=en&lr=&id=ifl7qoUNUgcC&oi=fnd&pg=PR7&dq=mentalization+Allen+2006&ots=0VlTk5maoi&sig=UXQlv0FejYd246nUs QsiuhgGzDQ#v=onepage&q&f=false
- Fearon, R.M.P., Target, M., Sergeant, J., Williams, L., Bleiberg, E. & Fonagy, P (2006) Short-term mentalizing and relational therapy: an integrative family therapy for children and adolescents. In Bleiberg, E. & Fonagy, P (Eds). *Handbook of Mentalization-Based Treatment.* Chichester, UK: Wiley.
- Fonagy, P., Gergely, G., Jurist, E. L., & Target, M. (2002). *Affect Regulation, Mentalization, and the Development of the Self.* London: Karnac.
- Slade, A. (2005) Parental reflective functioning: An introduction. *Attachment and Human development,* 7*:* 269-281.

Mothers
Recommended Reading:
- Klaus, MH & Kennel, JH (1995) *Bonding: Building the Foundations for a Secure Attachment.* Addison Wesley USA
- D Fairbrother, N & Woody S.R. (2008) New mothers' thoughts of harm related to the newborn, *Archive of Womens Mental Health* 11:221–229
- Giardino, J., Gonzalez, A., Steiner, M. & Fleming, A.S. (2008). Effects of motherhood on physiological and subjective responses to infant cries in teenage mothers: A comparison with non-mothers and adult mothers. *Hormones and Behaviour*, 53**:**149-158.
- Stern, DN (1995) *The Motherhood Constellation*, London: Basic Books.
- Winnicott DW (1956) Primary maternal pre-occupation. In: *Through paediatrics to psychoanalysis,* pp. 300-306. London: Hogarth Press.
- Winnicott DW (1960) The Relationship of a mother to her baby at the beginning. In: *The family and Individual development*, pp15-20. London: Tavistock.

Additional reading
- Baraitser, L (2006) Oi Mother, keep ya hair on! Impossible transformations of maternal subjectivity, *Studies in Gender & Sexuality*, 7:217-38
- Chodorow, N (1978) *The Reproduction of Mothering- Psychoanalysis and the Sociology of Gender,* University of California
- Raphael-Leff, J. (2008b) Maternal Subjectivities. Studies in the Maternal, 1 (1) http://www.mamsie.bbk.ac.uk/back_issues/issue_one/Joan%20Raphael-Leff_1000%20words_new.pdf.
- Welldon, EV (1988) *Mother Madonna Whore, the Idealization and Denigration of Motherhood*, London: Karnac

Neuroscience
- Balbernie, R (2001) Circuits and circumstances: the neurobiological consequences of early relationship experiences and how they shape later behaviour, *Journal of*

Child Psychotherapy. 27:237-55

- Karmiloff-Smith, A (1995) Annotation: The extraordinary cognitive journey from foetus through infancy, *Journal of Child Psychology & Psychiatry.* 36:*1293-1313*
- Panksepp, J (1998). *Affective Neuroscience.* New York: Oxford University Press
- Pollock, SD (2005) Early adversity and mechanisms of plasticity: Integrating affective neuroscience with developmental approaches to psychopathology. *Development & Psychopathology.* 17: 735-752
- Steinberg, L. (2009). Should the science of adolescent brain development inform public policy? *American Psychologist*, 64:739-750.
- Schore, A. (2001) Effects of secure attachment relationships on right brain development, affect regulation and infant mental health. *Infant Mental Health Journal*, 22 7–66.
- Watts-English, T, Fortson, BL, Gibler, N, Hooper, SR, & De Bellis MD (2006) The Psychobiology of Maltreatment in Childhood, *Journal of Social Issues,* 62:717-736

Observation

Recommended Reading:

- Bick, E (1964) Notes on Infant Observation in Psychoanalytic Training, *International Journal of Psychoanalysis,* 45:558-566
- Hopkins, J (1990) The Observed Infant of Attachment Theory, *British Journal of Psychotherapy*, 6:46
- Salzberger Wittenberg, I (1997) The family, the observer and infant observation group in S. Read (ed) *'Developments in Infant Observation - the Tavistock Model, London:Routledge.*

Additional reading:

- Freud, A (1953) Some Remarks on Infant Observation *Psychoanalytic Study of The Child* 8:9-19 [*The Writings of Anna Freud. Vol. IV, 1945-1956, New York: International Universities Press*].
- Freud, S (1920) 'The child playing with the reel' in *Beyond the Pleasure Principle,* SE 18, pp.14-17.
- Grier, F (2003) Amanda: observations and reflections on a bottle-fed baby who found a breast mother, Chapter 11 in *Parent-Infant Psychodynamics – wild things, mirrors and ghosts,* J Raphael-Leff (ed), London:AFC, 2009, pp 209-230
- Raphael-Leff, J (2003) Cannibalism & succour: is breast always best? (thoughts on 'Amanda'), Chapter 12, pp. 231-243, ibid.
- Miller, L *et al* (1989) *Closely Observed Infants*, London, Duckworth
- Reid, S. (ed)(1997) *Developments in Infant Observation*, London: Routledge

Parenting

- Brazelton, T. & Cramer,B. 1990: *The earliest relationship.* Reading, MA: Perseus
- Gergely, G & Watson, JS (1996) The Social Biofeedback Theory of parental affect-mirroring. *International Journal of Psychoanalysis,* 77:1181-1212
- Klaus, M and Klaus, P. H. 1998: Your amazing newborn. Reading, MA: Perseus
- Leach, P (2009) *Child Care Today,* Cambridge: Polity Press
- Rayner, E (2005) Parenthood, Chapter 12, in *Human Development: An introduction to the psychodynamics of growth, maturity and Ageing,* Rayner, E., Joyce, A., Rose, J., Twyman M., & Clulow,. D., *London:Routledge,* 2003 231-259

- Slade, A (2005) Parental reflective functioning: An introduction. *Attachment & Human Development*, **7**:269 – 281 To link to this article: DOI: 0.1080/14616730500245906 URL:http://dx.doi.org/10.1080/14616730500245906
- Slade, A. (2007). Reflective Parenting Programs:Theory and Development. *Psychoanalytic Inquiry, 26(4)*. http://www.reflectiveparentingprogram.org/pdfs/Reflective%20Parenting%20Programs%20PDF.pdf
- Winnicott, D.W. (1986) *Home is where We Start From. Essays by a Psychoanalyst: By D. W. Winnicott.* Compiled/edited by C. Winnicott, R. Shepherd, and M. Davis. New York/London: W. W. Norton & Co., Inc.

Perversions
- Welldon, E.V.(2011) *Playing with Dynamite,* London:Karnac

Play
- Emde, R, Kubicek L & Oppenheim, D (1997) Imaginative reality observed during early language development *International Journal of Psycho-Analysis* 78:115-133
- Greenacre, P (1959) Play in Relation to Creative Imagination. *Psychoanalytic Study of the Child* 14:61-80
- Mayes, LC & Cohen, DJ (1992) The Development of a capacity for imagination in early childhood. *Psychoanalytic Study of the Child,* 47:23-47
- Meares, R.(1993). *The Metaphor of Play: Disruption and Restoration in the Borderline Experience.* Northvale, NJ: Jason Aronson.
- Raphael-Leff, J. (2010) The 'Dreamer' by Daylight - Imaginative Play, Creativity, and Generative Identity in *The Psychoanalytic Study of the Child*, 64:14-53.
- Sinason, V. (2001). Children who kill their teddy bears. In B. Kahr (ed.) *Forensic Psychotherapy and Psychopathology: Winnicottian Perspectives.* London: Karnac Books. pp. 43-49.
- Target, M. and Fonagy, P. (1996). Playing With Reality: II. The Development of Psychic Reality from a Theoretical Perspective. *International Journal of Psychoanalysis* **77**: 459-479
- Winnicott, D.W (1942) Why children play, in *Collected Works: Through Paediatrics to Psycho-Analysis,* London: Hogarth, 1975
- Winnicott, D. W. (1971), Transitional objects and transitional phenomena. In: *Playing and Reality*. pp. 1-30
- Freud, S. (1908a). Creative Writers and Day-dreaming.S.E.9, pp.141–53.

Postnatal disturbance
Recommended Reading:
- Fraiberg, S., Adelson, E. and Shapiro, V (1975) Ghosts in the nursery: a psychoanalytic approach to the problems of impaired mother-infant relationships. *Journal of the American Academy of Child Psychiatry,*14: 387-421. Chapter 8 in *Parent-Infant Psychodynamics – wild things, mirrors and ghosts,* J Raphael-Leff (ed), London: Anna Freud Centre, 2009, pp.87-117
- Oates, M et al, (2004) Postnatal depression across countries and cultures: a qualitative study, *The British Journal of Psychiatry* 184: s10-S16
- Raphael-Leff, J (2001) 'Climbing the walls': puerperal disturbance and perinatal therapy, in *Spilt Milk -perinatal loss and breakdown.* J.Raphael-Leff (ed), pp.60-81, London: Routledge

Additional reading
- Brown G.W.& Harris T.O. (1986) Stressors, vulnerability and depression: a question of replication, *Psychological Medicine* 16:739-744.
- Fonagy, P., Steele, M., Moran, G., Steele, H. and Higgitt, A. (1994) *Measuring the Ghost in the Nursery.* Bulletin of the Anna Freud Centre, 14: 115 - 131.
- Murray, L (1997) The effect of infant's behaviour on maternal mental health, *Health Visitor* 70:334-5 [Chapter 20 in *Parent-Infant Psychodynamics-wild things, mirrors and ghosts,* J Raphael-Leff (ed), London: Anna Freud Centre, 2009, pp.262-267]
- Green, A (1960) The dead mother complex, In Green, A. *On Private madness,* 1986, Rebus Books. [Chapter 13, in *Parent-Infant Psychodynamics – wild things, mirrors and ghosts,* J Raphael-Leff (ed), London:Anna Freud Centre, 2009, pp162-174]
- Raphael-Leff, J (2000) (ed) *Spilt Milk - Perinatal Loss and Breakdown*, Routledge

Pregnancy
- Pines, D. (1988). Adolescent Pregnancy and Motherhood: A Psychoanalytical Perspective. *Psychoanalytic Inquiry* 8: 234-251
- Raphael-Leff, J(1991) *Psychological Processes of Childbearing*, 4th edition, London: Anna Freud Centre, 2005
- Raphael-Leff, J (1993) *Pregnancy - The Inside Story*, London/NY: Karnac 2001
- Burton, G.J., Barker, D.J. P. & Moffett, A.,*(2011) The Placenta and Human Developmental Programming,* Cambridge University Press

Psychodynamic & Perinatal Psychotherapy
Recommended Reading:
- Baradon, T. Broughton, C., Gibbs, J, James J., Joyce A.& Woodhead, J. (2005) *The Practice of Psychoanalytic Parent-Infant Psychotherapy: Claiming the Baby.* London:Routledge
- Bergner, S, Monk, C., & Werner EA (2008) 'Dyadic intervention during pregnancy? Treating pregnant women and possibly reaching the future baby',
- *Infant Mental Health Journal* 29/5:399-419
- Cramer, B. G. & Stern, D. (1988). Evaluation of changes in mother-infant brief psychotherapy. Infant Mental Health J., 9:1.
- Daws, D. (1999). Parent-infant psychotherapy: remembering the Oedipus complex. *Psychoanalytic Inquiry.*, 19: 267-78
- Emanuel, L & Bradley E (2008) *'What Can the Matter Be?'* –Therapeutic Interventions with Parents, Infants and Young Children. The work of the Tavistock Clinic Under Fives Service,* London: Karnac
- Lieberman, A. & Pawl, J. (1993). Infant-parent psychotherapy. In Handbook of Infant Mental Health, ed. C. Zeanah, Jr. New York: Guilford Press, pp. 427-42
- N.T. Malberg, N.T.& Raphael-Leff, J. (2012)*The Anna Freud Tradition: Lines of Development - Evolution of Theory and Practice over the Decades*, London: Karnac

Additional reading:
- Cooper PJ., Murray L., Wilson A. & Romaniuk, H (2003) Controlled trial of short- and long-term effect of psychological treatment of postpartum depression, *British Journal of Psychiatry,* 182:421-9
- Holmes, J. (2009) *Exploring in Security: towards an Attachment-informed*

Psychoanalytic Psychotherapy. London:Routledge.
- Tronick, EZ (2003) 'Of Course All Relationships Are Unique': How Co-creative Processes Generate Unique Mother—Infant and Patient—Therapist Relation-ships and Change Other Relationships. *Psychoanalytic Inquiry*. 23: 473-491

Toddlers
Recommended Reading:
- Lieberman, A (1995) 'Who is the toddler?', Chapter 2 in *The Emotional Life of the Toddler*, New York: The Free Press, pp.6-20
- Joyce, A. (2003) One to two year olds: junior toddlers, chapter 5 in *Human Development: An introduction to the psychodynamics of growth, maturity and ageing*, Rayner, E, Joyce, A, Rose, J, Twyman M & Clulow 4*th* edition, London:Routledge, 2003 pp. 71-95
- Joyce, A. (2003) Two to three year olds: senior toddlers, Chap. 6 *ibid*, pp.96-119

Additional reading:
- Emde, R (1994) Three roads intersecting: changing viewpoints in the psycho-analytic story of Oedipus. Chapter 6 in M. Ammaniti & D. Stern (Eds.) *Psycho-analysis and Development*. New York: New York University Press, pp 97–110.
- Freud, A (1965) The concept of developmental lines. In *The Writings of Anna Freud*, Vol.6 New York: International Universities Press, 1973, pp. 62-92
- Freud, A. (1981). *Psychoanalytic Psychology of Normal Development*. London: The Hogarth Press and the Institute of Psycho-analysis.
- Freud, S (1908) *On the Sexual theories of children*: S.E. 9 pp. 205-226
- Freud, S. (1909) *Analysis of a Phobia in a Five-Year-Old Boy, S.E.10, pp.1-318*
- Lyons-Ruth, K (1991) Rapproachment or approachment: Mahler's theory reconsidered from the vantage point of recent research on early attachment relationships. *Psychoanalytic Psychology*, 9:1-23.
- Tyson, P (2004) Points on a compass: four views on the developmental theories of Margaret Mahler and John Bowlby. *Journal of the American Psychoanalytic Association*, **52:** 499-509.
- Zaphiriou Woods, M & Pretorius, IM (2010) (eds) *Parents and Toddlers in Groups: a Psychoanalytic Developmental Approach,* London: Routledge
- Zaphiriou Woods, M (2011) From dependency to emotional self-reliance: the
- Anna Freud Centre parent-toddler group model, in *The Anna Freud Tradition Lines of Development - Evolution of Theory and Practice over the Decades*
- (eds.) NT. Malberg & J. Raphael-Leff, London: Karnac, (pp.340-356).

Trauma
- Lyons-Ruth, K. And Jacobitz, D. 1999: Attachment disorganization: unresolved loss, relational violence and lapses in behavioural and attentional strategies. In Cassidy, J. and Shaver, P.R P.(eds) Handbook of Attachment Theory and Research.New York Guildford Press.
- Main, M and Hesse, E. 1990: Parents' unresolved traumatic experiences are related to infant disorganization attachment status: is frightened and/or frightening parental behaviour the linking mechanism? In Greenberg, M. et al. (eds) Attachment in the preschool years. Chicago:University of Chicago Press.
- O'Connor TG, Bredenkamp D. & Rutter, M (2000) Attachment disturbances and disorders in children exposed to severe early deprivation, *Infant Mental Health Journal* 20:10-29.

APPENDICES

Appendix 1: **AIDE MEMOIRE FOR PRESENTATION OF A CASE**
Leezah Hertzman *

A. **Context**
- Describe your work place setting and your role in it
- Introduce us to the young parent/s and baby
- How long have you been working with them?
- How did they come in to your service? (self referral, health visitor, GP etc)

B. **Relationships**
- Provide a Genogram of the family if possible
- Brief personal history of the parent/s - including feelings about the pregnancy (planned or unplanned?) and the baby
- Quality of the baby's mother and father connection (and plans if known)
- Father's attitudes to the mother, the baby, parenthood etc
- Wider social network such as extended family, friends, other non-professional support and brief evaluation of the quality of these connections
- Relationship to school, college, workplace

C. **Details of the case**
- Why are you choosing to present this case?
- What aspect do you feel you need help with thinking about?

D. **Observation** – descriptive report of the interaction:
- emotional quality between parent/s and baby (harmonious, playful, tense)
- physical proximity, holding, facial expressions, tone, etc
- baby's capacity to self-soothe
- age appropriateness

Focus on:
- attention to detail and its recall
- Choice of sequence of events to report
- Awareness of counter-transference issues
- Appreciation of different perspectives
- Accurate and descriptive reporting (with appropriate levels of detai)l
- Appreciation of issues of confidentiality

E. **Applying Psychoanalytic Concepts/Ideas**
- How does this young person make you feel (unedited)?
- Why do you think they make you feel this way?
- Are there any personal resonances for you with this young person, their family or circumstance?• Are these influencing how you interact with them?
    - What are your own fantasies and expectations about this young person?
    - How do other people react to him/her: professionals, family, partner, friends?
    - How do you think the young person views you?
    - What psychoanalytic ideas/theories may seem applicable to this young person and their interaction with their baby (e.g. defences,

oedipal issues, psycho-analytic concepts of adolescent development, representations etc).

---

* **Leezah Hertzman** is a Psychoanalytic Psychotherapist and Clinical Lecturer at the Tavistock Centre for Couple Relationships (TCCR) and Clinical Lead for TCCR's 'Parenting Together' Service. She has a wide range of experience working with families, in different assessment and therapeutic paradigms. Previously, as Research Psychotherapist at the Tavistock & Portman NHS Trust, she was involved in developing and investigating interventions for vulnerable parents and children. She was also Child Mental Health Adviser to the Department of Children, Schools and Families, advising Government on the development of policies and practice in the area of young people's mental health. Leezah has a private psychoanalytic psychotherapy practice for individuals and couples in North West London, alongside teaching and supervising.

Appendix 2: **HOW THIS TRAINING WAS CONSTRUCTED:**
Joan Raphael-Leff *

The original training course *'Adolescents becoming Parents'* consisted of eight study-days over 16 weeks. Each of the course components was closely evaluated by all participants every study day, and the training amended according to this feedback. Three months post-course Focus Groups were conducted with selected clients – and an independent follow-up was conducted nine months later.

To accommodate work schedules and budget restrictions the second pilot training was condensed down to the current length, of five half-study days, at two weekly intervals. The third and fourth pilot groups of *'Adolescence as a Second Chance'* had the training delivered over two weekends (Friday afternoon and all of Saturday) at a week or two week interval.

Learning Outcomes

- Evaluation by all participants provided detailed feedback on each of the components of the course every study day.
- Mid- and end-of-course evaluation allowed for amendments of content and structure during the running of the course.
- Effectiveness was assessed by comparing each participant's pre- and post-course reflective functioning measures.
- The increasing sophistication of pre- and post-training case report/write-ups with observational material provided additional measures of course efficacy.
- These, plus a post-course focus group and an independently conducted end-depth qualitative follow-up with a subsample of individual participants nine months after the course ended, confirmed that due to the training participants –
- showed increased knowledge and deeper understanding of the subjective experience of their adolescent clients (during pregnancy and/or early parenthood) and ways in which parent/s' emotional needs intersect with those of their children.
- acquired better listening skills, an 'observational stance' and clinical strategies conducive to enhancing family interactions.
- were more aware of the importance of psychodynamic forces operating within their clients, themselves and in the institutional work context.
- learned to detect and understand the meanings of antenatal and postnatal parental disturbances and identify symptoms.
- were better equipped to critically evaluate claims, theories and evidence regarding contemporary teenage parents and their experience

Positive Feedback:

- All the 112 course participants lauded the course. At follow-up nine months later the original group noted persistence of their –
- appreciation of having had time to reflect on their work practice
- greater awareness of the capacity of babies to feel and to communicate feelings
- enhanced confidence in working effectively with teenage parents and their toddlers
- increased insight and continued interest in their own psychic processes
- improved social networking and understanding of how workers in different roles approach work with young parents.
- greater self awareness, personal growth and confidence in finding new internal and external resources.

Evaluation: 'Adolescents Becoming Parents'

The *quantitative data* of feedback, evaluation and follow-up was enriched with *qualitative data* collection, focusing on less conscious feelings/ fantasies/ motivations as well as overt knowledge, understanding and relational and psycho-social dynamics). This approach is in keeping with the psychodynamic nature of the training and feedback included many open-ended questions, feedback during the course itself, and post-course group- and individual in-depth interviews.

Some feedback had an *action research element* and input was utilised to improve the pilot course, which then ran a second time in its altered form. Some measures (such as pre- and post-course reflective functioning; evaluations of participants' early and late case-history write-ups, and change in observational capacities) tapped the *course efficacy* in terms of individual progress.

However, because of ethical restrictions, the impact of the course on the client was not measured directly, but followed up through self-report by the course participants. Ideally, when evaluating roll-out of the training, trainers will negotiate with managers to interview a sample of local clients before and after delivery of the course to their practitioners (see attached questionnaire).

Joan Raphael-Leff, Psychoanalyst (Fellow, British Psychoanalytical Society) and Social Psychologist is Leader of UCL/Anna Freud Centre Academic Faculty for Psychoanalytic Research. Previously was Head of University College London's MSc in Psychoanalytic Developmental Psychology, and Professor of Psychoanalysis at the Centre for Psychoanalytic Studies, University of Essex. For the past 40 years has specialised both clinically and academically in Reproductive and Early Parenting issues, training primary health workers on six continents, and has over 100 single-author publications, and ten books in the field including: *Psychological Processes of Childbearing; Pregnancy - The Inside Story; Parent-Infant Psychodynamics - Wild Things, Mirrors and Ghosts; Spilt Milk - Perinatal Loss and Breakdown; Ethics of Psychoanalysis; Between Sessions and Beyond the Couch;* and most recently, *Female Experience: Four Generations of British Women Psychoanalysts on Work with Women* (coedited with RJ Perelberg) and *The Anna Freud Tradition - Lines of Development. Evolution of Theory and Practice over the Decades* (co-edited with Norka Malberg).

Appendix 3:
RUNNING REFLECTIVE WORK GROUPS
Joan Raphael-Leff

These regular small groups provide time for participants to reflect on the course input and apply this to their own practice.

The method of inquiry differs from ordinary supervision in that group members are invited to reflect: to investigate their own thinking and imaginatively explore emotional responses evoked by the material, their own and that of colleagues. Through the **group process** a new kind of understanding begins to emerge, bringing with it a gradual *personal change in one's ability to listen psychodynamically, and to tolerate not knowing* – staying with, rather than evading discomfort and pain.

These groups bear in mind the general topic of the day in discussion of problems brought up by members of each small group, with examples from their own case-loads.

Aims:
- To further knowledge and a capacity for *self-reflection.*
- To enhance work-skills that inform practice in work situations within this high-risk field.
- To deepen understanding of the *psycho-dynamic processes* of adolescence, pregnancy, parenting and the emotional needs of infants and toddlers to help professionals to break the trans-generational 'cycle of disadvantage'.
- To identify *risk factors* associated with parental immaturity, including non-attunement, inconsistent or ineffectual parenting, neglect, violence or trauma leading to cognitive deficits and emotional disturbance in the child.
- To explore issues of *cultural diversity* and to foster awareness of anti-discriminatory practices.

Learning Objectives:
- The small group experience allows for exploration of dynamics and the institutional forces within which we operate developing better multi-agency team cooperation and intra-agency team collaboration.
- Rich discussion of problematic cases enabling members to develop self-awareness and the capabilities needed to confront the disturbing feelings this work entails.
- Reflection enables members become aware of the importance of unconscious forces operating within both clients and ourselves.

Group Composition:
Group members are selected with a multi-disciplinary mix of group participants in mind. This fosters understanding of the rationale behind the ways other professionals work It Develops a common language, pooled information, skills and competencies across disciplines

Method:
At the beginning of the course each participant will have prepared *a case* for discussion that includes a *brief observation* of an interaction between teenage parent/s and their baby. This may have been conducted at their place of work, in the baby's own home or elsewhere. *An 'Aide Memoire'* (Appendix 1) is available to help write up this report.

- Hopefully, all participants will have a chance to present their case to their small group for discussion and comments. In time, they may wish to rewrite the initial report in line with what has been learned.
- Each session is based on a presentation by one group member of an individual case brought from her/his own case-load.
- In each session, time is also allocated for other members of the group to provide updates on previously presented cases and/or difficulties they have encountered.

Conducting a Refective Work Group:

Group leaders must encourage the group to 'gell', and enable members to talk freely, relying on in-group confidentiality and support. It is crucial that members feel free to reveal their failures as well as successes. It is important to discuss the problems that arise in localities where group participants work together on a particular case, and where some information might be privileged. These particular issues of case confidentiality are intricate. It is hoped that through discussion of them, and the feelings they arouse in different members of the team, participants will become aware of the intentions and thinking process of colleagues, and also of the tensions and reactive dynamics that are set up when one practitioner decides (on good grounds) to withhold information from another.

When several groups run simultaneously, **meetings of the leaders** before and after the groups are useful in assessing the prevailing mood across groups, indicating problematic issues in the training.

The group's ongoing focus includes examination of inter-generational transmissions, issues of containment, expectations, counter-transference feelings aroused by the material, and addressing the father (present or absent). The interdisciplinary nature of the small group promotes awareness of different perspectives in team work with troubled and vulnerable young families in a variety of work settings.

Reflective Work Groups
Form for Group Leader:

Reflective Work Group: *This is for the Group Leader's own comments*
Date:_____Who presented:_____

Notes on
The presentation, leading the group, encouraging discussion
Level of engagement, quality of participation
Enhancing self-awareness, containing anxiety
Other issues
Encouraging inter-displinary & multi-agency team work.
Hidden hierarchies, Readiness to pool experience
Difficulties
Thoughts about what needs to be done differently next time

Appendix 5:

THE PRINCIPLES OF OBSERVATION
Joan Raphael-Leff

Objectives:
To enhance the capacity for observation which is the core to a practitioner's work-skills.

Contemporary understanding:
In recent years there has been a major conceptual shift in observational studies. It is now acknowledged that even in Science, there is no such thing as an aloof observer.[i]

- It is recognised that the observer's presence alters the situation even in 'naturalistic' situations that are neither pre-structured nor select discrete attributes for examination.

- The observer of human interaction can no longer be thought of as a 'fly on the wall' but is a *participant observer',* drawing on the commonality and similarity between him/herself and the 'object(s)' of observation.

- The idea of 'observer objectivity' has been replaced with a greater awareness of the inevitable *subjectivity of each observer* who experiences the world through her/his own sensorium, primed by conscious and unconscious personal experience.

- One's own psychohistory and theoretical preconceptions colour not only what each observer sees, but how s/he recalls and reports upon it. Paradoxically, this bias can be reduced by awareness that one is not an impartial recorder.

- The presence of an observer introduces tensions. Even a hidden one-way observational booth arouses fantasies about the mirrored surface and what lies behind it, and we know that camera's increase self-consciousness.

- Recognition of the complexity of the mind and its unconscious as well as cognitive processes, alerts us to the fact that what we *see* in observations is merely the tip of an iceberg. The observed is a tiny and not necessarily representative fraction. And in the case of families a fragment of ongoing relationships.

- The advocated approach is one of open, receptive 'evenly hovering attention' rather than preconceptions, sentimentality or perfectionistic expectations.

Methods
With growing evidence of the interpersonal nature of development, developmental observations have now shifted from the previous mode of investigating a baby in isolation or studying the parent's influence on the child - *to ongoing observations of reciprocal influences.* Even so-called 'infant observation' in the baby's home used in many trainings for psychotherapists, the defined unit of observation is now the dynamic interaction between child and mother/father/carer, and/or siblings, peers and others (whose presence may be inferred even in their absence).

Purpose
Psychoanalytic understanding of childhood was initially gained from recollections of adult patients. However, it became clear that these were 'reconstructions' of events, from an adult's point of view rather than unembellished veridical accounts of them. Child and infant psychotherapy have afforded more immediate understanding of feelings, thoughts and fantasies as these arise within an intersubjective exchange. Observations of non-clinical populations, particularly those made in natural

surroundings, rather than laboratory settings have further enriched our awareness of ordinary everyday interactions, and in particular, those with family members or peers. In fact, fine-grained records of observation constitute the raw-material for understanding the formation of the self in infancy and childhood.

- Over the past twenty years, particularly with development of micro-analytic techniques, numerous studies have shown that from infancy, our minds are constituted *interactively*. Together with their carers babies co-construct both external and internal realities [see the reading list sections on Babies and Developmental Research, especially Intersubjectivity].

- This relational and intersubjective emphasis has shifted the focus from the individual and his/her intra-psychic processes to the *relational matrix*, both interpersonal and *inter*-psychic (see Glossary). Each particular observed twosome, family or group builds up a special pattern of interaction with unique dialectical patterns of exchange.

- However, the observer must be aware of the difference between observation and the inferences that may be draw from it. Similarly, of obstructions to observation caused by personal prejudices or expectations due to theoretical viewpoint.

Emotional impact:

Recognition of the implications of a 'participant-observer's' own subjectivity must also make us aware of the inevitability of the *impact of observation on the observer* as well as the observed. While attempting to maintain a non-intrusive but friendly presence and open-minded stance, an observer is vulnerable to influences from the matrix of observation.

At times, an observer is exposed to highly arousing situations. Intimate aspects of family life or children's interactions with their peers, or exposure to pain and nakedness during labour all can create an intense emotional impression that evokes disturbing feelings and primitive anxieties which reverberate with unprocessed feelings within us. When thinking about such situations, this may lead an observer or even a reflective discussion group to retreat into theorising to avoid the painful uncertainties provoked by the scene.

To cope with emotional responses and to enhance personal awareness of these, the practitioner may wish to chart her/his journey as observer in her/his Private Journal. If a course participant finds her/himself feeling overwhelmed by the observational encounter (or any other aspect of the course) it is suggested that they contact the Course Leader, to consider ways of alleviating distress.

Written Records

Observations of behavioural interactions should be

(a) as descriptive as possible, incorporating feelings aroused in the observer in response to what has been observed, and a commentary that reveals intuitive inferences which may have led to an interpretation of these happenings.

(b) reflect growing understanding of psychodynamics from lectures, workshops, observation, discussion and reading

(c) use self-reflection and awareness of the effects of subjectivity, expectations and anxieties.

Clarity about the parameters of the role enables the observer to maintain boundaries, to avoid pressures to act outside these, and to utilise his/her own feelings in the service of the observation resisting the desire to identify.

Observation Reports:

One way of evaluating the effectiveness of the course workshops is to assess whether these have been effective in enhancing observational capacities.

- The seminar leader keeps a copy of an initial *5 minute observation* made by participants <u>before</u> the course begins, and at the end of the course asks participants to hand in another 5 minute observation.

- These two observations will offer each participant a sense of the development of an observation stance and reflective work skills over the ten weeks of the course.

The pre-course and last written observations can be compared using the following criteria:

- Evidence of having developed a non-judgmental, impartial observational stance.

- Attention to detail and its recall

- Awareness of a plurality of perspectives including your own subjective biases and counter-transference.

- A capacity to report in a rich, descriptive and coherent way [beware of emotive language – meanings suggestively introduced through descriptive adjectives/ adverbs (i.e. 'yearning') in your report]

The second observational report should show to what extent the practitioner has managed to develop an 'observational stance' despite awareness of the difficulties inherent in this i.e. seeing what is happening as objectively as possible, separating one's own thoughts or feelings from what is observed and identifying the specific affects, both positive and negative, displayed by child and/or adult. When commenting on observations, which include the mother or another carer, special attention should be paid to the emotional content of the relationship and the extent to which the child can be seen to adapt to the carer's handling. Observations may focus on of how the parents and/or child experienced and responded to the observer and of the response of the observer to what has been observed, in so far as it illuminates the processes involved in the child's behaviour.

Over-involvement or inappropriate engagement with the observed infant and/or family or disregard for issues of confidentiality reduces the quality of the report. When observation write-ups are too vague, or if they provide too much detail to get an overall impression of the encounter, or show little or no self-reflection, one would have to conclude that you have not understood the observer role and stance.

It is suggested that the written observation report for this course should be no more than 750 words in total.

Ethical considerations

The issue of **confidentiality** is of the utmost importance. When presenting and writing up observations names of parents and children, as well as disguising any distinguishing or identifying facts such as home location or parents' occupation should be disguised.

Observation is a privilege. Although there are many situations in which strangers can be observed anonymously (on a bus or in a café), to undertake a systematic observation **permission** will need to be obtained to make people aware of the way in which your observation will be used. Even when permission has been granted, special **consent** may be required for particularly intimate situations such as nappy changing or breastfeeding in home or workplace observations and must abide by the relevant regulations of each organisation.

Appendix 5

PSYCHODYNAMIC PERINATAL PSYCHOTHERAPY
Joan Raphael-Leff

Therapy during the perinatal period offers an opportunity to break the cycle of cross-generational transmissions. In the therapeutic space, a person, couple or family can verbalise, process and integrate implicit emotional forces, memories and attachment experiences, however traumatic. This 'working through' takes place in the context of a caring attuned relationship with an empathic therapist who helps them voice and understand their feelings (an experience these people may not have had in their own infancies), which in time can be internalised as a basis for sensitive parenting.

The capacity for healthy nurturing is associated with the carer's realistic self-esteem, enabling appropriate management of sadness, anger and anxiety. As an expectant parent's self-confidence is enhanced through therapy obsolete defences may be shed. Negative forces subside as the past becomes more understandable, with more empathy for one's own parents and glimpses of more positive experiences with them. When this happens during pregnancy, modification of unconscious 'baby-carer representations' from their own childhoods alters expectant parent's expectations of the unborn baby.

However, to be effective, perinatal therapy must deal with the two interleaving parent-baby systems – the parent's internal representations of the past and their own current interaction with the real baby. As they recognise their own difficulties, they can become more forgiving of the conflicts, shortcomings and fallibility of their own parents.

Needless to say, deep-seated changes such as these cannot be expected to occur through brief intervention. A recent controlled trial comparing the effect of three different psychological treatments for post-partum depression delivered at home (in 10 sessions) found that although CBT (Cognitive Behavioural Therapy) and non-directive counselling produced short-term mood changes and relief in early relationship difficulties, only psychodynamic psychotherapy produced a significant rate of reduction in depression, however even this benefits did not persist beyond 9 months postpartum (Cooper et al, 2003). The need for more prolonged intervention and time to consolidate changes is one reason it is strongly recommended to begin therapy with people at risk early on, preferably during pregnancy. In the case of antenatal depression/persecution, a further reason is the hope of changing negative representations <u>before</u> these materialise in actual interactions with the new baby.

However, even brief parent-infant consultation can be therapeutic with the therapist 'gathering in' for the parents all the relevant aspects of a baby's life and its relationship to them. This consists of open-ended questioning about the nature of the presenting problem, a free-ranging inquiry into memories of the pregnancy, birth, and early weeks and questions about the parents' relationships with each other and with their own parents, to get a picture of the family context of this particular baby. However, for the interchange to have meaning it is necessary for the therapist to have 'real curiosity and to be attuned to the family' (Daws, 1999).

Appendix 6:   **READING WITH BABIES**
                              Susan Straub, Ph.D*

Reading books with the baby, may offer teenage parents a semi-structured interactive experience that facilitates reflective function, with emotional benefits for both. Many adolescents were not read to as children, and school may not have been a rewarding or successful experience for them. Using books with sparse text encourages poor readers to engage with reading, boosting confidence and fostering freedom to be creative and playful in telling a story. Reading picture books together provides opportunities for the young parent to revisit their own infantile issues in safety, and to become more sensitive to the baby's anxieties – about bedtime and other separations, day care experiences, being ignored or attended to, coping with frustrations…

Sharing such 'special time' with their babies also helps the teen to be more observant and to initiate conversations with the infant about emotional issues.

On the other hand, listening to stories stimulates the child's imagination, gives him/her an opportunity to initiate communication and games with the parent and initiates early literacy skills, enlarged vocabulary and enriched language structure which aids the child's later school success. In immigrant and ethnic minority families, books may be used to facilitate wider knowledge of their own origins as well as learning aspects of the prevailing culture.

Practice: *Practitioner workshops can break into threesomes with one reading a book to the others to*

- Experience the intensity of sharing a picture book with partners as an interactive, conversational pleasurable activity
- Exploring how books trigger memory of one's own childhood and provide both access to the dominant culture.
- Discuss how books prompt parents to interact with their babies? (Included in 'books' in the broadest conception of finger games, nursery rhymes, etc.)
- What is the value of nursery rhymes?
- What books work best with what ages? Why do parents seem to need their infants to perform in a particular way? What happens when the babies don't?
- Why are books so helpful when raising babies and young children?
- We know what the babies learn, but what about the parents? What issues do books raise for them in a way which allows access to thinking about them? *Practitioners can* encourage young parents to read to their babies at home, or in their own group activities, or engage a RTM project offers work-shops to practitioners or directly to young people providing a model for fostering reading. [www.readtomeprogram.org].

Objectives of a 'Read to Me' programme are:

- to offer reading as a resource to young parents for pleasure, and to enhance parenting skills, psychological insights and educational development;
- to stimulate imagination and initiate early literacy education;
- to improve the potential for healthy parent-child relationships.

This intervention endorses the goals UK Government's 'Every Child Matters' agenda by introducing themes which help young parents to understand the world of the child and help babies and toddlers to understand the world around them.

---

* Susan Straub, PhD is a clinical social worker specialising in work with children and adolescents developed RTM 20 years ago in the USA States..She kindly ran a RTM workshop for practitioners for the original *'Teenagers Becoming Parents'* course in April 2008 at the Anna Freud Centre.

EXPANDED NOTES:

<u>Expanded notes for Module 1</u>

MENTALIZATION BASED APPROACHES
IN WORK WITH TEEN PARENTS
AND THEIR CHILDREN.

Norka Malberg, Ph.D*

The main aim of Mentalization-based technique is to activate the capacity for *reflective thinking*. In its applications to the practitioner-client relationship, we would consider the capacity of the former to keep the young parent's mind in mind. Similarly, regarding the parent-infant relationship we would encourage the young parent to keep the baby's mind in mind – that is to think of the needs and wants of the child as separate from her/his own – to think of the other as a separate partner in the 'relational dance'.

This Handout introduces the concept of mentalization in the context of young parents, aware of the challenges faced by the practitioner when attempting to promote reflective functioning in teenagers who are experiencing developmental tasks for which they are not ready.

<u>The basic message</u>: *Interpersonal stress militates against mentalizing*

What is mentalizing?
We all have the capacity to mentalize - to understand the other's perspective, and be aware of one's own feelings – but our reflectiveness is affected by stress.
As a practitioner, be aware of the perception of your impact on the other.
Ask yourself: *I wonder how I make the client feel?*

Adolescents do have the capacity to mentalize, but some of the time this is *suppressed defensively*. There is a reason for this – and for their risk-taking behaviour. *Don't take away their coping skills*.

- This work can be very frustrating at times. You need to check with yourself (mentalize) about your *counter-transferential feelings* – why may I be feeling sad, angry or feeling like rescuing or nurturing, etc now?
- Be boundaried but thoughtful – prepare to share some of your relevant feelings/thoughts.
- Remember both sides of the equation in the intervention – not only how the teen feels but also how s/he makes others feel. And similarly, regarding your self.
- Capitalise on the client's curiosity, gradually introducing awareness of limitations – her/his own and others'.

<u>Mentalizing behaviour:</u>
Give young people a different language to think about their own feelings and an opportunity to think about their own mind. This may feel quite scary for them – especially those who never had such an experience. Don't try and be too clever – teenagers have many of those around. What is important to the mentalizing stance is

being aware of pitching things wrongly Have the capacity to acknowledge mistakes and to laugh at yourself.

Strategies for engaging the teenager:
- Be tentative in any interpretations of their behaviour.
- Be playful and lively, yet respectful of their mental states, and recognising that these are opaque.
- Practitioners should model 'grown-up' thinking rather than being too 'pally' and 'cool'.
- Engage in a mirroring process – and ask the teenager for help with appropriate interventions. *'I'm trying to understand –...'*
- Identify the feeling for the young person who is confused about their feelings.
- Help to put ambiguous feelings in simple words. *'You seem to be getting closer to that feeling of ...'*

Thinking about thinking.
- Acknowledge when you feel lost for words and ask for help in understanding.
- Provide an awareness of multiple perspectives
- Try to activate the attachment system, especially in very young parents, for the sake of the child – recognising their own needs as separate from those of the baby.

In the pregnant teenager or young parent the ordinary developmental processes of adolescence have been derailed. Practitioners can gradually awaken their awareness of capacities which have been defensively suppressed, revisiting the 'attachment system' in a new way.
- Validate the young person's experience, enabling her/him to feel heard, remembered and thought about – but be aware of his/her need for privacy.
- Express a genuine wish to get to know the young person but create boundaries.
- Understand why s/he may contact you at an inappropriate time but suggest a better alternative.
- When s/he feels safe in a relationship with you, you will get her/his rage at feeling ignored elsewhere – and you need to differentiate what actually belongs to you and what does not.
- Don't *tell* her/him – but invite the teenager to think about his/her reactions; how s/he is affected and perceived by others.
- Bear in mind - how the baby is intended to close a 'gap' in his/her life

Basic tools:
- *Check* to see if you have got it right. *'I get the impression that'*...
- *'Rewind'* back to the previous stage of interaction with you in this encounter which seems to have led to a misunderstanding. Explain this misattunement.
- *Think* about what happened – helping the teenager to internalise that capacity to 'stop and rewind' before things escalate.
- Help him/her *practice* phrases that can be used with others to avoid fights and confrontations.
- Be *empathic* to the client's world. *'If I was you I might be feeling'*....
- Teach a young person to question *'why this is happening right now'* – which is contrary to the impulsive ways of many adolescents.
- Distinguish between what is 'old' and 'new' and the way the old impacts on the current – *'who do I remind you of just now?'*...

- Give the young person the space to express their feelings but challenge any fixed ideas and confusions.
- Young people tend to ask what to do with their lives. The biggest temptation is to answer – yet the question is how to help without doing so, and to make interventions without being directive or bringing in jargon.
- Tentative wording: *'Is it possible that?'*, *'It seems that…'*

Impaired Mentalization

<u>Components of impaired mentalizing</u>

There are several ways in which mentalization may be impeded, which in turn generate, maintain, reinforce or exacerbate emotional, behavioural and/or interpersonal difficulties.

a) Generalised mentalizing difficulties

There may be trait deficits in mentalizing ability in one member of the family, for example in a child presenting with oppositional behaviour. Such behaviour typically represents a non-mentalistic, physical effort by the child to control his feelings and generate a response in others. Angry or violent outbursts have the effect of forcing caregivers to experience what the child experiences thus offering the child a sense that their feelings can have an impact. However, in the medium term, this immediate impact fails to secure effective support reciprocity, control or self-coherence. Instead the child's non-mentalistic, coercive behaviour evokes non-mentalistic efforts of behavioural control from the caretakers, with resulting self-reinforcing and self-perpetuating cycles of non-mentalizing, coercive interactions.

b) Concrete mentalization difficulties

These can manifest themselves in a general lack of attention to the thoughts, feelings and wishes others, or interpreting one's own behaviour in terms of the influence of situational or physical constraints rather than feelings and thoughts in oneself or in others around one. This often happens when family conversations invariably focus on concrete concerns, such as who did what and explanations of behaviour in terms of physical circumstances and influences (e.g. we always argue when we travel long distances in the car).

The typical features of concrete understanding or simplistic mentalization are:

1. *Difficulty in emotion recognition* – not understanding positive or negative emotions
2. *Confusing a feeling with a thought*, e.g. because I feel sad, the world is a miserable place (aim to be able to see that you can feel sad without drawing conclusions from it). This confusion may be because feelings are leading to automatic thoughts outside awareness, or because the child notices how he feels and decides that this is what it must mean
3. *Understanding behaviour in 'concrete' terms* (e.g. in terms of external circumstances or other behaviours rather than in terms of internal states; e had a fight because it was hot rather than being able to recognize that one was irritable and had difficulty in hearing the other person)
4. *Difficulty in observing one's own thoughts and feelings*, and in identifying changes in them
5. *Not recognizing the impact of one's thoughts, feelings and actions on others*

6. *Not being able to see how one thing has led to another*, e.g. a thought led to a feeling which led to an action, and a reaction from someone else

7. *Over-generalizing from mental states*, e.g. feeling that because one upsetting thing happened, everything has gone wrong

8. *Not being able to be flexible and to play* with different ways of thinking about situations

9. *Feeling that somebody else's thoughts are dangerous*, e.g. that if someone disagrees that means that your own point of view is obliterated or that they hate you etc

10. *Struggling to relate thoughts to reality*, so that the individual ends up going round in unproductive circles and only becomes more anxious

11. *Acting without thinking*, or avoidance of thinking.

In this category a parent-child relationship may be described as simplistic or concrete if the parent reacts to behaviour without being aware of the child's feelings or wishes, which are motivating the behaviour. There is an absence of mentalizing of the child. The parent may thus be angry, over-reactive, blaming, and prescriptive. The child's mental states are obscured and treated as unimportant. This may also happen when there is an identified problem, e.g. ADHD or a physical condition, and either the condition is ignored or every behaviour is explained on the bases of it. The child may be treated as an object, a machine, an extension of the parent's identity, without curiosity about or recognition of him/her as an individual. Another way this kind of situation can arise is when there is a passive resignation or withdrawal of awareness from the child and non-thinking over a period of time on the part of the parent. Thus as in the previous case, his/her approach has become unthinking, concrete and behavioural. The parent may be depressed or overwhelmed and too tired to focus on the child unless situations have escalated when the parent falls back on a stock response, without trying to understand the specifics. The child recognises that only amplified behaviour will get through the parent's preoccupation or distraction, so that the situation begins already in an exaggerated and distorted way.

c) Pseudo-mentalization difficulties

Pseudo-mentalization, perhaps more appropriately termed *'inaccurate mentalization',* refers to the type of difficulty where there is apparent thoughtfulness, but this lacks some essential features of genuine mentalization.It is a partial understanding, containing some truth and it is not intentionally abusive. Broadly speaking pseuso-mentalization difficulties manifest themselves by a tendency of the individual to express absolute certainty about the thoughts and feelings of others. We also find a limited or absent recognition of the inherent uncertainty about knowing someone else's mind or appreciation for what it is like to have someone else define what is on one's own mind. Furthermore, thoughts and feelings in others or the self are recognised as long as these are consistent with the individual's self interest or preferences. For example, in a separated family, each parent may feel confident that they know how the children feel and that the children prefer to be with them and dislike the other parent. The lack of recognition of ambivalence, or of the child's need to present a distorted picture of his or her feelings to please the parent, characterizes such instances of impaired mentalization.

Pseudo-mentalization can take a number of forms.

1. Preserving a developmentally early view of the child/parent: In these instances the parent/child continues to think of the other person in the dyad from an earlier perspective. For example, a parent may not be able to consider their adolescent's burgeoning sexuality and continue to view them from a developmentally earlier point of view.

2. Intrusive mentalizing: In these instances the separateness/opaqueness of minds is not respected within a family– someone thinks they *know* what another person thinks/feels. Sometimes elements of the parent's image of the child's mind might be correct (making it even more pernicious) but the subtle differences between what the parent expresses and what the child is likely to feel reveal that they are not in touch with the thoughts and feelings of the child. In any case they are unaware of the impact that being told what they think and feel can have on children's capacity to have their own mind.

3. Overactive inaccurate mentalizing: Often parents invest a lot of energy in thinking or talking about how people in the family think or feel, but this has little or no relationship to the other person's reality. There can be an idealization of 'insight' for its own sake. The child might come to feel that mentalization is obstructive and confusing and should be avoided whenever possible.

4. Completely inaccurate attributions: At the extreme end of this category there may be somewhat bizarre attributions ("you are trying to drive me crazy", "your grandma is in league with your father against us"), denials of objective realities ("you provoked me", "you fell down the stairs, I never hit you"), or denial of the child's feelings ("you enjoyed it when I touched you like that", "you don't care about whether your Dad is here or not", "you don't care about me", "you would be glad if I was dead"). In such cases a child may be so traumatized by the parent's misperception, and the threat represented by the carer's mental state that s/he will seek to inhibit his/her own capacity to mentalize. These more chronic states should be distinguished from the consequences of the more temporary loss of mentalization.

d) Misuse of mentalization

This refers to situations in which understanding of the mental state of the individual is not directly impaired, yet the way in which it is used is detrimental. While this may occur in the context of the parental relationship, what we are concerned with is the extent to which it is experienced directly by the child. Misuse of mentalizing may occur unconsciously, but nevertheless the way in which it is used will be motivated by the goals, wishes or interests of an individual, a dyad or the family as a whole. This can take the following forms:

1. Manipulative use of understanding of the child: The child's mental states are recognized but not used to understand the child. There is no mutuality and there is a coercive element where mentalization is used for something else, e.g. as ammunition in marital battle. In these situations the child might experience mentalization as aversive because "being understood" occurs in the context of being manipulated. For example, in the case of separated parents a mother argues with the father about his unreliability in collecting the children. "You are such a bastard. You never think about how the children feel when you are late! Johnny was really upset and disappointed because he had been waiting to show you his soccer trophy. When you did not come he felt you did not really care about him anymore. Maybe it would be better if you did not bother to come at all!" Here the mother's accurate perception of the son's feelings is used to support a case, which is even more threatening to the child than the disappointment had been. The lesson the child might learn is to try to hide his feelings and pretend that it is 'OK'. The father, rather than focusing on his son's mental state, might shut off concern with it in order to avoid noxious battles with his wife. He arrives on time but is less sensitive to his son's feelings and thoughts.

2. Self-serving distortion of the child's feelings. Here the children's feelings are exaggerated or distorted in the interest of the parent's unspoken intention or attitude. For example, the father criticizes and complains to his wife that her taking a job means that the children feel neglected and rejected and unimportant to her. He only makes this complaint in weeks when he was required to do more chores but does not make the complaint when she has an au pair there to assist him.

3. Coercion against the child's thoughts. The parent appears to undermine the child's capacity to think by deliberately humiliating the child for her or his thoughts and feelings. For example, the parent exposes the child's sexual feelings in a family gathering or even individually to the child but in a belittling and insensitive manner. It is often an abuse of power; the child might have confided in the parent or the parent was given the information by virtue of their position of responsibility.

---

*Norka T. Malberg, DPsych. Child and Adolescent Psychotherapist, worked at the AFC as clinician, seminar leader and coordinator of collaborative outreach projects in schools and hospitals. Before that was Counselling Psychologist in USA, Chile, and Switzerland. Currently, Faculty of the Continuing Education Section of the Western New England Psychoanalytic Institute in New Haven, Connecticut. She is also clinical supervisor for the Child FIRST programme at the Clifford Beers Child Guidance Clinic in New Haven, CT. She continues her role as clinical consultant to the AFC in London.

Expanded notes for Module III:

ATTACHMENT THEORY – AN OVERVIEW

Dana Shai, Ph.D*

Attachment Theory

The founder of the field of attachment theory was John Bowlby (1958). As a trained psychoanalyst, Bowlby was in disagreement with Freud's view regarding the nature of mother-infant relationship. Classical psychoanalysis viewed the relationship between a mother and her infant as a result of the infant's dependence on his[1] mother to provide soothing of libidinal drives by means of feeding him. This hunger soothing produces pleasure, and this accumulative pleasurable experience, in turn, is associated with mother, eventually resulting in strong desire to be close to mother, independently from the need to be fed (Freud, 1910/1957).

Bowlby, on the other hand, viewed the intense emotional tie between a child and the mother as a need by its own right, rather than a derivative of other needs. Grounded in evolutionary thinking, Bowlby suggested that another possible explanation for the intense bond between a child and his mother is based on natural selection, and more specifically, to allow the enhancement of the individual's survival chances under mother's care (Bowlby, 1969/1982; 1973). Those infants who managed to maintain contact with their mothers had better chances of survival than those who failed to do so. Consequently, those who survived could pass down their genes from generation to generation, including those responsible for attachment behaviours (Belsky, 2005). Over many years, this cycle has resulted in the human species' capacity, from the earliest moments of postnatal life, to attract the attention, care, and proximity of the caregiver and to establish and maintain contact with the caregiver, thus promoting the parent's investment. This interchange of behaviours is, according to Bowlby, the attachment behavioural system.

The Attachment Behavioural System

Attachment behaviours, according to attachment theory, are those aimed at promoting and maintaining parental proximity and contact and thereby protection. These behaviours include crying, smiling, approaching, clinging, and seeking contact (Ainsworth, Blehar, Waters, & Wall, 1978; Bowlby, 1969/1982). In this way this biological attachment behavioural system is designed to function as a protective system, in which the parent is the child's primary protector and haven of safety. This attachment relationship is activated (or heightened) in times of distress and perceived threat to the child's physical and emotional well-being, which then promotes the parent and the child to keep in close proximity (Goldberg, Grusec, & Jenkins, 1999).

From an internal perspective, however, the system's goal is to enhance a sense of security in the infant (Bretherton, 1985). Sroufe and Waters (1977) used the term 'felt security' to capture the internal state associated with attachment relationship. 'Felt Security' refers to the sense of confidence the infant has that mother will indeed protect her/him, physically and psychically. The extent to which the child has an internal feeling of security influences the degree to which the child feels safe to explore the world, that is, to use his mother as a secure base for exploration (Goldberg et al., 1999). According to van Den Boom (1994), Felt Security "refers to the *emotional* core of a relationship with a specific caregiver which is characterized by

---

1 For the purpose of clarity, child will be referred to as 'he' and the parent/caregiver as 'she'.

feeling safe and protected in the presence of that person and by feelings of longing and desire to restore proximity and contact when that person is absent" (van Den Boom, 1994, p. 1458, italics added). Thus, the attachment behavioural system can be viewed as a homeostatic interplay between 1) maintaining a sense of security manifested in proximity seeking; and 2) exploring the world through information and stimuli seeking. The operation of the attachment system, mediating these two distinct forces, facilitates exploring the world under reasonably safe conditions (Bretherton, 1985). In other words, exploration of the world is a function of the degree of felt security the individual experiences.

Internal Working Models (IWM)

In early infancy, the attachment behavioural system is constantly active, appraising both the degree/extent of danger as well as the availability of the attachment figure. This appraisal of relative safety/danger does not, however, occur afresh every time. Instead, through repeated interactions with the world and attachment figures, the young child gradually comes to construct increasingly complex Internal Working Models (IWM) of the world, of the attachment figure, and of self (Bretherton, 1985). The IWM's are mental representations constructed from internalizations of the child's experience of the role of the attachment figure as a protector and of himself in the relationship with the caregiver and reflect the child's anticipation and expectation as to what extent the parent is responsive and available to signals of distress. Thus the IWM of the parent's responsiveness is closely associated with the child's model of self – to what extent does the child feel effective in eliciting an appropriate parental response and that he can engage in relationships where his needs can, and should, be met. Empirical investigations demonstrate these IWM's to be stable over time (Main, Kaplan & Cassidy, 1985), and once organised, they tend to operate outside conscious awareness (Bretherton, 1985). Nonetheless, they affect the way an individual interacts with others, how one perceives, anticipates, and interprets others' behaviours and reactions to oneself, what and how information is processed, remembered or repressed.

Assessment of attachment security in infancy: the Strange Situation Procedure

As we have seen, the attachment relationship is an affective tie of the infant with the primary caregiver, determining to what the degree the infant feels he can use the caregiver as a source of comfort and reassurance in the face of threats from the environment. Virtually every infant develops this tie by the end of the first year, yet the nature and effectiveness with which the caregiver can be used in this way differs across infant-parent dyads. In 1969, Ainsworth & Wittig developed a standardized laboratory-based procedure called The Strange situation Procedure (SSP) which examines to what extent the infant can use the mother as a secure base from which to explore (Ainsworth, Bell, & Stayton, 1971) and assesses the child's IWM of the degree of security or insecurity he experiences in his relationship at approximately one year of age. More specifically, the infant's *behavioural* reactions to a set of reunions with mother following brief separations (thus being times of heightened distress) are thought to measure the infant's IWM of the child's security of attachment, that is, revealing the child's expectations about the availability of the caregiver in a time of distress and difficulty. It is noteworthy that the classifications of security or insecurity of attachment of the child in the SSP are not a function of the child's level of distress, but importance is given to how the infant can use his/her mother to regulate his/her emotions and behaviour (Belsky, 2005).

Adolescence as a 'Second chance'

The classification of the quality of mother-infant attachment has been defined in terms of the infant's ability to effectively use attachment behaviours which enable using the mother as a secure base from which to explore and as a source of comfort in times of distress (Ainsworth et al., 1978; Sroufe & Waters, 1977). Thus it is <u>neither</u> the mother's bond to the baby or of their relationship in general that is being evaluated but rather the child's degree of experienced security of attachment to his mother. Three main categories of attachment security were introduced by Ainsworth et al. (1978):

1.   <u>Secure attachment (B)</u> - securely attached children feel confident of their mothers' availability and responsiveness (Crockenberg, 1981) and use their mother as a secure base for exploring the environment. Secure attachment indicates that the infant can rely on the parent as a reliable source of comfort and protection if the need arises, thereby promoting his ability to safely explore and expend his mastery of the environment (Weinfield, Sroufe, Egeland, & Carlson, 1999). When distressed, securely attached infants actively seek proximity and contact with the mother and are readily comforted by her (Belsky, 2005).attachment security is promoted by maternal prompt maternal responsiveness to infant's distress, with moderate and appropriate stimulation, as well as with warmth, involvement, and physical intimacy (for more details see Belsky, 1999).

2.   <u>Insecure-avoidant attachment (A)</u> - insecurely-avoidant infants engage in little affective sharing with mother, they show little preference to mother over a stranger, and actively avoid and exhibit dampened or neutral affect towards mother upon reunion (Belsky, 2005). These infants feel anxious about the parent's availability, fearing that the parent will be unresponsive or inefficiently responsive when needed. This results in being unable to direct attachment behaviours at the parent when appropriate (Weinfield et al., 1999). Maternal behaviours which have been found to promote avoidant attachment are intrusive, excessively stimulating, controlling behaviours of mother while interacting with her child (Belsky, 1999).

3.   <u>Insecure-resistant attachment (C)</u> – insecurely-resistant infants manifest impoverished exploration, are vigilant of their mother's whereabouts, are wary of the stranger, and tend to become very distressed during the separation from mother. When reunited with mother, these infants usually mix contact seeking with resisting contact with mother and have difficulty to settle. They actively seek mother's contact yet are unable to be comforted by it. Resistant attachment has been found to be related to unresponsiveness and under-involvement of the mother towards her child (Belsky, 1999).

Collectively, these three patterns of attachment are considered adaptive 'organised' strategies of attachment, which are based on the dyadic interactional history and allow the maximal proximity to the attachment figure whose responsiveness to distress is anticipated (Madigan, Moran, Schuengel, Pederson, & Otten, 2007; Main, 1990). In 1990, a forth pattern of attachment, labelled disorganised, was introduced by Main and Solomon.

4. <u>Disorganised/disoriented attachment (D)</u> – disorganised infants manifest lapses in the organisation of attachment behaviour which is suggested to develop when the attachment figure is not only the haven of safety for the child, but simultaneously also a source of fear. This paradox results in opposing behavioural tendencies to both approach and to flee the parent, preventing the development of a stable strategy to use the attachment figure as a source of comfort in times of distress (Main & Solomon, 1990; Madigan et al., 2007). A meta-analyses conducted by Van IJzendoorn, Schuengel, and Bakermans-Kranenburg (1999) led to the conclusion that the most

important precursors of disorganised attachment are maltreatment, parental unresolved attachment, and marital discord. Infants classified as disorganised/disoriented in the SSP exhibit conflicted or disoriented behaviours that indicate an inability to maintain a coherent attachment strategy when distressed. Such behaviours include freezing, stilling, contradictory behaviour, or direct apprehension and fear towards the parent.

In most samples studies around the world, including thousands of infants assessed on the Strange Situation Procedure, approximately 60% of children are classified as secure, about 15% are classified as insecure-avoidant, 15% are classified as disorganised, and about 10% are classified as insecure-resistant (van IJzendoorn & Kroonenberg, 1988). In teen mothers' population, the distribution of infant attachment security rather different: 40% are classified as secure, 33% as avoidant, 23% as disorganised and less than 4% are classified as resistant (Van IJzendoorn et al., 1999). Also in groups of mothers with alcohol or drug abuse deviation from the general population is noticed: 26% - secure, 15% - avoidant, 16% - resistant, and 43% - disorganised.

Predictions of individual differences in attachment security
Attachment theory proposes two major hypotheses regarding individual differences in attachment security. The first one regards the *antecedents* of attachment. A central hypothesis of attachment theory is that maternal sensitivity - the parent's ability to perceive and accurately interpret the infant's signals and communications, and given this understanding, to respond to them both appropriately and promptly (Ainsworth, Bell & Stayton, 1971, 1974) – is an important contributor to attachment security. As it has been demonstrated, through the history of care and interaction with parent, and the degree of that parent's sensitivity, the infant will form expectations of the caregiver's likely responsiveness to signals of distress, that is, internal working models.

The second hypothesis concerns the *consequences* of individual differences in attachment security for the child's development particularly that of personality and interpersonal relationships (Bowlby, 1973). These early experiences that result in expectations serve later behavioural and emotional adaptation, even in totally situations and with different people (Weinfield et al., 1999). Clearly, other factors in children's lives predict individual differences in adaptation as well. It is by no means suggested that attachment security is solely and directly responsible for socio-emotional adaptation in later life, but that attachment patterns in infancy are predictive of specific attachment-related aspects in later development. For example, it has been found that preschool children with securely attached histories were more "ego resilient" than children with insecure histories. That is, they were more able to respond flexibly to the changing requirements of a situation (Sroufe, 1983). It was also demonstrated that toddlers with secure histories were more ambitious, more goal-directed and achievement-oriented than children with insecure histories (Frankel & Bates, 1990; Matas, Arend, & Sroufe, 1978; Oppenheim, Sagi, & Lamb, 1988). Children with insecure histories are also more likely to express anger, negative affect, and aggression than children with secure histories (Sroufe, 1983). Additionally, children with avoidant histories were significantly more likely than other children to victimise and bully their play friends. Children with secure attachment were never victims nor did they victimise others, whereas children with resistant histories were likely to be victims (Troy & Sroufe, 1987). Also later on in childhood, children with secure histories were found to be more socially competent, being able to engage in turn-taking (Sroufe, 1983), to belong and adapt to a group (Sroufe, Bennett, Englund, Urban, & Shulman, 1993), and to exhibit leadership abilities (Englund, Levy, Hyson, & Sroufe, 2000). In regards to psychopathology, children with secure attachment are more resistant to stress (Pianta, Egeland, & Sroufe, 1990), whereas a history of resistant attachment was found to be related specifically to anxiety disorders (Warren, Huston, Egeland, & Sroufe, 1987). Children with disorganised histories exhibited aggression in school and dissociative tendencies later in life (Van IJzendoorn et al., 1999).

Adolescent mother-infant dyads have been found to be particularly exposed to developmental risk, including early school leaving, unemployment, early parenthood, and violent offending (e.g. Furstenberg, Levine, & Brooks-Gunn, 1990; Jaffee, Caspi, Moffitt, Belsky, & Silva, 2001). Moreover, adolescent mothers are significantly more likely than the general population to have experienced sexual and physical abuse (Boyer & Fine, 1992) and thus to be classified as *unresolved* on the AAI.

Attachment security as a developmental trajectory

According to attachment theory, individual differences in attachment security are viewed neither as linear traits inevitably manifested over time, nor as indefinitely elastic, which can easily altered by every new experience. Rather, attachment security is viewed as a developmental trajectory that influences the individual's course of development. Put differently, following a particular developmental pathway constrains the probable degree and nature of change, resulting in changes that are lawful to the developmental history rather than unpredictable (Weinfield et al., 1999). In this way, based on their attachment histories, individuals select, elicit, and interpret particular reactions from the environment that are consistent with their experience based history of adaptation (Sroufe, 1983).

Assessment of attachment security in adulthood: the Adult Attachment Interview (AAI)

The main method of assessment of internal working models of attachment in adulthood is by means of employment of the Adult Attachment Interview (AAI) (George, Kaplan, & Main, 1996). The AAI consists of 18 questions regarding the individual's relationship with his mother and father during childhood and the individual is instructed to provide specific biographical episodes to validate global evaluations (Hesse, 1999). The interview is designed not so much to evoke the adult's actual experiences in childhood, but, rather, the representation of those experiences and what they mean to the individual (Belsky, 2005), that is, to the interviewee's internal working model of his attachment relationship with his parents. The tape-recorded interview is rated by trained evaluators on a series of rating scales, and special importance is also given to the general sense of coherence, organisation and integration of the individual's recalled memories and description of his childhood experiences.

Attachment security classifications on the AAI are as follows:

1.   Autonomous (secure) – autonomous individuals value their attachment relationship and regard attachment-related experiences as developmentally influential. When interviewed, these individuals appear self-reliant, balanced in their descriptions, and not defensive. Autonomous people either convincingly describe a history of emotionally supportive experiences or that they have come to terms with lacking elements of their childhood.

2.   Preoccupied (insecure-resistant) - these adults demonstrate a continuing involvement and preoccupation with their parents. They appear confused, incoherent, and might exaggerate the influence of the relationship with their parents on their development. These people exhibit unresolved anger towards their parents and it occupies a major aspect of the relationship with them. These individuals seem to be caught up in their early relationships with little ability to move beyond them.

3.   Dismissing (insecure-avoidant) – those classified as dismissing have a tendency to deny negative experiences and emotions or to dismiss their developmental importance. These people find it very difficult to remember childhood experiences and cannot relate to them emotionally. They might present an idealised portrait of their parents but then recall memories which are quite inconsistent with their positive and global appraisals. Dismissing adults present themselves as strong, independent people, for who closeness and attachment means little.

4.   Unresolved (disorganised/disoriented) – unresolved attachment classifications are assigned when discourse related to loss, abuse or neglect suggests lapses in reasoning. These adults display mental disorganisation and disorientation by means of odd and bizarre lapses in their narratives or dissociative fragments in their speech.

References

Ainsworth, M. D. S., Bell, S.M.V., & Stayton, D.J. (1971). Individual differences in Strange Situation Behaviour of One-year-olds. In H.R. Schaffer (Ed.), *The origins of human social relations* (pp. 17-52). New York: Academic Press.

Ainsworth, M. D. S., Bell, S.M.V., & Stayton, D.J. (1974). Infant-mother attachment and social development: 'socialisation' as a product of reciprocal responsiveness to signals. In M.P.M. Richards (Ed.), *The integration of a child into a social world* (pp. 99-136). London: Cambridge University Press.

Ainsworth, M.D.S., Blehar, M., Waters, E., & Wall, S. (1978) Patterns of Attachment: A Psychological Study of the Strange Situation. Hillside, NJ: Lawrence Erlbaum.

Ainsworth, M. D. S. & Wittig, B. A. (1969). Attachment and exploratory behaviour of one- year-olds in a strange situation. In B. M. Foss (Ed.), Determinants of infant behaviour IV (pp. 111-136). London: Methuen.

Belsky, J. (1999). Interactional and contextual determinants of attachment security. In J. Cassidy and P.R. Shaver (Eds.), *Handbook of Attachment: Theory, research, and Clinical Applications* (pp. 249-264). New York, NY: The Gilford Press

Belsky, J. (2005). The Developmental and Evolutionary Psychology of Intergenerational Transmission of Attachment. In C. S. Carter, L. Ahnert, K. E. Grossmann, S. B. Hrdy, M. E. Lamb, S. W. Porges & N. Sachser (Eds.), The 92nd Dalhen Workshop Report, *Attachment and Bonding: A New Synthesis*: MIT Press.

Bowlby, J. (1958). The nature of the child's tie to his mother. *International Journal of Psycho-Analysis,* 39: 350-373.

Bowlby, J. (1969/1982). *Attachment and loss: Vol. 1.* New York: Basic Books.

Bowlby, J. (1973). Attachment and loss. Vol. 2: Separation: Anxiety and anger. New York: Basic Books.

Boyer, D., & Fine, D. (1992). Sexual abuse as a factor in adolescent pregnancy and child maltreatment. *Family Planning Perspectives,* 24: 4-11.

Bretherton, I. (1985). Attachment theory: retrospect and prospect. *Monographs of the society for research in child development, Vol. 50* No. 1/2, Growing points of Attachment Theory and Research, 3-35.

Crockenberg, S. B. (1981). Infant Irritability, Mother Responsiveness, and Social Support Influences on the Security of Infant-Mother Attachment. *Child Development,* 52: 857-865.

Englund, M.M., Levy, A.K., Hyson, D.M., & Sroufe, L.A. (2000). Adolescent Social Competence: Effectiveness in a Group Setting. *Child Development, 71*(4), 1049-1060

Frankel K.F. & Bates J.E. (1990). Mother-Toddler problem solving: Antecedents in attachment, home behaviour and temperament. *Child Development,* 6: 810-819.

Freud, S. (1910/1957). Five lectures on psycho-analysis. In: J. Strachey (Ed and Trans.), *The Standard Edition of the Complete Psychological Works of Sigmund Freud,* Vol. 11 (pp. 3-56). London: Hogarth Press.

Furstenberg, F., Levine, J., Brooks-Gunn, F. (1990). The children of teenage mothers: Patterns of early childbearing in two generations. *Family Planning Perspectives,* 22: 54-61.

George, C., Kaplan., N., & Main, M. (1996). Adult Attachment Interview Protocol (3rd ed.). Unpublished manuscript. Unpublished manuscript, University of California at Berkeley.

Goldberg, S., Grusec, J. E., & Jenkins, J. M. (1999). Confidence in protection: Arguments for a narrow definition of attachment. *Journal of Family Psychology,* 13:475-483.

Hesse, E. (1999). The Adult Attachment Interview. In . J. Cassidy and P.R. Shaver (Eds.), *Handbook of Attachment: Theory, research, and Clinical Applications* (pp. 395-433). New York, NY: The Gilford Press.

Jaffee, S., Caspi, A., Moffitt, T., Belsky, J., & Silva, P. (2001). Why are children born to teen mothers at risk for adverse outcomes in young adulthood? Results from a 20-year longitudinal study. *Development and Psychopathology, 13:* 377-397.

Madigan, S., Moran, G., Schuengel, C., Pederson, D.R., & Otten, R. (2007). Unresolved Maternal Attachment Representations, Disrupted Maternal Behavior and Disorganized Attachment in Infancy: Links to Toddler Behavior Problems. *Journal of Child Psychology and Psychiatry, 48*(10), pp. 1042-1050.

Main, M. (1990). Cross-cultural studies of attachment organization: recent studies, changing methodologies, and the concept of conditional strategies. *Human Development,* 33:48-61.

Main, M., Kaplan, N., & Cassidy, J. (1985). Security in Infancy, Childhood, and Adulthood: A Move to the Level of Representation. *Monographs of the society for research in child development, Vol. 50* No. 1/2, Growing points of Attachment Theory and Research, 66-104.

Main, M., & Solomon, J. (1986). Discovery of a new, insecure disorganised/disoriented attachment pattern. In T. B. Brazelton & M. Yogman (Eds.), *Affective development in infancy* (pp. 95-124). Norwood, NJ: Albex.

Main, M., & Solomon, J. (1990). Procedures for Identifying Infants as Disorganized/Disoriented during the Ainsworth Strange Situation. In: M.T. Greenberg, D. Cicchetti, & E.M. Cummings (Eds.), *Attachment in the Preschool Years: Theory, Research, and Intervention* (pp. 121-160). Chicago: University Of Chicago Press.

Matas, L., Arend, R., & Sroufe, L.A. (1978). Continuity of adaptation in the second year: The relationship between quality of attachment and later competence. *Child Development,* 49:547-556.

Oppenheim, D., Sagi, A., & Lamb, M. (1988). Infant-adult attachments on Kibbutz and their relation to socioemotional development four year later. *Developmental Psychology,* 24:427-433.

Pianta, R., Egeland, B., & Sroufe, L.A. (1990). Maternal stress in children's development: Predictions of school outcomes and identification of protective factors. In: J.E. Rolf, A.Masten, D. Cicchetti, K. Neuchterlen, & S. Weintraub (Eds.), *Risk and protective factors in the development of psychopathology* (pp. 215-235). New York: Cambridge University Press.

Sroufe, L.A. (1983). Infant-caregiver attachment and patterns of adaptation in preschool: The roots of maladaptation and competence. In: M. Permutter (Ed.), *The Minnesota Symposia on Child Psychology: Vol. 16.* Development and Policy concerning children with special needs, (pp. 41-83). Hillside, NJ: Erlbaum.

Sroufe, L.A. (1987).

Sroufe, L.A., Bennett, C., Englund, M., Urban, J., & Shulman, S. (1993). The significance of gender boundaries in preadolescence: contemporary correlates and antecedents of boundary violation and maintenance. *Child Development*, 64:455-466.

Sroufe, L. A. & Waters, E. (1977). Attachment as an Organizational Construct. *Child Development*, 48:1184-1199.

Troy, M. & Sroufe, L.A. (1987). Victimization among preschoolers: The role of attachment relationship theory. *Journal of the American Academy of Child and Adolescent Psychiatry,* 26:166-172.

Van den Boom, D. C. (1994). The influence of temperament and mothering on attachment and exploration: An experimental manipulation of sensitive responsiveness among lower-class mothers with irritable infants. *Child Development,* 65:1457-1477.

Van IJzendoorn, M H. & Kroonenberg, P M (1988) Cross-Cultural Patterns of Attachment: A Meta-Analysis of the Strange Situation. *Child Development*, 59:147-156.

Van IJzendoorn, M.H., Schuengel, C., & Bakermans-Kranenburg, M. (1999). Dosorganized Attachment in early Childhood: Meta-analysis of Precursors, Concomitants, and Sequelae. *Development and Psychopathology,* 11:225-250.

Vondra, J., & Barnett, D. (1999). Atypical Patterns of Early Attachment: Theory, Research, and Current Directions. *Monographs of the Society for Research in Child Development,* 64:3 (258).

Warren, S.L., Huston, L., Egeland, B., & Sroufe, L.A. (1997). Child and Adolescent Anxiety Disorders and Early Attachment. *Journal of the American Child and Adolescent Psychiatry,* 36:637-644.

(Weinfield, N.S., Sroufe, L.A., Egeland, B., & Carlson, E.A. (1999). The nature of individual differences in infant-caregiver attachment. in: J. Cassidy & P.R. Shaver (Eds.), *The handbook of attachment: Theory, Research, and Clinical Applications* (pp. 68-88). New York: The Guilford Press

* **Dana Shai**, MSc, Ph.D, undertook her postgraduate degree in Psychoanalytic Developmental Psychology, at UCL and the Anna Freud Centre, and her Ph.D. in Psychology, Birkbeck College, University of London under the supervision of Profs. Jay Belsky and Peter Fonagy. Her Ph.D. title was: 'Beyond Words: parental Embodied Mentalising in parent-infant interactions and its links with maternal sensitivity and attachment security'. She was a Child and Adolescent Psychotherapist Assistant in Central and Northwest London Foundation Trust, and Internal Evaluator on 'Adolescents becoming Parents' training course at the Anna Freud Centre in 2008, and is currently Research Associate at the School of Psychology Interdisciplinary Center (IDC) Herzliya, Israel. Dana's research and teaching focus is on parent-infant relations, particularly nonverbal interactions, embodiment, movement, and mentalizing.

ENGAGING TEENAGE MOTHERS
AND USING VIDEOED OBSERVATIONS
IN WORKING WITH THEM AND THEIR CHILDREN

Maggie Mills, Ph.D*

Engaging teenage mothers is relentlessly difficult: both getting them to attend and getting their attention. You cannot take it for granted that helping them make a relationship with their baby is going to interest them. At their age infants often lack sustained dramatic interest and they may have little idea what kind of an organism a baby is. Mellow Parenting's method of working with teenage mothers is to show them videoed vignettes of interaction between mothers and babies or toddlers, and then get them to practise and experience things with their own baby/toddler while they are in the parenting programme. Ideally, one takes videotaped interaction of them and their baby during lunchtimes, with their agreement and gives them feedback in a positive way, acknowledging that they are the experts on their own children.

But before you can do any of this work you have to get the mothers involved and interested. The programme has to make them feel nurtured, valued and respected.
Some ways of promoting programme involvement might include:
1. The group process – using the name game (*how did you get your name?*), life stories, warm ups with 'Hello' magazine etc.
2. Sympathy and acknowledgment for the difficult task of looking after a little one: accepting the tedium of it all with the hassle game
3. A quiz about infant development. What is the world like for an infant and what DO babies do all day? What things change in the first year or so of development?
4. Provide support and sympathy for the mothers when they are feeling low
5. Indulge them in looking after themselves and take interest in their concerns about their bodies.
6. Talk about sometimes feeling as though they are on *'shark island'* and needing a cuddle (and of course, reflexively why the babies do.)

Along with this emotional understanding and empathy for the mothers themselves which should get them enjoying the sessions more, and wanting to turn up for them, you can now introduce filmed interaction clips. Ideally one uses the mothers' own interaction but you may not be able to, in which case provide useful clips from other observations. While looking at the clips parents are asked to do a kind of *football commentary* on what the child is doing.

Then one can introduce some styles of interaction that are particularly relevant for the *youngest age group*; for example, helping the baby to aanticipate changes and warning the child about what will follow; talk about providing warmth and responsiveness, with special attention to *safety* aspects of the physical involvement. With *toddlers* would come the introduction of cooperation, constructive boundary setting, what to do about aggression and frustration etc.

Through the *DVD clips*, behaviour that flags up risk and signs of maladaptive patterns can also be covered, such as the mother holding the baby outwards and away from her body to minimise interaction; calling the baby 'it'; using a negative tone to a baby, and dismissive comments that are critical of the baby, implying malevolent intentionality on the baby's part, and screening out crying without attempting to find a solution.

Attention to specific parenting concepts helps practitioners and parents alike to address the intentionality in the clips and understand what typically goes on between any given mother and baby. After all if you don't have a grasp on that, how can you help mothers to change their behaviour? *The knack is always to identify the positives when you are giving feedback* on viewed interaction. Never take a critical or judgmental stand as that will lose them immediately (you will get to what they find difficult soon enough because they themselves can never see the good things they are doing).

If you are working in a group, get the other teenage mothers to suggest alternative ways of handling problematic behaviour…what they might try. So that the group gives ideas on how to solve a handling problem. But always, always leave it to the mother herself to decide what she might try to introduce into her own interaction with her child or do differently. Then the group can help her come up with ways to *practise* at home during the week until the next session and encourage these efforts, and she can report back when the group reconvenes.

The practitioner's aim is first to get the parent to notice what is going on, and what she is doing, and then move to the feelings: *wondering what it feels like for her and ideally what it feels like for the child.*

Mothers find observed interaction on screen quite compelling. The practitioner's role is *not* to know the answers – indeed it is helpful sometimes to say you don't understand what is going on when viewing a tape, but to facilitate the process for the teenagers to discuss their feelings and concerns about their parenting but in a structured way.

Along with observations, you need to encourage actual interaction between each mother and her child. The task with a baby is always to get the mothers to get to *know* the baby (ie what 3 words best describe your baby? what makes him/her sad?).

It is important to get mothers to *follow* the baby, to attend to what s/he is doing - to watch when the baby is awake and content, and to imitate the noises or to respond in some way and report what the baby did in response.

That way *talking* to the baby starts to happen and baby massage, musical games, songs and a favourite toy to talk about and to play with together, can start to happen.

Research evaluation for positive changes in teenage parenting (using the CARE-Index sensitivity scale details) show improved behaviour as 'paying more attention to each other' by making more eye-contact, taking turns, sitting closer, talking more, stroking and holding.

Dimensions of Parenting from 'Learning to Observe'
Maggie Mills /Christine Pickering www.mellowparenting.org Observing interactions between mothers and their baby/children and providing feedback: *What practitioners can see and how to discuss it with very young mums,* with the aim of working towards good-enough nurturing on a number of dimensions.

- Anticipation
- Autonomy
- Responsiveness
- Co-operation
- Emotional Containment and Distress
- Control/conflict and Child Management

Anticipation

- The child is prepared for changes in activity or caretaking by facilitating a known routine, giving prior warning, providing information or distracting the child so that the parent's agenda is easier to achieve, accomplished with the least possible friction.
- We look out for the parent making activities involving them and the child easier or more acceptable to the child.
- There may be lapsed or negative anticipation where the parent fails to set up the child for some activity and then complains about it.

Autonomy

- The parent shows an awareness of the child's individuality, wishes, needs and is sensitive to timing in acknowledging feelings.
- The child is allowed to exercise choice and to behave spontaneously while the parent monitors ongoing activity.
- The parent can offer encouragement and help the child when trying things out and heeds the child's protests or complaints
- Poor practice occurs when autonomy is not granted in these ways, where the parent is intrusive or the child's protest is ignored or dealt with in a negative way

Responsiveness

- When parent and child are responsive to each other, act in a reciprocal way, have fun together and share each other's world.

Note how (positive or negative) affect is expressed in a behavioural, verbal, tone of voice or physical activity, especially when shared:

Positive (Reflective Functioning)

Parent link: enlarges understanding;Relates to Child's activity or preceding topic

Child responds/follows; Playful shared Affect

Negative (Behavioural Problems)

- Criticism of child - not of his/her action; implies inadequacy or rejection; negative tone or affect.

Cooperation

- Where the parent and child are compliant or able to negotiate
- The parent finds a positive way to influence the child's behaviour and to gain co-operation
- Poor practice occurs when requests are ignored or with negative responses, like threats or forcible compliance

Distress

- Where comfort and support is offered to a crying child who is upset, hurt or miserable. Distress is 'mopped up'

- Poor practice occurs when distress, whining and crying are ignored, precipitated, responded to negatively with unsupportive reactions.

Control and Conflict

- The parent intends to achieve compliance from the child and gets the child to do what they want. Handling can be appropriate or inappropriate; Nice or nasty.
- Does control escalate? Does it end in child compliance or parent ignoring and giving up, or a 'strategic ignore'. Is interaction positive afterwards or is there nagging and/or child distress?

---

* Maggie Mills, PhD Psychoanalyst, Fellow of the British Psychoanalytical Society. Formerly, lecturer in Developmental Psychology at RHBNC (London); Consultant Clinical Psychologist in the NHS running a Psychodynamic Psycho-therapy service (Shanti) for women from ethnic minorities in Brixton. Currently Director of the Mellow Parenting programme, helping disadvantaged families in difficult circumstances to parent their young children. Published on maternal depression, family relationships, psychotherapeutic change, domestic violence. Co-edited *Psychoanalytical Ideas and Shakespeare* (Karnac 2006).

TODDLERHOOD: THE BATTLE FOR AUTONOMY – IMPLICATIONS FOR TEENAGE PARENTS

Marie Zaphiriou Woods*

Toddlerhood
Toddlerhood is a crucial time in a person's development.
Fundamental issues to do with autonomy, attachment, separateness, and intimacy are negotiated during this developmental phase. And the foundations of managing feelings and impulses (aggression and sexuality) and developing an imagination are also laid down, having been already started in infancy.

When is toddlerhood?
Toddlerhood begins when an infant takes his first faltering, but independent steps. At *around one year*, independent walking ushers in a surge in the developmental advance towards being separate and autonomous. During toddlerhood, the thrust towards independence culminates in the toddler achieving sufficiently stable, positive inner images of his mother, and of himself in her absence to manage a half or whole day away from her. This usually occurs at *around 3*, the age at which most children in England start nursery school and marks the end of toddlerhood. (For the sake of clarity and convenience, the toddler is referred to as 'he' and the parent as 'she')

Outline of Toddler Development
Margaret Mahler's concept of *separation-individuation* is the central organiser.

Practising
Mahler and colleagues (1975) observed that when the toddler begins to walk, he is often elated, embarking on 'a love affair with the world'. A recent study suggested that a practising toddler spends up to 6 hours a day on play activities.
The young toddler's apparent freedom to range is predicated on the parents' continued physical and emotional availability; the parents are 'the external secure base that anchors the child's comings and goings' (Lieberman 1993, p.3).
The parent's enjoyment of her toddler, her sensitive attunement to his exhilaration and excitement, strengthens his attachment to her and confident approach to the world. With most mothers working nowadays, continuity and security have to be provided by a sensitive and graduated handover to a carefully chosen substitute caregiver (nanny, child minder or nursery worker).
'The most important emotional accomplishment of the toddler years is reconciling the urge to become competent and self reliant with the longing for parental love and protection' (Lieberman, 1993 p.2).

Rapprochement
The toddler's relentless researches inevitably bring him up against experiences which challenge his illusion of magical control.
He begins to realise that his mother is a *distinct person with a mind of her own*.
The growing awareness of separateness and difference punctures the young toddler's prevailing mood of elation.

He becomes frightened of losing his beloved parent, and sleep difficulties may occur as he struggles against relinquishing her and falling asleep.

He seeks "rapprochement" i.e a renewed closeness from the parent as someone with whom to share discoveries and to play.

Anality

This rapprochement is disrupted by further maturational developments.

About half way through the second year, the toddler becomes more aware of anal and urethral sensations. He may begin to take an active pleasure in soiling, wetting and messing, and perhaps even in touching, smelling, and looking.

He may become contrary, saying "no" at every opportunity and resisting attempts to bathe and dress him. This awkwardness serves him in his struggle for autonomy; it is as if he reasserts his separateness from his mother by being opposite.

It is often difficult for parents to manage their feelings in the face of such provocation which may touch on *their* unresolved issues to do with anality, sexuality and aggression. The 18 month old is often volatile, struggling with powerful contradictory impulses from within, and difficult realities without as the adults around him increasingly restrain him, by setting limits to keep him safe, and to socialise him.

One research study quoted by Schore has shown that at around 20 months, three quarters of parental interactions with their toddlers are prohibitions of one kind or another (compared to just 5% in the practising phase).

The parents need to be able to manage their own feelings in order to stand firm in the face of their toddler's ambivalence and contradictory behaviour.

Their resistance to his attempts at omnipotent control contribute to the toddler's growing awareness that the people he loves have a separate existence and are not part of the world he has made up. Their readiness to repair the relationship following inevitable disputes reassures him that he is not omnipotently destructive.

Moving on from rapprochement

Towards the end of the second year, certain developments help toddlers and parents to move on:

1. the toddler's increased command of communicative language
2. his growing ability to play symbolically
3. his growing identification with his parents

Through playing as well as talking, toddlers and parents can communicate in a pleasurable way while also learning about their essential separateness and difference.

Becoming like their beloved parents is a way for toddlers to hold on to them internally, to cope with increased separation, while also learning new skills and building their sense of identity.

Clear consistent expectations that the toddler can meet and a tolerance of failure facilitate the development of a benign aim giving superego or conscience.

Consolidating individuality and moving towards emotional object constancy

During the third year of life, the toddler ideally consolidates these earlier developments according to his individual temperament, his particular life experiences and especially his relationship with his parents.

He builds up an increasingly complex, solid and discrete sense of himself and of the important people in his life. They will have inevitably been perceived as both good and bad, but if positive experiences have dominated, and the parents have been able to contain their own as well as their toddler's ambivalence, his aggression will have been modified by his loving feelings and his image of himself and his parents will have become integrated into predominantly positive (loveable and loving) self and object representations.

These need to be sufficiently robust to survive short absences or times of frustration and rage, and will then contribute to his ability to maintain self esteem, to be alone and eventually to manage longer separations.

Ownership of the body
The older toddler's increasing awareness of and investment in his body tends to bring with it the determination to own and control it: "I do it myself".

The parent who, for over 2 years, has been almost totally responsible for the care and protection of her child's body has to negotiate a graduated handover in accordance with the toddler's growing wish and ability to manage independently.

Failure to do so can result in bitter battles for ownership and control over essential bodily functions such as feeding, sleeping, and toileting, which may spread to other areas such as dressing and bathing or showering.

Gender Identity
The attitude of both parents to their toddler's gender, and their feelings about their own and eachother's bodies and sexuality will affect how their girl or boy toddler feels about his or gender and genitals.

Starting Nursery School
By 2 ½ to 3 years, most toddlers are ready to manage a half or whole day away from home and to take advantage of a good nursery experience.

To do so, the toddler needs to have reached sufficient object constancy to be able to hold on to a positive inner image of his mother in her absence.

The ability to express himself effectively in both words and play, will help to regulate some of the intense affects aroused by the separation.

He also needs:

- to have reached some independence in managing his bodily needs (eating, toileting, and keeping safe)
- to have moved on from experiencing his peers as a threat, to beginning to play alongside them and even enjoying them as playmates in their own right. (See Anna Freud 1965)

The toddler's parents
The teen parents' flexible and sensitive responsiveness and availability in the face of the toddler's ever changing developmental needs is crucial.

A teenage mother has to move from experiencing him as part of herself to perceiving him as a unique individual, separate and different from herself.

Misattunements and misunderstandings are frequent and inevitable, indeed necessary if the toddler is to learn to tolerate anxiety and frustration, transform his aggression and feel properly separate. At the same time, disruptions in the attachment relationship will need to be repaired, so that communication can be resumed, and the toddler is reassured that he is not omnipotently destructive, and that mother or the relationship with her is not permanently damaged.

This is difficult for any parent. Their own history, personality, perhaps their external circumstances, may make them vulnerable to the turbulent feelings and fantasies their toddler arouses in them. *It is particularly difficult for teenage parents because the toddler's struggles for separateness and autonomy so closely mirror their own.*

Relevant Reading:

Bergman, A. (1999) *Ours, yours, mine: mutuality and the emergence of the separate self.* New York:Jason Aronson

Freud, A. (1965) *Normality and pathology in childhood.* Penguin University Books.

Furman, E. (1992) *Toddlers and their mothers.* New York:International University Press

Lieberman, A.F. (1993) *The emotional life of the toddler.* New York: The Free Press.

Mahler, M.S., Pine, F., & Bergman, A. (1975) *The Psychological Birth of the Human Infant.* New York: Basic Books.

Stern, D. (1985) *The interpersonal world of the human infant.*

Stoker, J. (2005) *You and your toddler.* London and New York: Karnac.

---

*__Marie Zaphiriou Woods__ is a Child and Adolescent Psychotherapist and Adult Psychoanalyst (Fellow, British Psychoanalytical Society). Previously worked at Brixton Child Guidance Clinic and Brent Adolescent Centre. She was the Psycho-analytic Consultant to the Anna Freud Centre Nursery, then managed the Parent-Toddler Group Service at the Anna Freud Centre from 1999-2008. Now Clinical Group Leader, Child Psychotherapy Service, AFC. Publications include 'Preventive Work in a Toddler Group and Nursery' [*Journal of Child Psychotherapy* vol. 26/2, 2000] With Inge-Martine Pretorius she co-edited *Parents and Toddlers in Groups: a Psychoanalytic Developmental Approach,* (Routledge, 2010).

<u>Expanded notes for Module V:</u>

GROUP AND INSTITUTIONAL DYNAMICS

Earl Hopper, PhD*

People working in organizations and particularly managers should be aware of various 'informal', unconscious processes, as well as more 'formal', conscious processes that are associated with the structure of their organisations. The former may be regarded as 'visible' and the latter as 'invisible', or at any rate visible only through their manifestations. Under certain circumstances the personnel tend to regress in response to their feeling various kinds of anxieties. They also develop interpersonal defences against these anxieties, and on the basis of projective and introjective identification [see Glossary] to develop particular kinds of relationships, cultures, forms of communication, styles of thinking and feeling, and forms of leadership and followership. Thus, the organisations lose their formal structures and become more like large groups with certain characteristic of their own.

Bion discussed these characteristics in terms of three *'basic assumptions* – of Dependency, Fight/ Flight and Pairing [see Glossary]. People in groups tend to get sucked into the roles that make up these basic assumptions. When basic assumption processes prevail, it is extremely difficult for group members to think clearly and be empathic to the needs of other people, and to fulfil work group tasks. As open social systems, organisations also import the dynamics of events that occur in their environments.

A fourth basic assumption is proposed in the unconscious life of social systems. It is called Incohesion: Aggregation/Massification, or **(ba) I:A/M,** which allows people to protect themselves from a fear of annihilation brought about by the traumatic experience of failed dependency. The fourth basic assumption of Incohesion is especially apparent in organisations such as hospitals, prisons, clinics and residential facilities for the care and treatment of highly dependent, immature and emotionally fragile people. Incohesion is magnified and amplified within societies in which traumatic experience has occurred.

When 'Incohesion' characterises the unconscious life of an organisation, managers and others tend to oscillate between aggregation (becoming bureaucratic and emotionally detached) and massification (becoming overly involved and merged) with one another. A better alternative would be to try to stand back from the heat of these processes and to think about the tendencies to be alienated, on the one hand, and enchanted, on the other, and then to try to get the balance right between being very neutral and objective, on the one hand, and encouraging and enthusiastic, on the other.

This is why an understanding of Incohesion is so relevant to those who work in facilities for the care of young mothers and their babies who have so often been traumatised. It is rarely necessary for managers to do more than try to contain and hold the organization and its participants, and to create spaces in which they can think about what is going on, sometimes trying to discuss the situation openly in an attempt to actualise a democratic style of management.

Some psychoanalysts and group analysts regard social systems such as organisations as though they were organisms, and think about unconscious processes that develop within them as aspects of what they call the 'social unconscious'. Some organisational consultants refer to the 'organisational unconscious'.

From this point of view, the study of basic assumptions is really a study of the so-called 'social unconscious'. However, there are many aspects of this concept and theories that underpin it. I prefer to think about the social unconscious with respect to the unconscious life of persons that has been caused and governed by socio-cultural factors and processes, rather than biological ones. I try to use the language of the social sciences when I am discussing properties of social systems. This help to distinguish the study of social systems, although these are, of course, closely related.

Relevant Reading:
Bion, W. R. (1961) *Experiences in Groups and Other Papers.* London: Tavistock

Hopper, E. (2003) *Traumatic Experience in the Unconscious Life of Groups: The Fourth Basic Assumption: Incohesion: Aggregation/Massification or (ba) I:A/M.* London:Jessica Kingsley Publishers.

Hopper, E. (2003) *The Social Unconscious: Selected Papers.* London: Jessica Kingsley

Hopper, E. (ed) 2011 *Trauma and Organisations.* London: Karnac Books Ltd.

Hopper, E. & Weinberg, H. (2011) *The Social Unconscious in Persons, Groups and Societies: Volume I: Mainly Theory.* London: Karnac Books Ltd.

Earl Hopper, PhD, Psychoanalyst, Group Analyst, and Organisational Consultant. Former President of the International Association of Group Psychotherapy, former Chair of the Group of Independent Psychoanalysts at the British Psychoanalytical Society. Supervisor and training analyst for IGA, BAP, LCP. Fellow of the British Psycho-analytical Society. Author of many books and articles.

Part 3: **TRAINING MANUAL**

Training motto: Teenage mothers and fathers are - Teenagers!

'Adolescence as a Second Chance' furthers the practitioner's *understanding of minds* to help young parent/s to relate to the child as a person with a mind. By improving our own capacity for *'mentalization'* – understanding our behaviour and that of others in terms of mental states (thoughts, feelings, beliefs, motivations and intentions) we can bring about *a meeting of minds*, helping teenage mothers and fathers to do the same for their child. The central tenet is that *inter-relations* (including those between practitioners and teenagers, or parents and their infants) are *co-created by both partners*. The practitioner's capacity for reflective thinking and emotional 'literacy' can encourage better understanding in young parents thereby fostering mental health (and decrease repeat pregnancies).

The Training

This training is designed with some flexibility in mind, to accommodate the particular needs of participants in different localities, and to enable each trainer to elaborate her/his own words and/or construct a power-point presentation from the templates which are included here handouts.

The training pack consists of

➢ an observational DVD of clips of teenage parents interacting with their children.

➢ the Theoretical Textbook which can be used for self-study by individual practitioners, as well as serving as an educational resource for all group participants.

➢ and this instructive Manual to support delivery of the training by a Trainer, conducting the interactive workshops and skill building seminars for a group of practitioners. For easy identification in the Contents, group activities and role play appear *in italics with this type arrow*, and in the Textbook itself, they and power-point type summaries appear in textboxes, as do messages and notes to the leader providing background information and detailed instructions in order to deliver the interactive and skill-based components of the course. Needless to say, trainers also must be familiar with the texts that participants read as part of their self-study.

Training Aims:

This training offers *an interdisciplinary programme* to increase shared knowledge among different practitioners. Each teenage parent has several practitioners dealing with her family, who do not always coordinate their provisions. A known aspect of working with teenage clients is their capacity to stir up powerful emotions in workers, and to pit one professional against another, exacerbating a tendency for splitting within multi-agency teams who have different ways of understanding emotional issues. By bringing together the variety of practitioners working with this complex client group in particular vicinity the training offers an opportunity to network, understand individual, group, and institutional dynamics, and to benefit from an integrative multi-disciplinary view of this complex clientele.

The training aims to
• shift our focus from the viewpoint of an external observer to awareness of the practitioner as participant and co-creator of the interchange.

- increase self-reflection and receptivity to subjective experience – our own and that of the client, honing the capacity for mindfulness.
- enhance understanding of perinatal emotional disorders, and recognition of distress signs, helping practitioners identify and target those most at-risk for timely referral of infants, young people and families in need of specialised therapeutic treatment.
- increase the practitioner's capacity to work with cultural diversity and socioeconomic adversity.
- appreciate psychodynamics relating to families, groups, teams and institutions, and how teenage clients can stir these.
- improve the participants' capacity for liaising with colleagues, sponsoring multi-agency efficiency, and appreciation of interactive psycho-dynamics.
- encourage efficient multi–agency work, recognising a tendency for splitting among practitioners who have different ways of understanding emotional issues.

Learning Objectives

To bring these changes about, the training programme provides

- A sound theoretical framework of psychodynamic concepts, relevant research and policy developments relating to pregnant teenagers, infants, toddlers and their young parents.
- An interactive learning opportunity to gain understanding of the developmental processes and maturational tasks of adolescents, babies and toddlers, and how these intersect.
- Exploration of contemporary social and parenting issues in a mixed population to facilitate work with teenage parents and/or child in ordinary, troubled or traumatised families, minorities, refugees and asylum seekers, in a variety of different work settings..
- Guiding principles for processing the impact on our everyday work of age, gender, race, religion, disability, class, culture, ethnicity and sexual orientation, to increase the practitioner's sensitivity to multicultural and socio-economic differences (including exploration of our own biased attitudes).
- Training in mental health issues, addressing psychological, behavioural and neuropsychological factors associated with the emotional immaturity of very young parents.
- Skill-building seminars to enable identification of disturbance, and detection of symptoms associated with emotional disorders, neglect, violence and trauma
- Interactive exercises to further understanding of interactive psycho-dynamics of dyads, threesomes, small groups, families, teams and organizations.
- Opportunities to hone the participant's interactive work skills through disciplined observational, listening and communication practice, experiential exercises and casework evaluation
- Self-study units and group assignments to encourage self-reflection and to elucidate how our own expectations, internal and external relations, prejudices and every other aspect of lives are both shaped by, and reciprocally influence, our interchanges with other practitioners and with our clients.

Mode of Delivery

The training is designed to be delivered by a trainer to a group of practitioners. But it can also be undertaken by individual practitioners who wish to enhance their work skills and understanding through self-study. To this end it is composed of different components.

Training Modules:

I. INTERRELATIONSHIPS
Interactive Workshop **Teen Clients - Expectations & Meaning Making**
Skill-Building Seminar **Co-constructed Interactions and Mentalization**

II. ADOLESCENTS
Interactive Workshop **Maturational Tasks of Early and Late Adolescence**
Skill building seminar: **Psychological Processes of Pregnancy & Teen Mothering**

III. BABIES IN TEEN FAMILIES
Interactive Workshop **Attunement, Attachment and Affect Regulation.**
Skill-Building Seminar **Babies - and Reflective Function in Teen Parents**

IV. TODDLERS & TEEN MOTHERS AND FATHERS
Interactive Workshop **Extending Boundaries: Attachment, Separation, Individuation & Imaginative Play**
Skill-building seminar **Contemporary Parenthood & Emotional Disturbance in Teen Parents**

V. FAMILIES, GROUPS & ORGANIZATIONS
Interactive Workshop **Family Dynamics & Psychosocial Narratives**
Skill Building Seminar **Teams, Groups & Institutional Defences**

Target Audience

This training is tailored for a wide variety of practitioners who work with pregnant teenagers and very young parents and their babies. Groups in any one geographical area can come together to encourage productive collaboration across disciplines and local agencies.

The multidisciplinary mix of participants may include:

Child protection and youth workers, personal advisors, parent-project coordinators, family support workers, counsellors, 'early years' professionals, specialist midwives, health visitors, nurses, supported housing staff, youth group leaders, young fathers workers, child and adolescent mental health practitioners, social workers, clinical psychologists and others.

Trainers

A professional with leadership qualities and knowledge of psychodynamic principles may lead the training which is psychoanalytically informed, also bringing in various related models such as attachment, group dynamics, intercultural and social theories. Because of the demanding nature of guiding an interdisciplinary group through complex and arousing material, it is important to recognise that the group leader too, may need support at times. It is vital to find someone in your own workplace or elsewhere who can act as a sounding board, and offer you advice, supervision or consultation during this course. Ideally, 'top-up' meetings with like-minded colleagues offer support, as do ongoing small reflective work groups do for practitioners.

Training Content

On addition to participants coming from many different types of discipline and practice the level of trainees may vary from people with minimal training but wide experience (e.g. hostel staff or youth workers, who may not have completed secondary education) to professionals with specialised qualifications, master degrees, or even doctorates. Participants in UK courses have come from all over the British Isles, and from as far afield as Australia, Holland, and Germany, but courses are also run in a variety of countries as dissimilar as Italy, Madeira, Morocco, Poland, and South Africa.

This variety of backgrounds means that the training must meet a broad spectrum of content relevance, without anyone feeling patronised, bored, or out of their depth. And provisions must be made for practitioners to benefit from their colleagues' varied experience. To accommodate these multiple needs the course is highly interactive, and *structured progressively* in both form and content: the nature of learning material and group exercises increases in complexity and depth from the beginning of each *session* to its end, and from the beginning of the training course to its end, with enough repetition to familiarise lesser known concepts and ways of thinking, to allow each participant to find their own 'comfort zone' and 'voice'.

Above all the training course provides *'containment'* – a safe work space in which to contemplate anxiety-provoking issues, and to imbibe some psychodynamic ways to continue thinking about these when engaged at 'the coal face'. Each study day is comprised of two interrelated sessions (an 'Interactive Workshop' and a 'Skill-building Seminar'), in which the large group of participants frequently breaks into smaller, less intimidating units of varying sizes for exercises and role plays.

Training Course Structure

The group training is comprised of *five half study-days* ideally to be run over a ten week period, but clearly, local conditions will determine the intervals and duration of training. These could be run weekly but an interval allows time to 'digest' complex and potentially troubling ideas. And to read further, or return to the sessions in the Handbook for explanatory 'refuelling'. Conversely, too long an interval between study days leads to less continuity, and a need to refresh and recapitulate before moving on.

In the intervals between study days, participants engage in 'Self study', the units of which include preparatory reading, internet lecture videos and self-reflective exercises. All trainees are asked to keep a private *Learning Journal* to chart their own emotional journey during training, including counter-transferential responses to their challenging teen clients, whose intense feelings often provoke strong reactions, involving irritation, concern, anxiety, and sometimes, secret admiration and envy.

Each of the five study days or modules include:
- **An Interactive Workshop**
- **A Skill-based Seminar**
- **Reflective Work Groups** – optional, but most important.
- **Self-Study Units** – preparatory reading, viewing, reflective exercises, Journal *[2-4 hours during the two week interval between Modules].*

The overall purpose of these different modules is to encourage *self-observation, self-reflection and self-inquiry.*

· Training Components

The first two training compo*nents are 100 minutes* long but can be broken into two 50 minute or hour long segments as required. The natural break point is indicated by the item: *'interim conclusions'.*

1. Interactive Workshops:

lecture or power-point presentation by the Course Leader to familiarise participants with theoretical issues, enhanced by group exercises, observational material and role play. Interactions take into account that participants differ in degree of out-goingness. Discussion in twos, threes, small and large group formats ensure that everyone present can participate in exploring the meaning, and consequences of interactive behaviours. A flip-chart or white board is essential for writing down contributions from participants.

2. Skill-building Seminars

These focus on the particular theme of the module (i.e. Interrelationships or Toddlers, etc.) working through some of the issues that arose in the interactive workshop, and developing skills to address these in the work situation. Seminars aim to clarify learning, to elicit a dialogic exchange of ideas among participants intended to stimulate *curiosity* and *reflective thinking.* Each seminar provides guidelines to build up an intricate array of interactive skills for emotional understanding and addressing practical problems.

Observational skills are improved through detailed discussion after watching DVD material, followed by a re-showing of the same DVD clip, focusing on what had been missed. Noting potential meanings and possible motives underpinning interaction, while aware of their speculatory nature. Appendix 4 deals describes the process in detail.

3. Reflective Work Groups:

These consist of seven to nine participants in the training who meet regularly each study day as members of the same small group with the experienced leader to discuss their own cases, becoming more aware of some of the unconscious configurations, defensive mechanisms, and underlying fantasies that make up the human psyche
Group discussion of an individual case is accompanied by a brief update on previously presented cases

Practitioners bring cases from their own caseloads for discussion in a containing small group. These regular more intimate seminars provide time to reflect on one's practice among peers, from a variety of professional disciplines in a confidential setting with an experienced clinician.

If possible, therapeutically trained or experienced professionals should conduct these 'Reflective Work Groups'. Detailed elaboration, including instructions on running such a group are included in Appendix 3. Ideally, Reflective Work Groups continue to be held even after the end of the course (to provide thinking space, regular supervision, ongoing support and consolidation of training).

4. Self-study units:

This has a double meaning – study of assigned films, readings and lectures that takes place without a teacher; and – *self*-study, introspective examination of oneself. It is hoped that through various guided tasks the practitioner will gradually acquire insight into her/his own habitual interactive patterns and feelings, becoming more aware of an internal struggle between a desire to know more and resistance to change.

Learning Journal: As the training arouses feelings that can be troubling in the absence of counselling, every participant is invited to keep a personal diary of their learning journey throughout this course, expressing, clarifying and reflecting upon the feelings it has stirred up, and on the emotional impact the new understanding has had on them and their work. This remains private and for their own use alone.

- This private document also serves as a measure her/his own change. A *self-evaluation* resource for the participant which enables her/him to draw personal conclusions about why certain aspects of the course are more meaningful than others.

- The Journal facilitates *empathy* with clients by serving as a helpful reminder of one's own subtle reactions to new ideas, and biases experienced as the course unfolds, as well as responses in reflective work group discussions.

- It helps acquire greater awareness of one's own personal strengths and insight into habitual defence patterns and resistance during the learning process.

- It offers a means of integrating comprehension and insight; and avoiding enactments and boundary transgressions.

Ideally the practice of keeping the Journal will persist beyond the end of the course.

Training Principles:

Wherever the course is delivered the leader will aim to –

- Provide a supportive lively setting in which emotional learning can take place.

- Promote and model sensitive interaction being neither too remote nor too close or intrusive; neither too lax or neglectful, nor controlling.

- Encourage lively curiosity, and open dialogue with respect for different opinions among participants, combined with critical thinking, and self-reflection.

- Facilitate different levels of discussion and more effective communication processes through varied small, medium and large group formats.

- Enhance understanding of psychological processes to help practitioners promote attuned emotional care of the baby, and appropriate use of local services.

- Help participants develop the capacity to contain and stay with difficult feelings without becoming overwhelmed by them or shutting down, and sustaining difficult situations without resorting to action (Wasp!).

- Encourage use of the Learning Journal to increase awareness of feelings and the work of making sense of them – recognising anxiety, projections and counter-transferential arousal.

- Enable practitioners to explore the interdisciplinary nature of the course itself, discuss multi-agency organisational dynamics, and to appreciate the importance of inter-professional liaison with colleagues involved with this complex client group.

- Facilitate an in-depth exchange of ideas and casework experience in the intimate work-discussion module, enabling participants to apply the concepts being studied to their own work practice.

Overview of the Training:

Each Module is comprised of two sessions in which at times, the large groups break into smaller groups of varying size. The third component, the Reflective Work Group has a regular small membership. The nature and content of learning material and exercise permutations increase in complexity and depth from the beginning of each session to *its* end and from the beginning of the course to its end.

Experiential exercises

In addition to theoretical understanding of the emotional needs of teenage parents and their children, the workshops use a variety of experiential strategies to –

- Explore the unique psychodynamics of working with young clients.
- Examine diverse cultural values and life-styles.
- Investigate our own psychosocial values and how our personal beliefs and attitudes influence the way we interact.
- Enhance understanding of the principles of interactive communication and ways in which minds intersect.
- Develop a set of work skills to help us reflect and communicate our impressions more effectively in face-to-face work with young clients and their children, and with other professionals.

Cross-Module Themes

- All modules involve psychodynamic thinking about *interactive processes,* and *reflective functioning.*
- Every component includes an emphasis on *self-awareness, observation & listening* skills, including exploration of observer bias and practice of sensitive responses.
- Every workshop is informed by *psychosocial and intercultural issues* and awareness of the need to involve *fathers,* as well as issues of *consent, confidentiality, ethicality and child protection.*

'Take-home messages':

- Teenage parents are teenagers.
- Difficult feelings can be thought about rather than enacted.
- …'we do not deal with the happenings in the external world as such, but with their repercussions in the mind' (Anna Freud, 1960:54).
- In adolescence unresolved emotional issues from the past are reactivated, with a *'second chance'* to rework them. In early parenthood too, our own early issues are reactivated by 'contagious arousal' through intimate contact with the baby and primal substances. We argue that this dual arousal offer a second 'second chance' to work-through conflicts belonging to the past, while processing current demands.

Key Lesson:

Our own feelings and biases affect our work, necessitating self-reflection and peer-supervision.

Emotional repercussions.

The course offers learning opportunities which lead to internal reorganisation. This arouses both inflated anticipatory hopes as well as resistance to change. However, it is *not* a therapeutic experience. Some participants may find the course disturbing. They should be encouraged to meet with the Group Leader if they feel the course content is personally too arousing. If this cannot be resolved through use of the private journal they should be made aware of counselling/therapy provisions in the locality, to work through their issues in a confidential space.

When the trainer becomes aware of unspoken feelings circulating in the group, the trainer will need to contain these, and to explore them if appropriate, enabling participants to name and to process their own feelings. Inevitably some members of the group will deflect their arousal by becoming cynical, hyperactive, obstructive or use diversionary tactics or 'flight' (joking, texting, responding to phone calls, leaving the room, etc). Recognising these for what they are – defences for dealing with the anxiety aroused – will help the leader to prevent their disruption of the group work. Tact is required but to facilitate the ongoing group activity, anxieties will need to be addressed for all those involved.

DELIVERY OF THE TRAINING

THE GROUP LEADERS' PACK

- **Theoretical Textbook** with instructions for leading interactive workshops and skill-building seminars [including large and small group exercises, role plays and discussion points]
- **Teaching Manual** with detailed practical points and specified ethos
- **Power-point Templates**
- **DVD of Observation material** to be administered and discussed
- **The Principles of Observation** (Appendix 4)
- **Reflective Work Group Leader's instructions** and **note page** (Appendix 3)
- **Expanded notes** (expanding on key topics. e.g. Mentalization, Attachment)
- **Feedback sheets** for participants
- **Student evaluation** - pre and post training, plus follow-up.
- **Reading Lists**
- **A Glossary** of relevant psychodynamic terms
- **Handouts** [which serve as templates for power-point].
- Access to Oscar winning short film **'Wasp'** [Director Andrea Arnold].

Ground Rules

1. The Manager is requested to safeguard time in the practitioners ongoing work schedules for the delivery of the training, and thinking space for participants to do their homework

2. It is important that after the end of the course, Reflective Work Groups continue to be held indefinitely (to provide thinking space, regular supervision, ongoing support and consolidation of training).

3. The course is highly experiential. Participants are encouraged to interact, bearing in mind that however well they may know each other from other situations, this is a new experience.

4. While the leader utilises the group exercises to bring out participants' reactions, it is not a confessional. Each participant tracks his/her emotional experiences during the course in a private journal.

Suggested Timetable:
Interactive Workshop (100 minutes or two sections of 50 minutes with a five-ten minute 'comfort break' between them)
30 minute *refreshments and socialising*
Skill-building Seminar (100 minutes)
Hour long *lunch [Optional. Otherwise, start next session after another interval]*
<u>**Reflective work group**</u> (90 minutes)
TOTAL: 5 hours excluding lunch

Group Size

There is no upper limit to the large group, and ideally it should aim to include *all* local practitioners working with this clientelle. Two of the pilot groups consisted on 45 participants each. Reflective Work Discussion groups are composed of five to nine people. In this multi-disciplinary course, it is important to ensure a good mix of disciplines in each group. Confidentiality of cases must be ensured.

Venue

Plenary sessions for all the participants should be held in a *training room* with power-point and DVD facilities. Between sessions, refreshments (and if possible, lunch) should be provided, with opportunity for 'networking'. *Breakout rooms* are required to accommodate small Reflective Work Groups. When large groups break into smaller groups, these happen in the large room. Groups of 3-6 remain in their seats, relating to people either side and in front.

Induction

The first Module begins with *a short induction session* to welcome participants, to facilitate introductions, and to help the group 'gell'. Even if all participants know each other by sight do not assume that they know each other's names. Supply name badges or stickers, and in a very large group, it is useful to give each participant a grid of photographs of everyone, with names and work positions. Encourage people to sit with those they do not know well.

Participation

To enable participants to recognise the complexity of any experience they are engaged in, group discussion is generated by asking questions rather than making statements: and small dialogue-work must be open-ended. A flipchart approach recording people's tentative ideas as they arise illustrates this multilayered complexity.

After every *role-play activity* the leader explores what each active player felt (while still in role), and how the observing group experienced aspects of the enacted relationship. Then the must be de-roled.

Homework

Many participants may not have access to a professional library, or access to electronic journals online. Where possible, homework consists of reading or watching items that are freely available on the internet.

Many classical and vital papers papers that are not accessible elsewhere have been collected in a Course Reader: ***Parent-Infant Psychodynamics – wild things, mirrors and ghosts***, J Raphael-Leff (ed), London: Whurr, 2003; Wiley, 2006; Anna Freud Centre, 2009.

This book comprises a carefully chosen collection of classic and commissioned papers. [Available from Karnac books online http://www.karnacbooks.com].

The course encourages self-motivated study. Participants check what reading and watching is required well before each Module, as it may be complicated and require some digesting. The trainer may provide a reminder about what is expected for the following time.

Pre-Training preparation:
Depending on the length of notice, the trainer may wish participants to prepare in advance of the training:

1. Case:
Participants can be requested to prepare the brief outline of a case for possible presentation in the confidential small reflective work group.

2. Pre Course Viewing:
Bonding Difficulties: http://www.channel4.com/programmes/help-me-love-my-baby/4od#2918381 [Help Me Love My Baby]

3. Pre-Course Reading:
Margot Waddell (2009) 'Why adolescents have babies parents? This book, p.216.
Also in *Infant Observation* 12:271-281
[This paper was written for presentation to the original AFC training course and is reprinted here with kind permission of author and publisher].

Course reading which participants should do during or before the training.
All are to be found in the Course Reader *Parent-Infant Psychodynamics – wild things, mirrors and ghosts*

Introduction **Joan Raphael-Leff** (2003) On wild things within - an introduction to psychoanalytic thinking
Face to Face – Containment and Early exchange
Chapter 1: **Ken Wright** (2003) 'Face and façade – the mother's face as the
    baby's mirror.
Chapter 2: **Donald W. Winnicott** (1967) Mirror role of Mother and Family in
    Child Development. [Originally in *Playing and Reality,* London: Penguin
    1971, pp.130 -138]
Chapter 3: **Colwyn Trevarthen** (1974) Conversations with a two month old.
    [Originally in New Scientist, May 1974]
Chapter 4: **Edward Z. Tronick** (1989), Emotions and emotional
    communication in infants. [Originally *American Psychologist* 44:112-119].
Chapter 5: **Joan Raphael-Leff** (2003) Where the wild things are
Chapter 7: **Wilfred R. Bion** (1961) A theory of thinking (Originally in
    International Journal of Psycho-Analysis 43:306-10; also in *Second
    Thoughts*, London: Karnac, 1984)
Unprocessed Residues - Introduction
Chapter 8: **Selma Fraiberg, Edna Adelson & Vivian Shapiro** (1975)
    Ghosts in the nursery: a psychoanalytic approach to the problems of
    impaired mother-infant relationships. [Originally in *Journal of the American*

206

*Academy of Child Psychiatry,*14:387-422, 1975. This later version is from *Clinical Studies in Infant Mental Health –The First Year of Life*, Tavistock publications]

Chapter 18: **Isca Salzberger-Wittenberg** (1970) Psychoanalytic insights and relationships. [Originally in Psycho-Analytic Insights and Relationships London: Routledge & Kegan Paul].

Learning Methods:
On this training course learning takes place in various ways:
1. Filtration (four-tier modelling):
- Responsive awareness of the particular stresses on course participants is modelled by the trainer (and small group leaders).
- The trainer contains within-group tensions, and promotes greater awareness of the complexity of interactions among participants.
- Practitioners who develop increased psychodynamic understanding can be more appropriately responsive to the needs of teen clients.
- This responsiveness to emotional states enhances client's sensitivity to their babies' experiences, and in turn, promotes mutual satisfaction.

2. Multi-level interaction
Group discussion, small dialogues, interactive games, role-play and direct observation of DVD material, and its replay –
- Increases the accuracy of observational skills (in practitioners)
- Fosters *a dialectical approach*
- Facilitates better listening skills (in practitioners and through them, in teen parents)
- Improves mentalization and a set of skills to enhance face-to-face effective communication in a culturally diverse environment.

3. Experiential Self-Reflection & Learning Journal exploration
- Helps practitioners to contain anxiety, powerful projections and emotional arousal, avoiding enactments and boundary transgressions.
- Promotes exploration of their own judgemental attitudes towards teens.
- Fosters cultural sensitivity and greater awareness of own blind-spots and subtle prejudice in our attitudes towards sex, race, class, and sexual discriminations.

These can be supplemented with discussion in pairs or threesomes - examining one's own judgemental attitudes [towards teen sexuality; pregnancy; birth rituals; feeding; teen lifestyle: music; appearance, piercings/ tattoos, hairstyles; clothes; hygiene; risk-taking behaviours, eroticism] and, issues affecting mixed-race babies.

Assessment:
'Adolescence as a Second Chance' involves a variety of evaluative procedures [see Appendix 2, and the various Evaluation and Feedback forms].

1. Study-day feedback from participants on training components of each module to evaluate relevance, efficacy of delivery and ways of improving mode and content *(feedback forms in the Appendix):*

2. Evaluation of the course as a whole: midway and at course-end

3. The trainer's own evaluation of each session
- Written notes to him/herself that may be helpful in administering the training in the future.
- Providing comments and valuable suggestions to the Anna Freud Centre on ways to improve the Training Course. jrleff@gmail.com

3. Assessment of student progress (this is optional)
- The Mentalization vignettes can be administered before beginning, and after completing the training.
- Writing up a case history before the training and elaborating on it post-course.
- Comparison of write up of an observation made before, and after the training.

4. Learning outcomes
- Qualitiative follow up to assess the long term influence of the training on *practitioners*.
- A questionnaire is appended to enable interviews and/or self-administered reports.
- Focus groups of selected clients – [three-four months post-training].
- Individual open-ended interviews with participants [eight-ten months post training].

5. Impact on Clients
- how the new learning is applied to the work environment
- what is the influence of practitioners' enhanced psychodynamic understanding on practice – the indirect effect of the course on the *clients*:

This is a sensitive area and a creative approach would be required to enable clients to document their own observations of any change in their practitioner, or themselves, to demonstrate the filtering-down impact of the course on client groups. In some settings, creative projects may demonstrate this greater understanding (i.e. paintings, clay models of one's own family or distribution of disposable cameras to parents, to create exhibition in a Children's Centre or elsewhere with accompanying narratives, to raise group/public awareness of the training project and of issues relating to teen parent/child emotional health.

FEEDBACK FORMS

Adolescence as a 'Second Chance'

1. MODULE FEEDBACK
Devised by Joan Raphael-Leff & Dana Shai*

Participant's Feedback

Module no.____

1. What do you think was most important aspect of today's training?
_____

Why? _____

2. What do you think you gained from today's Interactive Workshop?
_____

Why? _____

3. What do you think was the most meaningful aspect of today's Skill-building seminar? _____

Why? _____

4. Was there anything today you feel was particularly unhelpful?
_____

5. What could be improved?
_____

To what extent do you feel you have already gained from the course
(Please score these from 1 – 'not at all' to 5 – 'very much')
- Increased knowledge   [ ]
- Enhanced skills and clinical strategies   [ ]
- Time to reflect on work practice   [ ]
- Insight into psychodynamic processes/an internal world   [ ]
- Social networking with other course participants   [ ]
- Enhanced confidence in working effectively with teenage parents   [ ]
- Better emotional understanding   [ ]
- Self development   [ ]
- Sharing work concerns   [ ]
- Refined communication skills   [ ]
- Other (please specify)_____
How would you rate today's workshop? [1 – poor to 5 – excellent]   [ ]
How would you rate today's seminar? [1 – poor to 5 – excellent]   [ ]
How would you rate today's Reflective work group   [ ]

_____

* For Dana Shai's biographical details see Expanded notes on Attachment.

Adolescence as a 'Second chance'

2. **Pre and Post Training self-evaluation**

REFLECTIVE FUNCTIONING VIGNETTES
Devised by Dr. Norka Malberg*

Self-Study/Group participants: Fill this out BEFORE the training.

Repeat the exercise after the END of the training.

1. Samantha is very excited today because it is her 15th birthday. But nobody at home seems to have remembered as they are all so involved with her one month old baby daughter. At breakfast, her mother complains about the untidiness of Sam's room, reminding her of her duties as a new mother. Sam would usually say it is true, her room is untidy. This time she replies: "This is MY room, my baby, OK? I like it untidy. Just leave me alone!"

Please read below the different theories about why Sam might have said this and rate the answers below from 9 (most accurate in your opinion) to 0 (least accurate in your opinion). [You can use the same rating more than once on different answers]:

> a) Sam feels invisible and that she doesn't matter much to her family especially since her baby was born.
> Score _____
> b) Instead of wishing her Happy Birthday, Sam's mother has said something to annoy her on purpose.
> Score _____
> c) Sam's mother doesn't care much about Sam; she didn't even offer to help her with cleaning up her room like she used to.
> Score _____
> d) Because it is her birthday, Sam feels she has the right to be left alone and have the day off like most girls her age.
> Score _____
>
> e) Nobody remembered Sam's birthday and her mother is just complaining about her room because she is still angry over her pregnancy.
> Score _____
> f) Sam is disappointed and angry but for some reason doesn't want to mention the real cause of her anger.
> Score _____
> g) Sam tried to give her family a clue so that they would remember her birthday to make them feel guilty about having forgotten it.
> Score _____
> h) Sam was offended and insulted because her mother is more concerned with her untidy room than with making her happy on her birthday.
> Score _____

2. Helen's friend has invited her to his party on Saturday. Most of her school friends will be there and Helen has asked her parents if they can babysit so she can go. Her parents say they can't babysit, and suggest that instead, she goes with them to her grandparents' house. After all, this is more appropriate for

the mother of a baby. Helen tells them she hates her grandparents home and runs off to her room.

Please read below the different theories about why Helen might have acted the way she did and rate from 1(most accurate in your opinion) to 9 (least accurate in your opinion).The same rating can be used more than once on different items:

a) Helen feels her parents don't trust her anymore because she got pregnant. They don't allow her to do anything on her own anymore
Score _____

b) Helen's parents don't respect her freedom as a young person and are over-protective, and inconsistent treating her like a child YET reminding her of her responsibilities as a mother when they feel like it.
Score _____

c) If Helen doesn't go to the party her friends will think she is a loser and she will feel even more embarrassed and the odd one out.
Score _____

d) Helen's parents are selfish and don't understand that Helen needs to be with her friends as she can't enjoy herself around adults, regardless of her grown up responsibilities as a mother
Score _____

e) Helen is frustrated by her parents' decision and would rather not go anywhere if she can't go to the party. She feels her life as a teenager is over
Score _____

f) Helen doesn't want to ruin her friendship with the friend who invited her to his party, after all she is still single.
Score _____

g) Helen is hoping to make her parents feel guilty for forcing her to do something she doesn't want to and for ruining her possibility to have some fun which she doesn't since the baby was born.
Score _____

3. Sheila bought her friend Natalie a CD for her birthday. A few months later, when Sheila is at Natalie's house she sees the CD inside a box with several other things. "What's all this?" Sheila asks. Natalie replies: "I'm trying to get rid of some useless stuff. I don't even remember how I got these things". She then asks Sheila if she would like a coke. Sheila is thirsty, but says: "No, I'd rather go now, actually".

Please read below the different theories about why Sheila might have acted the way she did and rate from 1(most accurate in your opinion) to 9 (least accurate in your opinion),. The same rating may be on different items:

a) Sheila doesn't want to be friends with somebody who doesn't like her.
Score _____

b) Natalie is openly disrespectful of Sheila's feelings and has intentionally created a barrier between them by trying to make Sheila feel unimportant.
Score _____

c) Sheila has had enough to drink this afternoon and doesn't need any more.
Score _____

d) Sheila feels abandoned and lonely and that Natalie doesn't like her.
Score _____

e) Sheila was upset to see her gift being thrown away as "useless".
Score _____

f) The CD is symbolic of their friendship; Natalie has shown that she doesn't want or need Sheila to be her friend any more.
Score _____

g) Natalie wants to get rid of Sheila like she got rid of her gift.
Score _____

h) Sheila feels let down and hurt by her friend and doesn't want to be with her at the moment.
Score _____

Thanks!

Mentalizing Rating Sheet (for evaluator)

The vignettes above can be administered before the Training begins and after the last Module ends. It provides a means of assessing change due to the course in each participant's capacity to mentalize.

Instructions for Coding:

- The options below should be coded according to their degree of *mentalization*, i.e. how well they accurately and explicitly identify the mental states (e.g. wishes, thoughts, emotions, intentions) of each story's main character as the reason for the main character's behaviour in the story.

- Please note that justifications involving non-mental, physical states, labelling or ethical judgments, and inappropriate inferences as the reason for the main character's behaviour, as well as errors about the facts given in the story, should be considered as mainly non-mentalizing.

- Answers that involve inaccurate/implausible assumptions about the main character's or any of the other characters' mental states should also be considered as non-mentalizing.

Scoring Guide:

General Failure of Mentalization:	0
Concrete Mentalization:	1-3
Pseudomentalization:	3-5
Misuse of Mentalization:	5-7
Good Use of Mentalization:	7-9

---

* Norka T. Malberg, MS,EdM, MSc, PsyD
Member of the Child and Adolescent Psychotherapy Association and the British Psychological Society. Norka has worked with adolescents, as a psychologist in the USA, Latin America, and the UK as a child and adolescent psychotherapist. She focused on developing prevention projects targeting young women at risk in Chile in a collaborative effort between the Department of Health and Education and the Ford Foundation. Was a staff member of the Anna Freud Centre developing outreach prevention projects in secondary and primary schools, and in the SMART project providing a short term family intervention based on mentalization theory. Research interests include: Development and Assessment of Short Term Group Interventions for Adolescents in Outreach Settings (Hospitals and Schools), Clinical Applications of Developmental Therapy, Adolescence and Chronic Illness, Prevention of School Exclusion.

3. FOLLOW-UP FOR TRAINING COURSE PARTICIPANTS
6-9 months after the initial course:
Adapted from **Laurence Dumont**, MSc*.

This questionnaire can be the framework for an Interview or given as a self-administered (anonymous) questionnaire prefaced with the words below:
The aim of this follow-up is to obtain some feedback on the training course and to see whether it has influenced you in your practice and if so how.

I. Work practice:
1. Describe the work you are doing now:
How long have you been doing this work?
What would you say is the most important part of your role?

II. Course impact on you:
2. How has the training impacted on you personally?
3. How has the training impacted on you professionally?
4. What aspects of the training course do you feel are most helpful to you in your daily work/tasks? Example?
5. What aspects of the course do you feel did <u>not</u> help you in your daily work/tasks?
6. Do you think you are any different now compared with before attending the course? Example?
7. Do you think you have acquired *new skills* (or that you have become aware of skills you were already using without giving it particular attention)? Examples?
8. Has the training affected the way you *relate* to your clients? Example?
9. Has it changed or influenced the way you *communicate* with your clients? If so, how?
10. How has attending the course changed or influenced the way you *think* about young parents?
11. Has it influenced the way you *understand* young people, their behaviour, verbal and non-verbal communication? If so, how?
Looking back, what *concepts*, if any, have you found especially useful and how?

III. Course impact on the work environment
12. What influence, if any, would you say attending the course had on your relationship with your colleagues?
13. Is your relationship with colleague who attended with you any different from the relationship with your other colleagues? If yes, how?
14. How have you communicated what you learned on the course to colleagues who did not attend?
15. If so, how were your ideas received by your colleagues?
16. How much support or resistance have you have from work?
17. What do your colleagues or managers say about you? Have they made any comment about any changes in the way you work?
18. Has it influenced the way you work with other professionals?

IV. Hindsight:
19. How was the quality of the course for you? (too short/long, shallow/deep; enough/not enough to acquire new skills etc.)
20. What were your expectations before the course?
Were these fulfilled?

21. If you had to give advice to someone about to start this training, what would you say?

22. If you could do the course over again what would you like to be different?

23. If you had to sum up in a few words what the course represents for you, what would you say?

24. What was the most memorable aspect?

25. Do you remember the 'Secret History' exercise on the first day? What were your impressions of that session?
What did you learn?

Do you have any other comments you would like to make about the training?

To what extent do you feel you gained from the course
(Please score these from 1 – 'not at all' to 5 – 'very much')

- Increased knowledge   [ ]
- Enhanced skills and clinical strategies   [ ]
- Time to reflect on work practice   [ ]
- Insight into psychodynamic processes/an internal world   [ ]
- Social networking with other course participants   [ ]
- Enhanced confidence in working effectively with teenage parents   [ ]
- Better emotional understanding   [ ]
- Self development   [ ]
- Sharing work concerns   [ ]
- Refined communication skills   [ ]
- Other (please specify)_____

---

* **Laurence Dumont** MSc. in Psychoanalytic Developmental Psychology, UCL. Dissertation as independent Evaluator of 'Adolescents Becoming Parents' 2008-9. Worked in a Refuge in London for children under 16. MA in Social Work at Goldsmiths College: dissertation on parenting children with Foetal Alcohol Spectrum Disorder looking at strategies of adoptive parents.

4. Questionnaire for Assessment of
INDIRECT INFLUENCE OF COURSE ON CLIENTS:
Joan Raphael-Leff

In the weeks <u>before</u> the training begins trainers instruct practitioners to administer the anonymous questionnaire below to their current clients, specifying their own professional affiliation where it mentions 'practitioner'. The same questionnaire is administered in the weeks after the practitioner has participated in the training course.

Self-report Questionnaire for clients:

1. What expectations did you have of contact with your practitioner?

_____

2. How helpful do you find your contact with the practitioner?

_____

3. What difficulties have you encountered?

_____

4. Do you feel you are being listened to, and understood?

_____

5. Do you feel your contact with your practitioner has been *(tick one)*:
Excellent__   very good__   satisfactory__   poor__   other _____

6. What would you say was most helpful thing s/he did?

_____

7. What did s/he NOT do that you would have liked?

_____

IN CASE OF CONTINUITY:
8. Have you noticed changes in your practitioner's approach?

_____

Any other comments?

_____

Today's date:_____

KEY PAPER
'Why teenagers have babies'
Dr. Margot Waddell

This paper was written specifically for this training in 2008. It is reprinted here by kind permission of the author, and Taylor & Francis publishers of Infant Observation, the Journal in which it was subsequently published.

Margot Waddell , PhD(Cantab), MACP, MBPAS is a psychoanalyst and consultant child psychotherapist in the Adolescent Department of the Tavistock Clinic. She has written extensively on adolescence, including on groups, gangs and scapegoating, and is author of *Inside Lives: Psychoanalysis and the Growth of Personality* (2002) and *Understanding your 12-14 Year Olds* (2005). She writes, teaches and provides psychotherapy to troubled adolescents and their parents.

Infant Observation
Vol. 12, No. 3, December 2009, 271–281

Why teenagers have babies

Margot Waddell*

In trying to determine some of the factors which underlie teenage pregnancy, this paper offers a brief recapitulation of the nature and function of the adolescent process. It stresses the significance of the mother/baby/dyad in the light of the renewed infantile emotional states of the teenager. Special emphasis is put on the quality of early containment and on the internal world experiences of being parented as well as the external pressures of the adolescent world.

Keywords: the adolescent process; containment; puberty; Oedipus complex

Introduction

Adolescence is inevitably a tumultuous time. The normally regressive tendencies of the teenager are often especially pronounced when very early mother/infant relationships have failed to establish a strong enough sense of identity or a secure enough basis for managing the complex tasks that attend these transitional years. Such tasks include those of separation and individuation, of loss, of choice, of dependency, and the difficult process of moving from a place in the family to a place in the outside world. What tends to happen is that old conflicts, especially those of early attachments in infancy and of Oedipal struggles are being reworked – conflicts which test the quality of early containment and the internalization of principles and values which foster the development of the personality rather than hinder, or even arrest, the process of growing up.

If the ordinary struggles of the first five years – especially those involving passionate feelings towards one parent and intense hostility towards the other (including alternations between the two) – have remained largely unresolved, it may be that with the revival at puberty of these original feelings, now intensified by biological changes, extreme measures will be resorted to, to try to manage these new and untried responses. Sexual activity may represent an escape, through physical arousal and excitement, from the tumult of change and uncertainty. Un-resolvable internal conflicts are enacted externally. Thus, fears of abandonment and the loss of childhood relationships drive young people defensively into premature sexual activity.

*E-mail: mwaddell@tavi-port.nhs.uk

ISSN 1369-8036 print/ISSN 1745-8943
© 2009 Tavistock Clinic Foundation
DOI: 10.1080/13698030903299425
http://www.informaworld.com

In seeking to understand something of the determinants of teenage pregnancy, I shall begin with a brief recapitulation of the nature and function of the adolescent process itself. I shall then focus, in more detail, on what specifically may underlie any particular teenage pregnancy – a pressing issue currently in view of the ever-rising number of these in Britain. I shall be thinking, in some depth, about the developmental picture, about the impact of the infantile emotional states and personal dynamics which tend, in the normal course of things, to be renewed during the teenage years. I shall especially be stressing the significance of the mother/baby dyad and also that of the complex triangular relationship which develops between mother, baby and 'other'. These matters will, hopefully, be clarified with a variety of vignettes and observational material.

I shall begin with a few brief, but instructive, vignettes. A 25-year-old young man, Dave, reported that he had a baby with his then girlfriend when the two of them were 17. They had stayed together for about a year and then broken up because his girlfriend couldn't bear his parents' unremitting hostility towards her. He was devastated because he now scarcely saw his son in whose care he had been taking a big part. His parents' objections were apparently about race and class. Dave described them as both snobbish and racist and felt that, certainly, a component in his risk-taking, sexual behaviour at the time, was his intense opposition to them and what they stood for. Although he had not seen it like that at the time, he said, he thought that somehow or other the pregnancy was deliberate, almost a choice.

Sharon said that many years ago, when she was 15, she had some unfamiliar tummy pains. Her general practitioner took some tests and a few days later called her back to the surgery. Looking grave, he told her that he had very, very bad news for her, very bad indeed. Effectively this would ruin her life. Stricken, Sharon waited for him to explain her fate. 'You're pregnant', he said. Furious, Sharon had apparently jumped up, shouted at him that it might change her life but it wouldn't ruin it, and ran out, slamming the door behind her. It was certainly tough, she said, but she never regretted giving birth so young.

Nineteen-year-old Sally told me that the only thing she felt bad about was *how* she had got pregnant, not *that* she had got pregnant. She had got her boyfriend drunk and had done nothing about contraception. She had just been desperate to have a baby. All her life she had felt this great 'empty hole' inside her and had 'known' that having a baby of her own was the only way it would ever be filled.

Two 15-year-olds, Tom and Susan, looked at me as if still in shock. Susan said that she'd noticed putting on a bit of weight but she'd also starting feeling somehow weird. Her doctor told her that she was six months pregnant. 'It's our General Certificate of Secondary Education year. This is a catastrophe', she said. 'We used to drink far more then', Susan added, 'and I suppose I often really didn't know what was happening'.

These brief, and I am sure wholly recognisable comments, establish a central point: that teenage pregnancy stems from a wide range of motivations. Far from being simply the result of ignorance, stupidity or accident, pregnancy is often an expression of complex impulses and feelings, whether conscious or not. It is an expression of a 'choice' of sorts. I shall give a further, longer example, before exploring in psychological terms some of the determinants of the kinds of internal, as well as external processes and pressures which characterise this age group and its typical stresses and vulnerabilities. For working with the emotional needs of pregnant teenagers and very young parents involves a sense of the specificity of adolescent concerns, so that we can, in each case, derive some idea of what this particular pregnancy means to this particular person.

I have chosen to describe 14-year-old Christine, at greater length than a brief account elsewhere (Waddell, 1998/2002), because her dilemmas and conflicts are typical of many young teenagers and are suggestive of the themes that I shall be exploring later. Christine had been referred for counselling because of her increasingly challenging behaviour, her moodiness and rapid swings between infantile and pseudo-adult states of mind. She had long been a troubled girl, tending to act on impulse rather than to think. She had become a problem to herself as well as to those around her. The last straw, as far as her mother and her school were concerned, was when Christine started stealing, mainly objects belonging to her mother or grandmother – a wedding ring, earrings, a watch, and, in the most recent incident, a large sum of money. She had spent most of the money on grown-up, sexually-alluring clothes which she ostentatiously wore in what seemed like an invitation to be found out.

Christine had been brought up by her single mother who had become pregnant by a casual boyfriend when she was 16. Christine had never met her father. Her mother, whose own father had died when she was very young, had had several relationships during Christine's childhood, though none of them serious until recently, when newly-met Paul unexpectedly moved in. It was at this time that the stealing had begun. Christine's behaviour rapidly deteriorated and arguments flared. By her own account, she would try to drive a wedge between her mother and Paul and, for the first time, her attitude towards her mother became sulky and oppositional. She would wander around the house in a state of semi-undress; when her mother objected, Christine would tell her that she was only jealous because she was becoming a fat old bag. Her mother, a trim and attractive 30-year-old, was described by Christine as being alternately in tears about 'losing my daughter, my baby girl', and furious about her daughter's indiscipline and provocations. Paul was deemed unreasonably angry and possessive of his new partner and was said to have shouted at Christine, 'We'll have to throw you out if things go on like this'.

Christine outlined to the counsellor her plans to move out of her own accord. She would get a flat, do it up and have a baby. But, she added, suddenly tearful, she would need to have her Mum behind her: 'I couldn't do it alone'.

It is evident how vulnerable Christine was to actually getting pregnant. Her story brings together a number of factors that are typical of teenage pregnancies. Her own mother was a teenager when she first conceived; as a young woman who had herself been brought up effectively by a single mother. Christine's grandmother had done much of the caring for her immature, unhappy and rather volatile young daughter's baby while the daughter worked long hours in a local bakery. In other words, though loved, Christine did not enjoy the kind of consistent emotional attentiveness that contributes so much to a baby's getting to know him or herself, and to a familial climate of security and care. She had only had to share her mother with her grandmother and had certainly regarded both of them as her own exclusive possessions. She was quite unprepared for the impact of Paul's arrival on her mental equilibrium, and had few internal resources to control the anger and desperation that his arrival stirred in her.

What emerged in the counselling sessions was that underlying the intensity of the impact was the fact that Christine, as so many of her age, was also fearful of growing up at all, of separating, of becoming a woman, of finding a regular boyfriend, going out to work and leaving the dubious containment of what family she had for the unknowns of the world outside. She was especially terrified of being ousted from her relationship with her mother, to whom she had been only insecurely attached. The apparently robust and feisty young woman yielded to a frightened and insecure child part of herself, confused about where she really fitted in, lacking confidence or much sense of self-esteem.

It is of note that Christine started stealing soon after Paul moved in. At puberty, stealing is one of the most common manifestations of 'acting out'. It may represent any one of a range of meanings: perhaps of restoring what is felt to have been lost; here a mother/daughter relationship. It may be aggressive — that is, to deprive someone else of a treasured possession out of primitive envy and rage, or of precious things of which the person himself or herself feels deprived, and consequently impoverished. In Christine's case there may well have been feelings of guilt and a desire for punishment in relation to her attitude to Paul. Was this, in other words, a protest? Or was it a statement about something having been stolen from her to which she had a right (the commitment symbolised by the wedding ring was something which she now felt that she herself lacked)? Was the problem one of anxiety about her own attractiveness (it was feminine things that were stolen — a ring, a necklace, a purse, clothes, a watch)? Was there also a jealous attack on her mother and the desire to take her mother's partner away from her, a desire enacted by the flaunting of her own sexuality? Whatever the specific reasons there was clearly a general anxiety about change and growing up, about losing the relationships on which she was so dependent.

All these factors would naturally, though probably not consciously, contribute to the kind of infantile neediness and fear of being left out that is often central to the picture of teenage pregnancy. If there is a boyfriend in the frame, as was peripherally the case with Christine, there may be a fantasy of being able to create a 'real' family – a mum and dad and a baby scenario, the idealised realisation of what for three generations in her family had never been. Equally, there may be a fantasy, based on identification with the baby, of having the enduringly infantile part of the self looked after by the mother whom she probably never had in the terms that she needed. ('I want my mum behind me to bring up my baby at home'). The deprived child-like Christine seeks to recreate a situation in which she can continue to have her own infantile needs met by entrusting her own baby-self to her mother who is then also her partner in parenting. Thus any aspect of paternity is relegated to a functional and dispensable position. Christine wanted her mother to remain her mother and not be a sexual partner to Paul. So she set herself up in competition. There was no underwear, the counsellor was told, beneath the tracksuit that was sported around the house, and there were explicitly sexual garments bought with the spoils of Christine's forays into stealing. She feared that she could not count on her mother's continued emotional support for her daughter's necessary feminine independence and her need to establish a secure heterosexual relationship of her own. To feel, deep down, uncertain about being able to count on external and internal loving resources not only drove Christine to steal the symbols of commitment and femininity, the concrete representations of feared emotional deficit, but also, when the internal experience of deprivation was mobilized, as with Paul's arrival, to run the risk of enacting the most basic of internal scenarios – that of becoming pregnant in order to preserve, revive, repair or re-live the original mother/baby link.

The prevailing states of mind for teenagers tend to favour action rather than thought, and to provoke infantile rather than adult responses. For any young person, the integration of the mature sexual body into the unsettled experience of personal identity is a major feat. But for those who, like Christine, lack the internal and external experience of solid parenting, the pseudo-solution may well take the form of sexually risk-taking behaviour of a kind that unconsciously replicates, in actuality, precisely the situation of deprivation that cannot be consciously thought about. The teenage mother may interchangeably be identified with an idealised version of her own disadvantaged mother, or, equally, with the baby who is felt now to enjoy total maternal care, a source of infantile fulfilment, but also, often of envy for what never was. Almost every teenager who chooses to get pregnant will talk in terms of the desire for 'unconditional love', both for and from the baby. Sadly, the harsh reality of caring for a baby with such immature emotional resources seldom fulfils this imagined ideal.

Whereas the circumstances of each person's life are unique, nonetheless Christine's situation contains the elements and determinants of many stories of teenage pregnancy. To the personal, individual details must be added the cultural and political picture – not so much our immediate concern, but certainly one requiring a mention. For in this country, we need to bear in mind the backfiring of recent government policies of sex education. The idea that readily available and confidential contraception for teenagers would reduce pregnancy rates has taken an unexpected turn. As the press recently reported, Britain tops the league table of teenage mothers in Western Europe, despite also having a record number of school-age abortions. It seems that the availability of standard contraceptives and morning-after pills without parental consent is normalizing underage sex, and reducing the more ordinary disincentives and natural inhibitions. The press also points out the tendency for early single parenthood to be a generational matter, as was the case with Christine. When parent-led individual responsibility, for which the seeds are sown in the earliest years, is lacking, then internal primitive anxieties of the sort from which Christine suffered may well result in sexual activity. Some sociologists stress the decline of the conventional family structure in this country, by contrast with other parts of Europe, as being an important factor in the turning of a blind parental eye to the activities of the young.

In these circumstances, pregnancy may not be just an accident but rather a conscious or unconscious choice. Where the paternal presence has been peripheral or absent, there is often some considerable contempt, on the girl's part, for young men who themselves, perhaps, suffering from lack of self-esteem and from having inadequate role models, tend to privilege sexual conquest over intimate relationships and to regard contraception as definitely *unmanly*. Even if there is a sense of commitment between the young and immature couple, this tends to be of a somewhat 'dolls' house' kind in which reality is seldom consonant with the imagined picture. The kind of couple that adolescents manage to become, whether transitory or more lasting, whether destructive or developmentally helpful, is very much dependent on the kinds of couple, or absence of couple, that they have experienced from the first, as we have just seen with Christine. What we have also seen, both with her and with the young people described earlier, is just how tumultuous ordinary adolescence can be.

I shall now write, in more detail, about those normally regressive tendencies of the teenager which are often especially pronounced when early mother/infant relationships have failed to establish a secure basis for managing the tasks that attend these later years. If the ordinary struggles of the first five years, especially those involving Oedipal conflicts have remained largely unresolved, it may be that sexual activity constitutes an escape, through physical arousal and excitement. Unresolved internal conflicts tend to be enacted externally. Thus, fears of abandonment and loss of childhood relationships drive young people defensively into premature sexual activity.

These are years when there is a simultaneous drive towards both integration and fragmentation: years characterised by drastic defences against the psychic turmoil involved; years when there is a strong pull towards a pairing relationship of a kind which, it is important to say, can represent a vast range of diverse internal states which defy ordinary generalisations. For example, the establishing of an early 'long-term' relationship *may* indicate an unusually mature capacity for intimacy. But it may, just as possibly, signify an avoidance of adolescent disturbance by means of a pseudo-adult identification with 'being-a-couple'. By contrast, an apparently promiscuous approach to sexuality may represent just that – a reliance on multiple sexual experiences as a defence against a feeling of inadequacy and unloveability. But (to put the matter equally schematically) such an approach *may* indicate an exploratory and constructively experimental struggle to resolve the adolescent's dilemma. In which case, serial sexual partners could be a way of seeking a relationship not so much through mindless erotic adventures, but through the capacity to risk loving and losing in the name of fully engaging with life. There are, of course, innumerable positions beyond and between.

For the last part I want to concentrate on the two areas of infantile experience that I have already mentioned – the process of containment and the nature of Oedipal struggles, in order to link them to later developmental difficulties. Freud (1933) once wrote, 'If we throw a crystal to the floor, it breaks; but not into haphazard pieces. It comes apart along its lines of cleavage into fragments whose boundaries, though they were invisible, were predetermined by the crystal's structure' (p. 59).

The notion of planes of cleavage affords a way of thinking about the underlying operation of forces which often only become apparent later on, especially so in adolescence, when the stress of whatever undertaking it might be reveals cracks and fissures, vulnerabilities and weaknesses, which, though they may long have been present in the personality, have not been manifest hitherto. The nature of these underlying forces predominantly relates to the baby's early experience, particularly to the extent to which mental and emotional states were, as it were, held and understood by the mother or primary caretaker. It is these forces which shape people's inside lives, which influence the sort of internal picture that people build up of their parents which, as we all know, may bear little resemblance to the external realities.

I shall give a brief example of a picture exhibition in the gallery of a primary school in order to indicate how very differently a group of five-year-olds experienced a small flood which swept through their village when a dam further up the mountain burst and water came rushing down the hillside. Each child had a similar experience, obviously, of the depth of the water and the degree of danger, or lack of danger, involved. But the pictures they painted were fundamentally different. Very briefly, one child had depicted a church tower with a small huddle of people at the top and water almost reaching the parapet. The sky was dark and scary with clouds scudding by and no moon in sight. There were sharks and whales thrashing in the water and a look of terror on everybody's face.

The picture beside that was entirely different. It could almost have been a Bank Holiday. There were puddles on the ground, buckets and spades, a few rubber balls and plastic ducks. The sky was bright with a smiley sun up in the corner. There were red Wellingtons around and signs of water but, on the whole, simply rather small and shallow pools.

The third depicted a parental-looking figure with a sack marked 'Provisions' on his back, leading a group of children in crocodile formation up some half-flooded steps now above the water line. The line was drawn more or less exactly as it had been in reality.

A fourth picture was very precise, ruled with lines and measurements between the village square, the church, the butcher, and prolific labels, 'This is my house', 'This is where my Gran lives', 'This is my school' and so on.

A fifth picture was simply a black wash of paint with no figurative representation at all.

The first child clearly brought to the experience of the flood an anxious perception of things. Set-backs were catastrophes. The dangers that were perceived in the external world were a great deal exaggerated. Perhaps this child had anxious parents who *did* view set-backs as catastrophes and were not able to help their child with his or her unrealistic fears and fantasies. By contrast, the second picture was equally unrealistic. The flood, real enough in itself, had been wholly under-rated and turned into some kind of manic Bank Holiday atmosphere with a few puddles and, as I say, many Wellingtons. The third picture, as you will have realised, approximated much more closely the actual event. This child carried with him, or her, an internal picture of a parent who would always have foresight, who would provide, who had a realistic expectation of life, and who was able to protect and lead the children wisely to safety. The fourth child seemed to suffer from something quite obsessional, in that no ordinary imaginary expression of things was possible, simply quantification, labelling and exactness – a defence against anxiety rather than a capacity to express it symbolically. The fifth child was simply too utterly overwhelmed by the experience to find any symbolic means of representing it on paper at all.

Each of these children was demonstrating the nature of what we would call their 'inner world', a world which has been forming since the moment they were born – indeed, I would argue, well before they were born. Internal reality is by no means the same as external reality.

As I have suggested, two significant determinants of the culture of this inner world are the nature of the original mother/baby relationship and, later, the way in which a third term is introduced into that first dyad. Later in her life, Melanie Klein (1959) wrote conclusively that, 'nothing that ever existed in the unconscious completely loses its influence on the personality' (p. 262). She observed how we can gain insight into the way: 'our mind, our habits, and our views have been built up from the earliest infantile fantasies and emotions to the most complex and sophisticated adult manifestations' (p. 262).

Let us take a simple example from the beginning of the life-cycle: as a mind is observed encountering another mind, it is possible to identify both the seeds of those factors which may nurture, and also of those which may obstruct potential mental and emotional development. The following extract is from the quoted notes (Waddell, 2006) of an observer who, as part of her training in child psychotherapy, would spend one hour a week in an ordinary household watching the interactions between the baby and his or her family.

Fred at 4½ months

When I came in today, Fred was sitting in his bouncy chair in front of the washing machine, watching the drum going around. His mother was leaning back against the worktop facing him. Laughing, she said that he was going mad with it. He was indeed, very excited. As the machine rumbled and spun, so he waved his arms and legs. But the excitement peaked as his Mum, in imitation, made a low, rumbling sound deep in her chest. While she did this Fred's face was alert and watching, listening intensely to the sound. His mouth was open as if he was literally 'taking her in'. Every time she finished her performance, his arms and legs were released in a frenzy of activity: his legs stiffening and suddenly drawn back against his chest, his arms waving up and down, his hands alternately clenched and shooting open, all fingers rigidly extended. He made a variety of explosive noises: squeals, lip-bubbling, dribbling and spraying saliva, rich chortles which seemed almost like laughing. As if exhausted by these outbursts, he would lapse back into relative stillness while his face tensed in expectation, his eyes riveted to his Mum's face, waiting for her to take up the 'dialogue'.

When, for example, she turned to talk to me, to tell me that Fred had discovered the mouth-bubbling only this week, Fred remained tense, but his expression changed, as if a light had gone out. This happened two or three times. During these interruptions, Fred seemed to wait patiently, suspended, his face losing its animation but ready to re-engage as soon as she turned back to him, which she did quite quickly on each occasion. I found these interludes quite painful and felt relieved when she would turn back to him just before he could become too disappointed and therefore distressed. (She seemed to have a remarkable sense of precisely when this point might be and each time avoided it.)

This observational extract is suggestive of all sorts of possibilities – ones which may or may not be borne out as the pattern of Fred's relationships with his mother and family unfold, and the quality and intensity of the kinds of exchange so vividly described here can be gauged and reflected on over time. A baby's fascination with the visual effects and changing sounds and rhythms of a washing machine is a common enough sight. But, as it emerges, Fred's chair has been positioned not so much to distract and preoccupy, as an older child might, for example, be placed in front of a television, but rather in such a way as to be part of a richly shared relationship with his imaginative and intuitive mother. The observer, too, is sensitive to the specificity of the exchange. Fred's ecstasy and anticipation of fulfilment seems to involve the sense of a 'taking in', perhaps even of a 'drinking in', of a joyful quality of reciprocity and recognition – as if mother and infant is each conveying 'how wonderful you make me feel'. Fred is expressing his delight by every means at his disposal, the small degree of delayed gratification seeming only to add to the intensity of his eventual pleasure.

It is clear that when Fred has to share his mother's attention with a third – the observer – some significant psychic events are set in train. The observer finds herself painfully identified with Fred's distress, his disillusionment and disappointment at another relationship intruding on his feeling of perfect rapport. But she is also, nonetheless, able to appreciate that this mother has a capacity to register and understand what is within Fred's compass, and to re-focus her attention before its absence extends beyond him. In quite simple, yet subtle, ways we can trace how the minutiae of the observation of simultaneous external and internal emotional events suggest the beginnings of profoundly important patterns of developmental possibility. Movingly, the observer describes how the light seems to go out of Fred's world when he loses the passionate intensity of his mother's gaze and involvement. And yet he is able briefly to sustain the absence of the former exclusivity and to re-ignite lost pleasure as soon as he re-finds his mother because, as the description makes clear, she 'knows', and unconsciously 'times', the degree of frustration that her son can bear.

Here we see, in embryonic form, the beginnings of a baby being able to tolerate the introduction of a third party into the primary mother/infant dyad. In some analytic frameworks, this would signal aspects of the early Oedipal constellation. Freud took up Sophocles's version of one of the Greek myths in order to illustrate what he found to be a universal 'complex', as he called it, in human nature. He noticed, in himself and others, the tendency to love the parent of the opposite gender and hate the parent of shared gender. From a very young age the person struggles with feelings of love and hate within, and struggles, in particular, with not being the centre of the world of the person he or she loves. The Greek myth depicted parents who were worried by the Delphic Oracle foretelling that their newborn son, Oedipus, would kill his father and marry his mother. In fear of such a terrible eventuality they left him on a hillside to die. The myth describes how these events did come about and were felt, by Freud to depict universal phenomena in human nature.

In other psychoanalytic ways of thinking, the quality of early experience just described in relation to Freud might offer evidence of a mother's desire reciprocally to get to know her baby, thus allowing him, if it is a boy, to get to know her and himself in her, as a step towards knowing himself in himself. Thus the observer's reflections, inward as she seems to be with Fred's disappointment and with his mother's confidence, enable us to derive a sense of how this mother's understanding of her son's mental and emotional capacities contributes, in turn, to his own capacities to tolerate anxiety and frustration and to learn that disappointments need not be disasters. One infers that these very capacities to take in are already quite developed in Fred and that the gap between desire and satisfaction has long been bridged by a rudimentary form of 'mental holding' or 'reverie', as the psychoanalyst Bion puts it, which the observer is both witnessing and also experiencing and learning from. A modicum of anxiety, if contained, is part of getting to know oneself and of developing one's own resilience.

To go back to the picture gallery, we can see the consequences of the varying early experiences of the containment of anxiety amongst the young painters described – the range of defensive strategies clearly adopted very early on to manage anxiety in the absence of any properly secure internal structure for so doing. It is important to keep this in mind when thinking not just about infancy and young children but about the whole life cycle and, most especially, as I have suggested, the teenage years when these issues of frustration and anxiety, of loneliness and confusion, are so particularly evident. The adolescent who, as a baby, enjoyed the kind of experiences which were part of Fred's everyday life, would be much better able to withstand the stresses of this inevitably tumultuous time if able to draw on an internal version of a parent who can support extreme states of mind in the way that Fred's mother so clearly could, as could the parents of the third little painter whose emotional resources would seem to have resided in early experiences of wise and well-balanced parenting.

In my own practice, I have often come across teenage pregnancies occurring in the context of a mother having a last baby, to the absolute horror of her teenage daughter who had long believed that her parents no longer had a sexual relationship, in fact probably had never had intercourse since she herself was conceived! A mother's late pregnancy is an intense shock in most circumstances and it is not surprising that the response to it should be the child herself suddenly becoming sexually active and clearly at risk of getting pregnant, whether in competition with her mother, or in desperation at losing the previous mother/baby relationship (that between her mother and herself), or in a state of jealous destructiveness at the parents' ongoing sexual relationship. Whatever the reason, one can see the adolescent's difficulty in dealing with extreme emotional pain without seeking to enact some version of the pain, usually destructively.

To come back to our first examples, I hope that it will now be clear how central to the adolescent psyche are the two contributions to an understanding of human development just described, the theory of containment and that of the Oedipus complex. It is in the interrelationship of external circumstances and the internal weighting and freighting of the kinds of psychological mechanisms I have been tracing that the respective motivations, whether conscious or unconscious, for pregnancy among teenagers reside. It is here that we will be able to make those crucial discriminations between whether the original mother/baby relationship is being attacked, preserved, repaired, re-lived or revived. And these distinctions are of crucial importance for the present and future welfare of all those involved.

References

Freud, S. (1933). *The dissection of the psychical personality. Standard edition volume XXII.*

Klein, M. (1959/1975). Our adult world and its roots in infancy. In M. Klein (Ed.), *Envy and gratitude and other works. 1946–1963.* London: Hogarth.

Waddell, M.J. (2002). *Inside lives: psychoanalysis and the growth of the personality.* London: Karnac (Original work published 1998).

Waddell, M.J. (2006). Infant observation in Britain: the Tavistock approach. *International Journal of Psychoanalysis, 87,* 1003–1020.

'Adolescence as a 2nd Chance'
Devised by
Professor Joan Raphael-Leff ©
MODULE I:
INTERRELATIONSHIPS

1. Interactive workshop:
TEENS AS CLIENTS - Meaning
Making: Expectations &
Cultural Competence

Introductions:
*Leader and each participant says their name and position Now (or earlier) each fills out the Mentalization forms. Ask them to add initials after completion. [Throughout these Handouts, instructions in **italics** relate to group acivities, but can be used as guiding points for self-study].*

OBJECTIVES:
By the end of the study-day you will -
• be more aware of your own <u>subjective experience</u>
• have understanding of <u>inter-personal dynamics</u>
• see the unique aspects of <u>working with teen clients</u>
• be better equipped to help parents to think about their own **feelings, needs** and **effects** of their choices on the baby and others.

The 'storm and stress' of adolescence is
hormone driven but also due to uncertainty and
reactivated issues ▶ fluctuating between child-like
and adult feelings, while reworking their identity.
• **AS CLIENTS - ADOLESCENTS ARE**
NOTORIOUSLY DIFFICULT TO ENGAGE.
• Practitioners working with teen-parents struggle to
keep <u>thinking</u> in their presence - as young
parent/s do in the presence of their infant.
Their intense feelings, impulsive, risky behaviours &
enactments provoke strong **reactive feelings** in
us involving - confusion, irritation, concern, and…
possibly, our secret admiration and envy
HOW DO IMPROVE OUR UNDERSTANDING?

'Secret History'* [35 minutes]

*Large group divided in two. All participants on one side of room 'become' a **pregnant teenager**; those on other - **a midwife**. [use 2 Flip charts: one either side].*
Teenager: **Jane** aged 17 is 22 weeks pregnant. She
defaulted on her initial antenatal booking & comes
25 minutes late for the replacement appointment,
dishevelled & smelling of cigarette smoke. Seems
resentful when told she'll now have to wait for a gap.
*1. Members of Jane's group are asked about her
feelings, & later about her needs [No 'correct' answers]
Feelings & **needs** written in 2 columns on Jane's & Rita's
respective flipcharts]*

Leader turns attention to the <u>Midwife's group (saying)</u>:
Rita aged 38, is a divorced mother of two children
aged 4 and 6. She prides herself on managing her
large case-load, and answers to her staff nurse who
expects her to attend frequent staff meetings.
• *Rita's group are asked to shout out her feelings
(regarding Jane) and her own needs (use Rita's chart)*
• <u>Re</u> Jane: There's some confusion over her address.
A question of whether Jane belongs to the hospital's
catchment area or should go elsewhere.Her feelings?

*<u>After 20 minutes</u>, participants switch sides, physically
sitting in the others' chairs, <u>playing the other person</u>.*
• *Leader now adds <u>additional information</u>:*

When she told them she was pregnant, <u>Jane</u>'s parents
were shocked and distressed about her decision not to
have an abortion. Told she was an 'embarrassment' and
could no longer live at home, Jane was staying with her
boyfriend over the past 2weeks but yesterday, he beat
her up during a row, saying he was not the baby's father.
Jane slept over-night at a friend's house some distance
away. The journey to the clinic took longer than expected:
Leader asks for Jane's feelings? needs? [use flip chart]
Rita: She had a disturbed night with little sleep last night,
as her youngest child woke short of breath. He suffers
from croup, so Rita knows what to do, and spent some
hours with him in the bathroom, creating steam to relieve
his coughing fits. Very early this morning she had to
phone around to find someone to stay with him, as he
could not go to his nursery - but she still arrived on time.

*What is Rita feeling? What does Rita need? [Feelings &
needs are added to Rita's flip-chart list].*
*After 10 minutes participants change back to their
original seats, **leaving Jane** and **Rita behind.***
Are these unusual cases?
What was *new* in what we did today?
What have you learned?
Importance of listening & containing anxiety.
How do we protect our selves and yet remain
accessible and sensitive?
How can we enable clients to tell their 'stories'?

** This exercise is inspired by a training module used by Dr.
Simone Honikman, Director of the Perinatal Mental Health
Project in Cape Town, South Africa.   www.pmhp.za.org*

EXPECTATIONS:
- Faced with the unfamiliar, we dispel our uncertainty by **anticipating** what will happen, based on past experience
- This may make sense of why sometimes our clients treat us as other than who we are
- Each partner in an encounter is part of a complex **2-way system** - affected by own and other's expectations, feeling, thoughts and behaviour
- Expectations usually operate outside **our awareness** but are revealed in body language, speech rhythms, tone, facial expression, posture which affect the emotional atmosphere

ROLE PLAY 1: First appointment
*2 volunteers: Teen Client &'Experience': Leave room to
 discuss teen's expectations.*
*2 more:Referrer & Practitioner[what profession? previous
behaviour? presenting problems?]*
*Client & Practitioner **role play** (2 minutes) While still in-
role they tell about their expectations & feelings during
the exchange (2 minutes). Stop for group discussion (2
minutes). Replay: (2 minutes)*
NOTE: new strategies which have emerged
*DEBRIEFING – role players state their own name
leaving the role behind them.*
What are **the first steps** in changing the workplace
culture? (welcome clients; greet them with a smile; use their
name, eye-contact, etc…)

INTERIM CONCLUSIONS:
Client's expectations colour **perception** of you
These expectations are affected by her/his **past experience** with previous workers & carers
The client's expectations now affect **your behaviour**
And, you, the practitioner also have expectations (based on **your** experience with previous clients) which affect the way you **approach** this teenager.
These can **engender** the very behaviour you ascribe influencing the **give-and-take** & the client's collaboration with, or resistance to, the programme you are offering.
Together, you *co-construct* an '**emotional climate**'

Group discussion & examples of each of these points

BASIC PSYCHODYNAMIC ASSUMPTIONS
- A child's **INNER WORLD** is constituted in the family
- **FANTASY** & EMOTION accompany **cognition**
- Different **AGE LEVELS** coexist
- OLD feelings are transferred into NEW SITUATIONS ['**Transference**']
- **Unresolved/unprocessed** issues are REACTIVATED at times of vulnerability and **transition**
- **Transitions of Adolescence/Pregnancy/Parenting= receptacles** for anxieties & projections
- The baby is inserted into a **web of expectations** & *ascriptions which colour the way s/he is perceived*
- **Expectations induce responses** - bringing about the anticipated reactions/behaviours
- Each child evolves an **INTERNAL WORKING MODEL** of care-relationships. These representations form the basis of his/her **expectation** of future care

INTERACTIVE 'FIELD OF FORCES' :
• Worker & client's **expectations** may clash or dove-tail [client's rescue fantasies & practitioners desire to rescue]
• Both are pulled into **playing out an allocated role**
It is important to recognise how our preconceptions influence our perceptions
[prepare pens & paper]
EXERCISE (2 minutes): complete this sentence in writing [list 4 items]
In Purdistan women are forbidden to…

GROUP THINKING: *We were blind to racism, sexism, homophobia not long ago.* What are our blind spots today?

INTOLERANCE

Pre-judgements stem from ideas and value systems we imbibed <u>unquestioningly</u> in childhood & since

Groups identified by sex, age, race, ethnic categories, religious minorities etc. - are **generalisations.**

They do not take account of personal attributes

False hierarchies take on a social reality of their own, perpetuating oppressive and discriminary social arrangements.

Are we Victims, Perpetrators or BYSTANDERS?

Small group discussion: 4-6 members (2 minutes):
- *Think of a racist joke.*
- *What do you do when someone tells one?*

PREJUDICE

All forms of prejudice connect to *systems of belonging*
- We see **us** as 'good', and project what is 'alien' & 'bad' (or needy, greedy, mad...) in us - into **them**
GROUP THINKING (3 minutes): Do we unfairly condemn young people? **Discriminatory categories** reflect our own irrational beliefs and weaknesses. Statements may seem scientific, based in physical, sexual or genetic difference (♀='hysteria'; small brain size=lower IQ) but *any form of labelling* ['bastards' ;'unwed mothers'] *is a* **social** act. **Bigotry** can be personal or legislated (apartheid) disguised or blatant (bars: 'Gentlemen only'. 1950s Boarding House signs:'No children, no dogs, no coloureds!').

Our anxiety leads us to ► control, exclude, discriminate or subjugate others who are different from us.

The unquestioning person/group feels superior to others designated as **inferior or 'outsiders'**, by denying their subjectivity & 'sameness'
- We **project** aspects of our own **idealised** or **repudiated** selves into others (celebrities; 'enemy')

Projection: **expelling our own feelings or unwanted traits into another**
- **Projections** can **invoke the anticipated behaviour**
- Prejudicial concepts (of age, sex, class, gender, race, religion) are **internalised** - affecting self-image behaviour & performance *(Obama's election).*

Internalisation: *taking in something that becomes incorporated as part of <u>self identity</u>*

INTERACTIVE GROUP EXERCISE:

5 minute discussion in pairs: A client says her partner's mother insists she hang a chicken-bone above her (mixed-race) baby's crib to fortify his bones.

What do we say? *INVITED FEEDBACK to the group*
- MESSAGE: It a painful experience when we discover that our thoughts, feelings and interactions are riddled with prejudice. **WHAT CAN WE DO?**
- Take responsibility for our own *hostility*, even - and especially- towards the people we care for.
- Make a conscious decision to treat each encounter as **unique.**
- Help dispel some unthinking racist, sexist, ageist discriminatory practices.
- Monitor our own contribution to (co-constructed) relationships with clients.

GROUP EXERCISE: *How do we activate reflective thinking in teenage clients?*

5 minutes small group discussion (4-5 people) of this central question of the Course.
[5 minute feedback from a few small groups]

•Cultivate the teen's higher expectations and achievable ambitions for self and baby

• Increase the teen parent's 'reflective function' → her/his ability to think of child's needs as separate, complex & different from own

CONCLUSIONS:

SOCIO-CULTURAL COMPETENCE is the ability to understand and interact effectively with people 'different' to ourselves. This entails -
- **Knowing** one's cultural worldview & potential bias
- Honestly **re-examining preconceived ideas** on an ongoing basis, in peer groups & alone (Journal)
- A generally **receptive attitude** towards difference (age, gender, ethnicity, etc) and willingness to question our own assumptions.
- **Identifying detrimental procedures**
- Awareness of our bystander status - silence about known injustice is an act of compliance

REMINDER: Use **Private Journals** *to record and explore personal thoughts and feelings after today*

2. Skill-building Seminar:
The Effect of Relationships on Relationships –
Containment and Reflective Function:

OBJECTIVES: This seminar develops the practitioner's interactive skills - ability to engage teenage clients, activate the capacity for mentalization, develop the client's curiosity about their own and the baby's feelings…increase our awareness of our own 'baggage

THE PRACTITIONER-CLIENT RELATIONSHIP

*SMALL GROUP DISCUSSION [2-5 people: **What 'personal baggage' does the client bring to the interaction with practitioners? Group feedback** (3 mins)*

SKILLS:EMPATHY

To understand the emotional experience, thoughts and feelings of clients we **empathise,** trying to see things from **the other's perspective**

We reflect on effects of our own **personal 'baggage'**: do our responses relate to unresolved issues from our own adolescence? Are we over-identified with the teen's baby/toddler – reducing our empathy for the young parent/s' own difficulties?

The practitioner affects the client's (positive/negative) feelings transferred from the past into the present, by offering a **new experience**, building on a <u>work alliance</u> with that part of the client that wishes to change. FEEDBACK is essential to CHANGE.

GROUP DISCUSSION: *What are successful methods of engaging teenage clients?*(use flipchart)

A non-judgmental approach
• An informal invitation (texting reminders) yet maintaining upfront and clear boundaries
• Make it fun! Use drama/soaps; utilise their curiosity
• Focus on the teen NOT the baby (goody bags)
• Provide a familiar setting for first meeting (café?)
• Establish a support network of other teen mothers, be-frienders, advocates, etc.
• Engage fathers & other family members
• Encourage responsibility, empathy & containment
• Help the client out of poverty by increasing self-confidence (strengthen strengths; discuss options)
•**Provide tools - teach 'to fish' vs. feeding**

CONTAINMENT:

Before an infant can manage emotions, s/he is dependent on carers to reduce confusion.
A receptive parent, knows emotionally what the baby is experiencing, picks up the infant's unbearable anxieties - contains and 'de-toxifies' them, handing back a 'digested' version. When people have not been well contained in childhood – their anxieties are triggered in charged situations of **asymmetrical dependency** that remind them of childhood care situations
SKILLS: *this form of 'containment' can also be used by practitioners: <u>Role Play</u>: Practitioner and an adolescent parent who is scared her mother will 'hijack' her baby. [While in-role discuss feelings]*

INTERACTIVE WORK SKILLS: brainstorm *What does an adolescent client need?*[use flipchart for <u>suggestions & ideas</u>]

A trustworthy practitioner who can
• be honest; set boundaries; maintain values
• remain engaged without an agenda
• listen non-judgementally, igniting curiosity
• be empathic but not intrusive, over-involved nor over-identified with her/his issues
• be fair; won't 'take sides' in external/internal conflicts but rather **voice the core issues**
• remain 'uncorrupted' (especially if delinquent)
• foster awareness of the language s/he uses – as it expresses but also <u>shapes</u> our self-concept as agent, perpetrator or victim

---

INTERIM CONCLUSIONS:

Preconceptions affect one's perceptions
We try to avoid imposing our own feelings.
We get an intuitive 'feel' of what the client is experiencing emotionally by becoming aware of our **own emotional responses.**
But empathic awareness is **impaired** by **over-identification and collusion**
Professional growth depends on **self-reflection** and **responsibility** for our own feelings
Our aim is to offer the client an authentic experience of care, while being realistic given our caseloads and resources

RELATIONAL SKILLS: <u>CONTAINMENT</u>

- **Listen carefully. A**cknowledge difficulties of motherhood *[unpatronising praise; offer a role model]*
- identify some of the **underlying** *anxieties*: ask for best-case and worst scenarios'.
- be attuned to: *'who am I? what am I becoming?*
- **reflect back feelings** validating their importance
- **name conflicts** and help the young person to **take responsibility** for his/her own feelings
- **do not offer solutions** to family problems but **empower** the client to consider how thoughts, feelings & behaviour inter-connect within the family.
- help evolve **reasonable expectations** about the child and themselves

MENTALIZATION
is a form of imaginative mental activity:
an ability to **perceive & interpret human behaviour** in terms of **subjective intentional states** (goals, needs, desires, feelings, beliefs, purposes & reasons)…
Mentalization forms the basis of our capacity for relatedness

Reflective thinking:holding our own & the other's mind in mind
Attending to mental states in oneself and others
- Feeling curious about feelings behind behaviours
- Understanding misunderstandings
Seeing oneself from the outside – and others from the inside

SKILLS: REFLECTIVE FUNCTION

We all have the potential to 'mentalize' – to become **aware** of our own feelings and those of others.
- A carer's emotional responsiveness & intuitive ability to reflect back feelings helps the baby/child/adolescent to understand their own & others' behaviour in terms of <u>subjective mental states</u>: thoughts, moods, motivations
"You seem angry/sad…is it because of what I said?"
The goal is for practitioners to REFLECT on their own feelings and practice; to reflect the young parent's feelings & to encourage her/him to reflect the baby's
- to help teen understand more about the **effect** of their own feelings, so as to keep the baby's feelings in the forefront of her/his mind, while recognising that the child's needs are separate from his/her own.

SKILLS: ACTIVATING REFLECTIVE THINKING
1. **Practitioner signals** that **feelings** are i**mportant;** that feelings can be **thought about** (rather than enacted)
2. Provides **'containment'**: sensitive **feedback** that reduces anxiety & fosters client's belief that anxieties *can* be contained & processed.
3. Helps recognise how stress leads to *negative* views
4. Helps to learn from experience.
5. Promotes **mentalization:** The client internalises the worker's capacity to think/interpret her/his & baby's behaviour in terms of **underlying mental states** - feelings, thoughts beliefs & desires.
6. Client begins to reflect - for self and child.

Summary
'Mentalization' means interpreting our own behaviour and that of others in terms of underlying mental states, feelings, thoughts, beliefs and desires. It forms the basis of our capacity for human relatedness and 'mind mindedness' consists of
- Holding the other's mind in mind
- Understanding and repairing misunderstandings
- Attending to mental states in oneself and others
- Feeling curious about the feelings behind behaviours
'Seeing oneself from the outside and others from the inside'.

<u>CONCLUSIONS</u>:
By helping teenage parents to consider their own feelings and to wonder about and **reflect what is happening in the baby's mind**, the quality of their interaction is enhanced, providing both young mother (or father) and child with better conditions for growth.
- But the carer's capacity for **'reflective functioning'** is affected by current stressors (as well as negative past experiences).
In stressful situations we all need time and calm mental space for reflection.
- Feeling **contained** increases reflective functioning
To be supportive, we too must feel 'contained':
need for peer support groups and supervision.

Adolescence as a 2nd Chance ©
devised by
Professor Joan Raphael-Leff
MODULE II: ADOLESCENTS

3. Interactive Workshop
**MATURATIONAL PROCESSES
of ADOLESCENCE**

OBJECTIVES:
This workshop explores maturational processes in adolescence and the impact of pregnancy & parenting
By the end of the workshop you can expect to:
• be more aware of the complexity of adolescent reworking of old issues while consolidating new capacities
• see the young parent's perspective in the struggle to accomplish her/his own developmental tasks while fostering the baby's
• promote emotional understanding, coping skills and resilience

---

PUBERTY
Fundamental change = <u>actual</u> **potency/fertility:**
frightening new sexuality & strength: incestuous desires & aggressive impulses are now **realisable.**
Emotionally, this is a threatening experience as previous defences prove inadequate and there are breakthrough thoughts and ideas
Old issues resurface: love/hate/power, parent/child, male/female differences, sexuality, birth, death
Western Adolescence is regarded as a prolonged tran-sitional period of exploration, experimentation & play.
Puberty comes earlier [1860 x 16. 6 years; 1920 x14.6; 1950 x13.1; 1980 x12.5; 2010 ~ 11.7 years]

ADOLESCENT INCONSISTENCY
• Moodiness, irritability, unhappiness, intense reactions
• Silence, need for privacy, sensitivity to
                              external intrusions
↔talkativeness, loud music to block out
                              internal intrusions
Social withdrawal yet deep concern about relations
↕ Self-preoccupation and lower attunement to the feelings of others
• Confusion, impulsiveness, sadness, resentment, rage (some acting out)
• Panic attacks and lack of confidence coupled with ideas of 'invincibility' and super powers…

GROUP EXERCISE: **Early & Late** Adolescence:
[SPLIT large group into Early/Late: Subdivide to small units of 3-4 people] ROLE PLAY: parent & teen, and observer/s (In the case of fewer participants have two role plays – Early & Late for all to watch).

TASK: ***Parent & Teen discuss a Conflictual issue**
[5 minutes] S Then some observers report back to large group [5-10 mins]
Depending on time, possibly– get role players to exchange places and play the other role!*

What typifies early adolescence? *[5 mins with chart]*
Self study – write answers in your Journal

EARLY ADOLESCENCE (13-16)

Preoccupation with bodily changes, new somatic experiences and physical appearance
• Differences/similarities between the sexes
Tensions: exploring novelty & regressing to old patterns: intrusion of infantile processes
Boundary testing and search for control:
• Struggle w. parents/authority figures over limits/rules
• Mild antisocial behaviour peaking in mid-teens.
• Channelling the craving for excitement: competitive sports, dance, music - or more worrying risk-taking activities.

Group Discussion: what is typical for LATE ADOLESCENCE [16-24…)?

- Finding one's own 'voice' and value
- Separating from the parents while recognising them as complex people.
- Trust in own creative capacity (not having to prove fertility)
- Confronting own sexuality
- Position in peer-group hierarchy (or gang)
- Making more realistic plans for future

Feelings of
omnipotence
Struggle for
autonomy

tantrums
defiance
replay of
toddlerhood

Teenagers –
tired of being harrassed
by your stupid parents?!
ACT NOW!
Move out…get a job…pay
your own bills
Do it while you still
know everything!

MESSAGE:

- **Emotional fluctuations** during adolescence indicate a creative search for **change.**
- The upsurge of feelings, self-reappraisal and tendency to question authority →progressive 'out of the box' thinking, offer **an opportunity** to rework past conflicts and emotional deficits. **Adolescence is a second chance find new solutions to old problems and to achieve healthy authenticity in the present**

Troubled teens should be referred to specialist adolescent psychotherapists or counsellors for more intensive work.

EMOTIONAL DEVELOPMENT

- **Maturation**=self-reflection as opposed to acting-out
- Achieving a relatively **stable sense of self**
- Balancing tensions between **inter-dependence** and the desire for **self-sufficiency**
- Achieving **mindfulness** and management of his/her own feelings.
- LEARNING FROM EXPERIENCE!
- **Realistic self-esteem** = acceptance and integration of own mixed feelings and of multiple aspects of 'identity'

Group discussion of each point

SOCIAL DEVELOPMENT

- **Openness** to exploring the wider world (beyond family and school)
- Checking internal self-other relations externally
- Gradual disengagement from dependency on parents and elaboration of more complex relations to them
- Learning to control aggressive & sexual impulses
- Moving towards meaningful intimate relationships (more thoughtful discrimination)
- Awareness of other perspectives

Group discussion of each point

INTELLECTUAL DEVELOPMENT

- Curiosity and search for meaning
- Self-discipline and consolidating work patterns
- Self-motivation; responsibility for thoughts, actions and beliefs
- Awareness of the consequences of decisions
- Re-assessment of abilities and prospects
- Establishing interests, acquiring adult skills, knowledge and self-reflective skills

Group discussion of each point

PHYSIOLOGICAL CHANGES

Hormonal changes kick in: difficulty concentrating; emotional hyper-sensitivity
• **Altered sleep patterns** – teens need up to 12 hours sleep, from late at night to noon
Altered appetite patterns – growth is very rapid. 80% of growth hormone is released during sleep. On awakening, like a baby, the teen is very hungry.
Difficulty in affect-regulation and self-soothing. Experimentation with smoking, alcohol, illegal drugs [among friends less worrying than alone].
BRAIN: Gradual development of the medial prefrontal cortex [of reason, planning, executive function] but also, reversion to more 'primitive' brain areas which induces reactivity and impulsive decision making

SEXUAL DEVELOPMENT

NEW REALITY: New capacities – new physical strength; changing body shape & signs of virility/ fecundity (menstruation and emissions).
• Achieving coherent **body image** & **sexual identity** Making love=an intimate experience (vs.'link'; sex; physical activity)
• Becoming **a 'subject'** involves **agency:** self-respect and taking responsibility for one's own (sexed) body
Psychic representations (of femininity/female sexuality) can impact directly on physical development:
Teenage girls who resist growing up - **anorexia:** avoiding breasts and menstruation. Or, desire to out-do her mother may result in **precocious pregnancy**
Group discussion of each point

REAPPRAISAL OF GENDER

The experience of sexed subjectivity is dependent on meaning rather than anatomy.
We distinguish SEX: chromosomal status at birth & GENDER: a self-categorising psycho-social construct

Gender formation: a lifelong process based on identifications and internalised potentialities through interaction in primary relationships; intra-psychic representations of somatic impressions, and socio-cultural experience, in different contexts
Adolescence: gender re-evaluation; experimentation – 'ladettes', 'bending the mainstream';

GENDER COMPONENTS

1. **Sexual Embodiment** - gradual acquisition of a sense of maleness/femaleness
2. **Gender Representation** – of a masculine or feminine self-concept & psycho-social expectations of appearance and performance of roles & activities
3. **Erotic desire** – revisions of hetero/homo attraction, including fantasies which may or may not be enacted in sexual activity. **Peer-defined expectations** about permissible expression of erotic desire to love & be loved by a member of one's own or the other sex.
4. **Generative Identity** - self representation as a potential pro-creator which may be expressed through creativity or actual reproduction

---

Adolescent girls tend towards **'internalising'** behaviours (withdrawal, depression, anxiety and somatic problems) and **boys** towards **externalising** behaviours (anti-social behaviour and aggression)
GROUP DISCUSSION – WHY?
Possibly linked to most early care being female: Little girl's difficulty differentiating: (Self-harming may be disguised attacks on her mother). Boys dis-identify from female mother to become 'masculine'.
The early mother's disapproval, demands, anxiety, shame or rejection are retained as **procedural** (bodily) rather than cognitive memories, expressed by same-sex daughter psychosomatically.
What are the effects of 'hands on' nurturing fathers?

---

*WHAT ARE SIGNS OF **EMOTIONAL PROBLEMS** IN ADOLESCENTS? (group discussion)*

Eating disorders: obesity; strict dieting, anorexia, bulimia
Addictions: excessive daydreams, shoplifting, compulsive masturbation, drugs, alcohol, gambling, promiscuity
Self-harm: neglect, cutting, burning, hair extraction, suicidal attempts
• severe mood fluctuation or long periods of rage
• severe anxiety with panic attacks or phobias
• incapacitating obsessional rituals & defences

TEEN CONCERNS

- Balancing tensions between
    dependence & self-sufficiency
- Struggle with **authority** over limits/rules
- Intrusion of **infantile** processes into adult
- Vacillation between trust in own creative capacity & need to prove fertility
- Preoccupations with **bodily changes**
    somatic experience
    physical appearance

---

or need for punishment: **INTERACTIVE SKILLS:**
Exploring unknown territory
Explore client's explanatory theory
- Summarize her/his problems & anxieties
- Help to find her/his own solutions
- Help endure uncertainty, frustrations, obstacles
- Help her/him to create **a coherent life story**
- Don't collude with her/his desire to please you
- Provide a *model* – to use in her/his own family
- **Admit your mistakes: repair misunderstandings**

Some issues can be explored in the Reflective Work Group, including how to encourage teens to think about causes, explanations & solutions to their problems, to reduce their own feelings of grievance, anxiety, self-blame

---

CONCLUSIONS

Practitioners should be able to identify adolescent disorders, including severe anxiety, repeated relational failures, reluctance to grow up and defensive strategies, especially obsessionality, risky behaviours, depression and suicide risk.

When disturbances are severe and beyond the remit of the practitioner, tactful negotiation with the teen & referral to appropriate therapeutic services is crucial, especially when a baby is involved.

IDENTIFY YOUR LOCAL RESOURCES

---

4. Skill Building Seminar:**Psychological Processes of Pregnancy & Teens as Parents**

Compulsory Sex & Relationship Education: learning about contraception, sexually transmitted infections & relationships.

"Straight Talking = understanding of consequences of becoming a parent…then able to make responsible choices about their future".

But does not deal w non-conscious motivation

- Anna Freud:'we do not deal with the happenings in the external world as such, but with their repercussions in the mind'

MOTIVATION FOR CONCEIVING?? [5 mins-ideas?]
- 'invincibility' or 'dicing' with fate: denying consequences of unprotected sex; to keep a failing relationship
- a desire to prove his/her fertility (vs. 'getting' a baby)
- seeking identity, purpose, value
- loneliness, low self-esteem, disillusionment
- to find 'someone to love'/ 'someone to love me'
- peer pressures/sanctioning or social rejection
- to become 'fully adult'/ to emulate mother
- to get out of home, or to find a home/get a home?
- an unconscious 'message' to her own parents
- to flesh out a fantasy baby
- a desire to recapture lost aspects of her [baby-]self
- to repair or renegotiate incomplete developmental tasks
- to create the 'perfect family'/rewrite history
- to cheat Death (especially when life-threatening illness)

What components contribute to the experience of PREGNANCY?
Three intertwining systems
- **Physiological experience:** new sensations, symptoms, tests/ultra-sound scans, physical complications interpreted through
- **Personal representations:** fantasies, hopes, fears and wishes within a representational set of complex connections of
- **Socio-cultural expectations** about pregnancy and maternal identity, collective beliefs, and the actual experience of emotional/social support systems and teen interactive networks.

Preoccupations in the 3 TRIMESTERS?
Pregnancy, Fetus, Baby

Pregnancy is informed by **social conditions & attitudes which change over time**

Pregnancy is a state of transition which can lead to self-discovery

Some teenagers have a benevolent (internal) mother others a witch

PREGNANCY/BABY = RECEPTACLE
for memories, wishes, fantasies projections and… expectations

---

When pregnancy is juxtaposed with adolescence
► DOUBLE CRISIS:
- bodily transformations of puberty & pregnancy
- body <u>ownership</u> ↔ two people in her body
- <u>separation </u>from her own mother while becoming a mother
- individuation while vulnerable & caring for a dependent baby

---

PREGNANT ADOLESCENTS – WORRIES?
Pregnancy transformation+unfamiliar pubertal body
Anxieties about her appearance as 'obese'
Shame (and/or pride): shown up as sexually active
Alarm at the uncontrollable nature of hormonal fluctuations, emotional lability and the baby's movements inside her
Pressure to prepare for the baby while uncertain of her own identity and emotional resources
Demands of school work whilst preoccupied; or if she leaves school, exclusion from ordinary peer-group activities and social isolation.
Anxieties about her capacity to cope with labour pains, and the stretching of her vagina.
Doubts about her ability to mother a baby

TWO IN ONE BODY
- Blurred boundaries between
- Self & other
- Female & male (femininity yet male fetus? Sperm?)
- Past & present (carrying fetus as mother carried her)
- Dread baby knows/will reveal her hidden feelings
- Sexually abused girls: enforced intimacy of pregnancy reactivates issues of bodily invasion.
- Anxieties about vaginal or internal damage in labour, and fantasies of bursting, being torn apart or emptied out.

DISEQUILIBRIUM IN PREGNANCY
Mood swings, mixed emotions; vivid dreams, magical thinking and 'premonitions'. Also some depressive reactions, primitive anxieties, intrusive thoughts, hypersensitivity, paranoid feelings…
Most fall of these within the normal range – but teens have double dose!
Worrying only if associated with behavioural risks to herself or her unborn child: i.e. suicidal fantasies, severe eating disorders, nicotine, alcohol or drug misuse; phobias, incapacitating obsessional rituals, panic attacks, compulsive self-harm or elevated risk of domestic violence
► **Referral for psycho-therapeutic help**.

Skills: identifying antenatal warning signs
PLACENTAL PARADIGM –
maternal representations

Self-as-mother	Fantasy baby	
(archaic mother)	(baby-self)	Manifestation:
Mixed: +-	+-	healthy mixed feelings
Fixed:+	+	idealisation
-	+	depression
+	-	persecution
-	-	anxiety
+|-	+|-	obsession
+/-	0	detachment

Fixed ideas can be tactfully addressed, with a possible referral for perinatal couselling

MATERNAL DISTURBANCE –
has implications for the UNBORN CHILD

- **Antenatal depression:** poor antenatal clinic attendance, low birth weight & preterm delivery.
- Intimate Partner **violence** increase in pregnancy
- 20-40% of depressed mothers also report **obsessional thoughts** of harming the child

Depression, persecution, anxiety & childhood abuse are associated with unhealthy eating & smoking, alcohol, drugs, self-harm; risk-taking behaviours incl.suicide, & abusive enactments

---

SKILLS: SCREENING STATEMENTS
for persistent feelings of 1.depression 2. anxiety
3.persecution 4. obsessionality 5. detachment

1. *During this pregnancy I have: had thoughts of hurting myself/ felt quite sad without knowing why*
2. *I have felt anxious/had panic attacks without knowing why*
3. *The baby seems an intruder or parasite inside me*
4. *I have strange ideas about hurting the baby*
5. *I don't let pregnancy affect my life one bit*

Co-habiting EXPECTANT FATHERS, like mothers have **stage-specific changes** in **hormone levels:** 'Wake-up call' - F's cortisol level spikes 4-6 wks after being told, with higher concentrations of prolactin & cortisol just before the birth; in F & Ms lower postnatal concentrations of sex steroids (testosterone/estradiol) [pro-lactin stimulates milk-production; raised cortisol in Ms who bond & are more sympathetic to baby's cries].
- Fathers – during the first 3 weeks after the birth - **testosterone** drops by ⅓ (sex-drive; competitiveness, aggression). Seems an adaptive response, decreased 'fight or flight' behaviours, less demand for sex.
Hormonal shifts in men seem to be sparked by <u>exposure</u> to the pregnant woman's hormones and may similarly prepare them for parenthood.

SUMMARY: THE TRANSITION TO PARENTHOOD conflicts with ordinary teenage preoccupations
A young parent needs 'time out' from all-consuming demands of baby-care for their own development. Otherwise, unmitigated care for the child will generate resentment leading to defences, distortions & a desire to escape.
Shock at the irreversability: "what have I done?"

GROUP EXERCISE: 5 minute small group discussion [2-5 people] and 3 minute report back to large group on: 'What are the negative **hall-marks of teen-age parenting?'**

Discrepancy between fantasy expectations & reality
- High self-expectations & fear of being seen to fail
- Less life-experience; putting own needs first;
- The baby as an 'extension', treated as 'thing' or doll
- Daily struggle – re housing, money, relationships
- Deprivation – feeling they have 'no life'
<u>Positive features:</u>
- Flexibility, spontaneity, 'going with the flow'
- Enjoying the moment – pregnancy and parenting are not 'projects' to be studied
- Keen to learn
- Playfulness: treat baby like a sibling
Less sentimentality: can be brutally honest about their subjective experiences ['Breastfeeding is gross'…]

TEEN PARENTING
- Baby-care is an incredibly demanding task.
- Single parents, unable to share, or to debrief.
- Very young parents lack experience & maturity. Many teen parents feel harassed, over-whelmed by premature full-time responsibility for the physical welfare and emotional needs of a dependent infant.
- Receptivity is risky. The capacity for empathy & competent reflective functioning are undermined at times of stress and adolescent self-absorption.
- **Fight, Flight** (escape) or **Freeze** are common defences to reduce anxiety.

Self Study – Group: watch
the Oscar winning film 'WASP',
produced & directed by
ANDREA ARNOLD, 2002 *[23 minutes].*
[Allow a few moments' silence after this very shocking film, then encourage a GROUP DISCUSSION [15-20 minutes]:
WHAT FEELINGS DID FILM AROUSE IN YOU?
Self-study: write reactions in your Journal

Anxiety – sense of impending disaster; physical fear (edge of seat). **Anger** at mother. Poor aggression control; **Sympathy** for young Mother caught in a trap: sacrifices – education; social life; growth; in state of limbo since her school-days; few friends; unsupportive community. Incomplete maturational tasks.
Yet Maternal affection; joy, love, care, spontaniety; care; benign neglect; acknowledges mistakes. **Sadness** for all. Kelly=young carer, overly streetwise but empathic & reflective; All kids: adult-world exposure; developed survival skills.
Should the kids be in care? [if not] what would help? Contraceptive advice; Support; continuity of care; respite training? utilising her own network; involving child/ren's father/s? Other family members? Couple work?

PRECIPITANTS of TEEN PARENT DISTURBANCE?
Lack of emotional support; Sleep deprivation
Preoccupation with own developmental issues
Difficulties controlling own aggression and/or establishing limits Chaotic management
Lone mother more vulnerable since no partner or confidante to mediate
• Child is more exposed to maternal disturbance, intrusion and/or control.
• A sense of 'induced guilt' in the child who has curtailed the young mother's freedom.
Practitioners working with teenage parents have at least **two clients** – whose wishes & developmental processes may sometimes coincide or clash.

RELATIONAL SKILLS
• Empathise with parenting difficulties. "Making mistakes is OK; we can learn from experience"
• Help young parent to **confront their own short-comings, drop grievances** & 'forgive' own parents
• Teaching client about the capabilities and needs of babies helps establish a more meaningful relationship
• Client's curiosity/insight into the complexity of mixed feelings helps withdraw **projections** from the baby
• Assuming responsibility for one's own feelings engenders **changes in self-representation**.
• Practitioners use their **emotional responses** to identify/understand anxiety and distress in client/s
•

Difficulties in detecting signs of risk in teens?

Some effects are Psychosomatic (trauma can affect immunologic functions and endocrine activities - reflected in restlessness, irritability, sleep disorders, hyper-vigilance, and hyper-arousal) in traumatised child and adolescent.

Some symptoms are also common transient 'storm & stress' (somatisation, eating disorders, depression and impulsive suicidal behaviour, hyper-sexuality, gender identity issues and antisocial behaviour)

CONCLUSIONS:
Parenthood disrupts adolescence: teen parent have acute emotional, intellectual, social, sexual and develop-mental needs of their own which are often at odds with those of their child/ren.
When extended families are dispersed, support-systems and childrearing traditions are eroded, many young mothers continue to describe intense feelings of despair, bewilderment, incompetence & loneliness, over the first two-three years.
RESPITE is essential for **SELF-RENEWAL**
If ordinary support brings no relief, it suggests a deeply rooted disturbance, needing *specialised help*.
Referral for perinatal counselling, parent-infant, couple or family therapy.

Adolescence as a 2nd Chance © devised by Professor Joan Raphael-Leff
MODULE III: BABIES IN TEEN FAMILIES

5. INTERACTIVE WORKSHOP
ATTUNEMENT, ATTACHMENT & ORIENTATIONS

GROUP EXERCISE: 'HOME IS WHERE WE START FROM':

*Each person writes down **5 words associated with 'home'.***
Leader asks for examples of these – writing them on flip chart.
Show of hands for the most common of these –' security, predictability, warmth, comfort', etc.

HOME = 'SECURE BASE'

'hothouse' for infant to develop confidence/ belonging

Not **place** but emotional **'climate'** of *interactive processes* within which baby's mind is constituted

Ideally, baby is recognised and enjoyed

- With reliable responsiveness the baby becomes aware of the continued existence of carers even in their <u>absence</u>.
- **Emotional climate** is **internalised**
- Baby may create a **'transitional object'** (dummy, teddy, 'security blanket', etc) to represent safety.

OBSERVATION: It is useful but difficult to observe an interaction.
Partly because we only see a small bit and cannot be sure it is representative.
And partly because we are unreliable observers, even of something we look at frequently:

GROUP EXERCISE: *What is the Google colour sequence?*

GROUP OBSERVATION: *3 minute DVD [baby on sofa]*

- What did you see?
- *WATCH THE PIECE AGAIN – focus on your own 'counter-transference' feelings*
- What did you feel? What did the baby feel?
- What is her understanding of the world?
- What might you have said in the situation?

Interpersonal engagement promotes **a particular understanding of the world.**

BRIEF DISCUSSION on an 'observational stance'
  - being respectful and trying to be objective
  - aware the camera is an intrusion

*

CAREGIVING IS INTUITIVE

- Rooted in 'procedural' knowledge from having been babies ourselves - but
- <u>**Parents**</u> vary in attentiveness; ability to recognise cues; internal representation of the baby – as vulnerable, sociable or parasitic, benign or mean…
- <u>**Newborns**</u> vary in constitutional & temperamental factors, degree of alertness, clarity of cues

Unless processed, carers usually do what was done to them →*'Transgenerational transmission' of care*

Brain circuits & behaviour are shaped by caregiving patterns: emotionally damaging effects of parental depression, abuse and neglect are associated with **permanent maladaptive response patterns**.

COMMUNICATION:

Most carers speak a form of *'motherese'* – a high pitched, repetitive, rhythmic baby-talk.

Early 'proto-conversation' 'turn-taking' statement & reply becomes→ a **dialogue**

In DIALOGUES: Misunderstandings, disruptions & mismatched responses ALWAYS occur.

The crucial aspect is **REPAIR** (Tronick, 1989)

We apologise for and learn from our mistakes

Each mother-infant dyad co-create a unique emotional climate

A way of testing this - The Strange Situation: standard test of 1yr old's responses: to a **brief separation & reunion** with carer, and meeting **stranger]**.

ATTACHMENT

Bowlby: human babies seek **proximit**y to their carers as a means of protection against **danger** - through a series of innate behaviours [which??]

- **sucking, crying, smiling, following** and **clinging**.

The carer's **availability** & attentive **responsiveness** contributes to a baby's internal feeling of SECURITY giving him/her the confidence ability to tolerate brief separations, using the carer as a **'SECURE BASE'** from which to explore the (external & internal) world.

Prompt response in early months▶baby cries less later

SECURE ATTACHMENT = expectation that distress will be met by comforting. **Insecure:**coping strategies

Child behaves differently with different attachment figures

When distressed: A **'securely** attached' infant seeks **contact**; rapidly comforted by carer who 'holds' baby in mind.
• **Insecure 'avoidant':** if carer is *dismissive* of emotions, controlling, intrusive, rejecting or neglectful, the toddler defensively **deactivates** the need for attachment▶pseudo-independent (seems indifferent; avoids carer after a separation)
• If parent is inconsistently enmeshed & withdrawn, child exhibits features of **insecure 'anxious' attachment,** with heightened vigilance; little spontaneous exploration in carer's presence. When separated very distressed; on reunion **mixed** responses: **seeking/resisting contact.**
• If parent preoccupied with past issues of trauma or loss child: **'disorganized'** attachment **disoriented behaviour** freezing, approach-avoidance, dissociation, head-banging disorientation re carer's frightening/abusive responses.

Through cumulative experience the child evolves an inner representation of primary attachment figures: an **'Internal Working Model'** [IWM] forming an *expectation* of future relationships (Bowlby, 1969).

Security: learning to manage own sadness, anger & anxieties in a safe context with responsive carer who 'survives' without collapsing, retaliating or attacking.

In later life, this **secure inner core** offers protection at stressful times. **Adolescents'** 'romantic' contacts are shaped by their early attachment. Secure Teens = 'higher quality' love relationships (Roisman,2005).

Insecure practitioners work better with people of their same strategy vs. secure practitioners who can contrast with clients (Dozier, et al, 1993)

ATTACHMENT & MIND

Secure attachment: a **coherent** rep. of self-with-carer

Insecure attach: involves **inconsistent experiences** with caregivers▶relationship is split into unintegrated persecutory & idealized representations (Fonagy et al)

Secure attachment = confident exploration of external world + exploration of the 'internal world'= awareness of mental states: reflective capacity

vs. **Insecure** attachment either involves a defensive ignoring of the mental contents of the other's mind (avoidant attachment), over-involvement with the mind of the other (anxious-ambivalent attach), or hyper-attunement to other's mental states & neglect of own mental states (disorganized/disoriented)

What about young mothers?

21st century – INDIVIDUALISED PARENTING PRACTICES: now determined by subjective beliefs, conscious wishes & unconscious desires rather than childcare traditions

Choice of own **PARENTAL ORIENTATION**

A mixture of **collective experience** & **personal expectations**

incorporating the [expectant] parent's **'internal working model'** =self-perception, representations of the baby and of the relationship between them.

Predictable from antenatal representations

(Raphael-Leff, 2005)

FACILITATOR		REGULATOR
♀uniquely privileged		♂ are privileged
enjoys pregnancy		'necessary evil'
dual identification		resists introspection
	labour/birth?	
Natural birth		'Civilized' birth
exciting		humiliating
	identity?	
'MOTHER'		'PERSON'
Vocation	*mothering?*	Skill
Exclusive		Shared
Intuitive		Routine
M & Baby	primary unit	Sexual couple

FACILITATOR		REGULATOR
MOTHER ADAPTS		BABY ADAPTS
'baby knows'		'experts know'
gratification	aim	socialization
exclusive	care	shared
	security?	
Mother's presence		routine
	feeding?	
Permissive; frequent		*schedule*
late	**weaning**	*early*
	sleep?	
Parents' bed		*own room*
	crying?	
communication		'real' vs. noise

RECIPROCATORS

Parenting based on empathy [not identification like Facilitator or dis-identification, like Regulator]

Baby seen as similar because s/he has human emotions but different because still immature

Parental capacity to mentalize & tolerate uncertainty

▶ Flexible **negotiotions** (rather than adaptation)

FATHERS

Participator	Reciprocator	Renouncer
Primary care	Shared care	'Traditional'

---

2 Role Plays: six week point
2 sets of 2 volunteers [2 minutes each]

- *ROLE PLAY 1: A Facilitator talking about her mothering experience with a practitioner [group decides which professional]*

Feedback: *group, and role-players while still in role*

- *ROLE PLAY 2: A Regulator discussing her mothering experience with a practitioner [group decides on profession]*

UNCONSCIOUS FACTORS

FACILITATOR		REGULATOR
sociable	*newborn rep*	pre/anti-social
innate personality		bec.person later
recognises mother		undifferentiating
M's ideal self	*baby*	split-off weakness
'fusion'	*aim*	independence
Idealisation	*mother's defences*	Control
Vicarious gratification		Dissociation/detachment
fear of hating	*anxiety*	fear of loving

---

3 significant clusters: Fac/Reg/Recip

<u>Birth:</u> **Regulators** – more elected C sections

<u>PND:</u> **Regulator** increased risk PNP 1st 6 weeks: feel more anxious, less confident,deskilled, inadequate **Facilitators** PND due to enforced separation; birth interventions; complications ('perfect' start is spoilt)

<u>Night waking:</u>

More frequent in 1st born **Facilitator** babies linked to maternal separation anxiety. At 2 years child still requires/receives maternal intervention to regain sleep vs. Regulator's baby reported to sleep through the night by 5 wks.

Infants of **Conflicted** mothers take significantly longer to fall asleep (25 vs.11 minutes), wake later

LINKS WITH ATTACHMENT THEORY

Maternal orientation at <u>6 months</u> discriminates among Insecure & Secure infants (confirmed by Strange Situation at 1 yr).

Reciprocators+ moderate Fac & Reg **= SECURE**

Extreme **Facilitator** = enmeshed (baby **ambivalent**)

Ext.**Regulators**= dismissive control (baby **avoidant**)

Conflictual = preoccupied (baby **disorganized**)
(Scher 2001.JRIP, 19:325-333)

Discussion: CAN ORIENTATION CHANGE with next baby? WHY would it?

FACTORS AFFECTING ORIENTATION
PSYCHOLOGICAL?
Psycho-historical & current variables
Motivation for conception
Degree of emotional support/ confidante
SOCIOECONOMIC?
Age, employment/career status
Number of children & gaps between them
Partner? Social/economic pressures
Cultural expectations
Life events
PHYSIOLOGICAL?
Pregnancy/birth complications
Postnatal health, hormonal swings/sleep
EXPERIENCE OF PARENTING

'CONTAGIOUS AROUSAL' (JRL, 1991)

Reactivation of teen's own infantile emotions due to exposure to the **baby's 'primitive' non-verbal emotions** & to **primal substances** [amniotic fluid, milk, blood, urine, feces]. Old sibling rivalries revived

Exacerbated by

• **little previous contact with babies**
• **lack of preparation for emotional impact of baby**
• **Lack of emotional and practical support & developmental guidance**
• High risk of emotional disturbance if own mother had PND or died before teen's puberty (Brown & Harris)

REVIVED CHILDHOOD EXPERIENCE

The intimate non-verbal exchange revitalises the teen-parent's unprocessed feelings

Resilient people with insecure upbringing who process their deprivation become <u>Reciprocators</u>.

Some <u>Fac/Reg</u> actively utilise parenthood to rework & resolve old experiences, forgiving their parents.

For conflicted parents, parenting feels very threatening: The risk is controlled by **over-indulging the baby** and/or **maintaining emotional distance**. They need support & frequent respite if contagious arousal renders the mixed state of total-devotion and **persecution** overwhelming.

<u>Troubling cases</u>: need referral to joint-fostering or a mother-baby unit to support the healthier aspects of the relationship.

CONTEMPORARY TEEN FAMILIES

Western societies in a state of transition: USA/UK teen pregnancy 40+ per 1,000 under 18 [but not in Japan, Switzerland, Holland, Sweden, despite equally young sexual activity (less than 7 per 1,000)]. WHY?

Lower cognitive-linguistic abilities in the children of teen mothers: WHY?

high PND rates, homework, dis-regulatory effects of poor mentalization. Less dialogue. Possibly effects of pubertal brain physiology & biochemistry (Field, 1998)

Low educational achievement strongly associated with poorly paid jobs, child poverty & social disadvantage.

CONCLUSIONS

Babies need to be recognised as themselves – to be talked to, enjoyed & stimulated

<u>Secure babies</u> internalise a safe 'secure base' where distress is comforted & misunderstandings repaired.

<u>Insecure babies</u> develop defensive responses to an 'internal working model' of untrustworthy care

<u>Facilitator/Reciprocator/Regulator</u> orientations to parenting are based on the mother's subjective perception of pregnancy, birth, baby & mothering

<u>Parenting</u> reactivates unresolved infantile issues through '<u>contagious arousal</u>'

<u>Fathers</u>, too, manifest perinatal disturbances, including depression or violence

<u>Practitioners</u> can offer containment, support & referral

6. Skill-building Seminar
BABIES –REFLECTIVE FUNCTION IN TEEN PARENTS

OBJECTIVES
- Better understanding of the child's representational world
- Basic Mentalization techniques.
- Skills for enhancing attunement, emotional regulation and contingent responsiveness.

EMPATHY
From birth a baby is biologically 'wired' to be **a 'social partner'** – seeking and eliciting affection & a sense of belonging. By attributing **mental states** to their infant and sharing their own, carers help baby recognise his/her own feelings and those of others. Amazingly small babies both **communicate** feelings of pain, puzzlement joy & frustration and **register** the feelings of others, **feeling for them**: newborns cry on hearing another infant's cry. **'Mirror neurones'** allow **the baby's mind to mirror the minds of others** – resonating with feelings and imitating simple actions. The basis of HUMAN SELFHOOD is EMPATHY – compassionate resonating to the suffering of others, contagious laughter, anxiety, excitement, anger...

CONTAINMENT
- Our earliest experiences are bodily based, recorded somatically in states of arousal and quiescence.
- For the infant to represent these experiences in the mental realm - they must be received and processed by a carer who acts as a 'CONTAINER' for the raw, unmanageable feelings & transforms this nameless distress & confusion into tolerable, *thinkable* experiences. Other impressions remain somatic.
- By gradually 'internalising' the mother or father's capacity the child evolves a 'space' to think thoughts, and begins to process his/her own feelings (Bion,1962) *Infant mental health is a function of shared emotions and intentions within the **family system** as a whole*

If the parent is too depressed, preoccupied or over-whelmed to be receptive, the infant prematurely takes on the function of *self-containment* or even acts as *'container' for the parent,* becoming adept at fathoming feelings.
When abusive 'ghosts' from the parent's past intrude the baby is enlisted into old scenarios, unconsciously representing part of the self or a figure from the past

This **distorted dialogue** creates **deficits** in the child's ability to perceive his/her emotions, as s/he **absorbs** the parent's ascriptions & projections into own self-image, feeling guilty, dangerous, unworthy, despised... PRACTITIONERS also manage anxiety by <u>containing</u> their own feelings and <u>reflecting back</u> teen's & baby's.

SELF-CONTAINMENT:
The baby's exquisite sensitivity to his/her own subjective experience and resonance to what others are feeling can be **overwhelming.**
A newborn is dependent on the carer's capacity to **regulate arousal & to reduce confusion & anxiety.**

Carers who believe in the baby's mind & recognise his/her struggle to make sense of the world **'contain'** the baby's feelings & **feed back** a 'digested' version.
- Kept within tolerable bounds enables the baby to learn to 'contain' own positive & negative emotions.
- To **self-soothe** [inhibit crying; fall asleep; 'sing'] **& to regulate interactive** arousal [gaze aversion; calling].

DEVELOPMENTAL GUIDANCE: How do practitioners enhance parent-infant interaction?
- by helping carer recognise baby's **growing mind**
- demonstrating **early capacities**: innate sociability; human face preference; seeking contact; voice/smell recognition; mirroring; conversational pause/turn-taking; protective gaze avoidance...
- showing the importance of **emotional regulation, conversation** and **repair** of misunderstandings
- helping them note **two-way sequences** of interactive responses such as turning away; signs of separation anxiety; different emotional levels (alert inactivity to fussy, drowsy less attentive states of consciousness) which require different responses.
- encouraging better **attunement** & parental **reflective function** through moments of mutual gratification

Teen parents: 'REFLECTIVE FUNCTION':
• Carer's understanding of baby's behaviour in terms of **'mental states'** (thoughts, motivations) and their capacity to keep *the child's mind in mind:* thinking of the child's needs as **separate from their own**.
• Young people have difficulty recognising a baby's feelings when these parallel/clash with their own.
• Many young parents <u>don't believe</u> babies *can* feel sadness or fear, or sense parental moods, but do think infant's *should* control their emotions (although research shows this only occurs around 3-5 years!).
• Studies find that <u>teen mothers</u> *report* feeling sympathy but have **lower physiological arousal** to baby-cries (than older mothers), possibly due to brain neural immaturity

---

Family interaction provides the most basic form of shared understanding.
• With babies carers intuitively speak **'motherese'**– high pitched, repetitive, rhythmic. Spontaneously match/mirror the baby's prevailing emotional 'mood'.
• Exaggerated **'social biofeedback'** helps child to recognise his/her own emotions, distinct from the carer's (Gergley & Watson, 1996).
• The carer's **reflective function** helps child to develop a *'theory of mind'* - that s/he and others have a **'mind'** – of feelings, thoughts, intentions and expectations.
• The child practices, explores and gradually integrates feelings through 'pretend' play.
Dawning self-consciousness of being seen through the eyes of the other.

SKILL BUILDING: fostering parental reflective functioning
• being **'voice'** of the baby
• helping client think about the **child's viewpoint**: asking
For: - *'running commentary'* on the baby's thoughts
       - *their view of normal developmental patterns*
       - *best/worst case scenarios, etc.*
2 tier questions (for Practitioner):*'What do you think your client was thinking when s/he became scared/upset/angry? How did it make you feel? How would you have wanted this scenario to work out differently?'*
Fostering insight: *'In what way do you think your client's reaction was different or similar to your own?' 'Does this make you think of anything similar you might have experienced in the past?'* <u>NOW</u> apply to client & child
• Then promote more complex **systemic understanding**: *'What do you think your client/child thought you were feeling?*

EMOTIONAL CLIMATES
• each infant-carer dyad *co-constructs* the meaning, nature and quality of primary experience.
• the carer's *reflective capacity, attunement, emotional regulation*, and *contingent responsiveness* to the baby's needs are prerequisites for the infant's attachment & emergent representational world.
• internalised, this 'emotional climate' of in/security is drawn upon at times of stress.
• When what is internalised is a climate of **danger or confusion**, it is retriggered at times of high arousal, when others (including the baby) may be seen as persecutors

---

OBSERVATION & *discussion: young father putting on his son's trousers: Discussion: attuned? secure/insecure?*
• Baby's responsiveness & identification with the other's 'stance', facilitates a **temporarily shift of perspective**, with growing sensitivity to his/her differing view/ meaning of the same reality [clothes must be worn; I'm busy – not rejecting...] ►
enhanced self-awareness: being seen through the others' eyes
• Moments of **mutual gratification** secure positive aspects of their relationship, allowing feelings of love to develop between them, strong enough to survive healthy ambivalence, and inevitable passing irritation, frustration.

TECHNIQUES TO ACTIVATE MENTALIZATION
(adapted from mentalization-based therapy training)
<u>Always ask yourself</u>:
• *I wonder how I make the other person feel?*
• *How does the client's perception of me impact on the encounter?* (and vice versa).
<u>Give the client</u> an opportunity to think about her/his own mind (recognising that this may feel scary at first)
Capitalise on curiosity – our own and client's.
<u>Offer client</u> a language to think about her/his feelings
Admit mistakes and laugh at ourselves.
Pitch things at an appropriate level (don't be too clever)
The young parent who can express his/her own feelings can be enabled to think about **the baby's**

AFFECT REGULATION:
• Infant-Carer **reciprocal coordination** of inner & relational processes: *self-soothing & mutual regulation* **Influences** are 'bi-directional': co-creative processes produce a **unique dyadic baby-carer pattern** of 'expectancies' of being together.
• Baby's with little help in modulating affect▶ 1st year disturbance: hyper-arousal, excessive crying, feeding & sleep difficulties arousing parental hostility.
• Eventually, the unsupported baby becomes impassive, no longer expecting help.
• Carers who cannot monitor/modify their <u>own</u> negative feelings <u>create</u> stress & stimulus overload, leaving the baby with his/her own anxieties + an intrusion of chaotic feelings from the carer

FAILURES OF AFFECT REGULATION
Recent research suggests that **over-stimulation** (where parents allow experience to exceed the baby's threshold barrier), or **chronic deprivation** & unpredictable, **disrupted care** necessitate *continual over-activity* of the infant's own emotional systems. A child may then become **habituated to stress overload.** When carers do not help the stressed baby to recover, this may lead to a distorted bio-chemical baseline that may provoke neuronal loss. **Chronic states of intense arousal** in infancy have been linked to ADHD, over-vigilance, anxiety, panic disorders, depression, eating disorders, addictions and borderline personalities in later life.

INNATE 'ALARM SYSTEMS'
• **Overactive** or conversely, under perpetual bombardment, may **defensively shut down**, or are managed by **denial, dissociation** or **obsessional-compulsive defences**, including harm-avoidant preoccupations & rituals intended to control all unpredictable eventualities.

High levels of early stress accompanied by chronic feelings (such as sadness, wariness, alienation), lead to persistent personality traits (shyness, guilt, shame or low mood [203].

CONCLUSIONS:
• Baby-carer patterns of interaction form the basis of the child's **representational world.**
• **Representations of others** (as helpful, soothing, playful, or pressurising, frustrating, etc) derive from repeated experiences with carers.
• These coalesce into *'working models'* of expectations, peopling the child's inner world.
• **Representations of the self** as *an effective agent* arise out of the carer's responsiveness, allowing the baby to feel s/he is **influential**
Insecurity & powerlessness lead to abuses

Insensitively raised babies have difficulty in organising and modulating their own emotional states

When **misattunement** is a chronic situation, the baby cannot learn to develop a smooth transition between emotional states, living in a state of **hyper-arousal** with deficits in self-regulation.

Defences (hyper-vigilance or dissociation) are brought in as strategies to avoid unmanageable affects and ward off unpredictable intrusions.

Parental stress manifests as behavioural deficits, defence patterns & personality disorders in the child.

Note:
Self reflection applies to the practitioner as well. Ask yourself the same sort of questions as you would your client: *"What was I thinking when that situation arose? How did it make me feel? Would I have wanted it to pan out differently? In what way? Does it remind me of anything I experienced previously?"*
Write your comments in your private Learning Journal

Adolescence as a 2nd Chance ©
Project leader
Professor Joan Raphael-Leff
MODULE IV
TODDLERS IN TEEN FAMILIES

7. Interactive Workshop
EXTENDING BOUNDARIES
Attachment/Separation-individuation
Imaginative Play

OBJECTIVES:
By the end of the study day you will
• understand different phases of the '**Separation-Individuation**' process: Practice, 'Rapprochement' Oedipal conflicts and 'moving on'
• learn to identify different **underlying motivations** as reflected in changes in primary relationships
• improve your capacity to **observe** toddler–parent interactions and to identify **emotional difficulties** that may arise in teen-toddler relations
• become aware of the **young father**'s needs and consequences of his absence
• be better able to identify signs and symptoms of **parental disturbance**

Which 2 forces organize lifelong identity formation?
close **connectedness** (attachment) & *separation – individuation* (recognition of selfhood/separateness)

• The tension between these two poles is heightened during **toddlerhood** & again in **adolescence** (also set off by marriage, parenthood, immigration, meno-pause, etc), when **earlier developmental issues are revisited** - reworked and transformed into enduring, yet flexible organized structures within our minds, composed of multiple self-images, self-with-other representations and revised expectations…

---

a. **'PRACTISING' STAGE: ~11-15 months**
• New upright perspective & freed hands
• Toddler's *'love affair with the world'* (Greenacre)
• *Experimentation* ~ 6 hours a day of imitating and practising new physical and verbal skills (toddling, speaking, clapping, singing, pointing…)
• *Pleasure* in bodily sensations and new capacities.
• *Trial separations* - need for a **'secure base'**.
Exploration→ leads to **forbidden** activities/places.
Previously permissive parents now issue a prohibition every 9 minutes! (Schore, 1994)→Anxiety about loss of parent's love
'Social referencing' - 'checking' carer's face for encouragement; to see if activity is safe/repulsive, etc

---

b.'**RAPPROCHEMENT**': 16-24ms: awareness of limits
• **Self esteem** - pride in increased competence
• **Clash** between desire for omnipotent autonomy & carer's banning socially unacceptable habits.
• The previously 'invincible' toddler is saddened by own limitations and outraged by encroachments
• **Attachment/separation-individuation processes** arouse both defiance & anxiety (clinging), requiring empathic responsiveness to child's contradictory needs.
• **'Regressions'** are attempts at 'rapprochement' with carer: increasing **concern** & **remorse** with recognition that the attacked hated 'bad' carer & loved 'good' one are the same person. If non-retaliatory response→ **internal 'good-enough' carer.** Affirmation of trust. Mastery over intensified separation anxiety

---

OBSERVATION – a young toddler venturing out but needing 'emotional refuelling'
What did you see? Watch it again
CONCLUSION: to be confident a young toddler needs a 'safe base' for confidence and 'emotional refuelling' to keep going. When this is not sufficiently encouraging, s/he gives up.
Practitioners can encourage toddler and parent to **discover** pleasure in each other's company through **play**, **curiosity** and **humour** helping the carer to provide a safe base and sufficient 'refuelling' – both strengthening the attachment relationship and promoting separation and individuation.

TODDLER & ADOLESCENT = SIMILAR DYNAMICS:
Defiance & anxiety. A bid for separateness. Self-assertion coupled with powerful internal struggles.
Contradictory impulses of love/ hate, competition/ concern

Tasks: managing own body, rage & sexual feelings.
Similar anxieties: fear of separation yet also dread of merger. Own aggression↔loss of love; How to repair?
Teen parent/toddler have a bond of **mutual excitement**.
Yet **passionate reactions** of fury or despair and potentially **clashing goals**► BATTLE OF WILLS!

What typifies the 'TERRIBLE TWO' ERA?
Tantrums, bossiness; negativism if thwarted. Escaping, dawdling, choosing own clothes/ activities, refusing toilet training, playing with food/ faeces, resisting help.
TEENS &TOTS challenge & antagonise each other
Boundary setting may be difficult for a teen who is unable to do so yet for him/herself.
TEEN: loss of control→ emotional retaliation, sarcasm, threats, aggressive teasing, physical harshness, violence

TODDLER's response: defiant disobedience; running away or hiding; accident proneness; over-compliance or antisocial behaviour as a **defence** against further abuse and/or a means of expressing anxiety, anger & distress

---

c. 'Moving on': 3 ½ - 4 ½
Older child's greater ability & confidence in physical skills, bodily control: hop, skip, jump, run, swim, scoot, eat neatly, use toilet.
Oedipal conflicts – wanting parent's complete love
Both Toddler & Teen must recognise realistic limitations and **differences:** between child/adult needs; between the perspectives of different generations, genders, …

New social capacities: Language, symbolic thought.
More reflective imaginative play (including hidden feelings).
Gradual internalisation of constraints→ growth of an **internal conscience.** *Why?* Phase: concern with rules

---

Observation: Senior toddler – restraining himself (cake)
- Struggle to be 'good'. Needing parental help in self-restraint, and explanations of reasons for restrictions.
Needing forgiveness & reassurance when s/he fails.
- Learning through play
What is the importance of play?
- It fosters a variety of **crucial functions** for the developing mind. It offers opportunities for **learning & emotional expression**
- **Observation** – 2 toddlers (early & late) playing with shredded paper [NOTE: different levels of play between them] **What did you see?**
- Play provides an exciting activity that enhances social bonding
- Oulets for energy and mild aggression
- Way to test hypotheses and to fulfil desires.

Play: is an innate, primary emotional function of the mammalian brain

Play extends experience   [picture:playful animal/s]
Promotes neuronal growth
& mastery of behaviours

Animals play in response
to direct sensory stimuli but
human play can utilise
the **imagination** - to leap
beyond restrictions of the
immediate material reality

IMAGINATION =
the capacity to form a mental representation of an ABSENT OBJECT
[picture:cave paintings?]

Maternal attunement fosters an **illusion of omnipotence** that baby 'created the world'
Mother's **'graduated failures'** ►baby becomes aware of her absence & separateness
Baby learns to **play alone** in m/other's safe presence.
Later creates own **INTER-MEDIATE PLAY SPACE** between **internal/ external world,** illusion, imagination, fantasy, reflection [Winnicott]
BUT if **M Fails:** baby develops a **'FALSE' SELF** [insecure Attachment] ► **distortion/ inhibition of play**

Imagination grows through awareness of LACK

Baby creates A TRANSITIONAL OBJECT that symbolises their relationship

Linus blanket

In **BABYHOOD**: co-constructed & solitary play:
- innate *imitation (tongue extrusion–hours after birth; facial expressions & gestures [mirror neurones]; play acting, reciprocal feeding; baby-doll care).*
- *oral play (sucking, mouthing, biting, chewing, blowing bubbles, spitting, kissing, babbling).*
- *body-action games (tickling, suspense & surprise (repetitive rituals - 'round the garden'; masturbation?)*
- learning body parts *('this little piggy', 'head & shoulders, knees and toes)*
- mutual exploration of objects *(give & take (reciprocal offers, 'ta' handover, 2ndary subjectivity)*
- Later: games signifying *loss & being found (peek-a-boo, drop & recover, jack-in-box; hide-and-seek)* **control over separation and reunion**

Early Toddlerhood: ADVENTURE & DISCOVERY!
Greater mobility▶ greater *anxieties/ excitement of flight & reunion*

'PRETEND' PLAY: imaginative exploration of the **social world** – trying on different roles & new perspectives, practising activities; learning to express and control feelings

Increased BODY CONTROL – preoccupation with orifices, products & skills: *sensual messiness/order (self-feeding; food/mud play; finger-paints; categories)*

OEDIPAL PERIOD: Power & Limitations: *(domination; exhibitionism, voyeurism, magic, omnipotent building/ demolishing, super-powers, competitive board & electronic games).*

Mastery over disturbing experience by reality-testing

- Imaginative play can compensate for painful reality restrictions & frustrations.
- Fosters & restores self esteem
Increasing capacity for Reflective Play *(what I and others are feeling inside)*

'**Make believe**' respects both **internal/external** worlds

From imitation [phone to ear] to 'pretence' [banana = telephone], & 'psychic equivalence' [fantasy = reality] to imaginative play, around age 4 a child develops more **reflective** play (Fonagy & Target, 1996):
- Recognises that others have a different perspective
- Tries to envision what others feel & think
- Becomes aware that one's own mind is **private** → greater capacities for **secrecy, teasing & lying**:
- Judging how much to share; creating social alliances and forming discriminatory intimate connections.

IN SUM: imaginative play is **multifunctional**.
Used to:
- PROCESS anxiety-provoking situations & complex ideas
- COMPENSATE for painful frustrations
- RECOGNISE & ACTUALISE facets of the inner world in the external one
- CULTIVATE A PLURALITY of experiences through a variety of alternative conceptual narratives/roles of self and others
- increase UNDERSTANDING of **social** procedures – (modifying expression of sexuality & aggressiveness)
- PLAN ahead; rehearse possibilites
- DEVELOP INVENTIVENESS - by fostering new combinations & reformulation of his/her personal world.

---

*SKILL BUILDING: **WATCH, WAIT AND WONDER***
- *Practitioner invites teen mother to sit on the floor with her infant/toddler for 10 minutes, to watch and simply **responsively follow his/her lead**, without taking over or guiding the play activity.*
- *In parallel, the practitioner's role is to watch, wait, and wonder about **interactions** between mother and child without intervening or commenting.*
- *Later, **discussion with mother** about her feelings, anxieties about non-structured play and risks of following the infants' lead.*

TEEN PARENTS CAN BE FUN!!!

However, those who have **missed out on play** in their childhoods or currently feel **deprived of their own play-time** may resent or not know how to provide a joyful play experience for their child.

How does parent's non-engaged play manifest?
in repetitive games; intrusive play; overstimulation.
A managerial attitude controlling the child's play (constantly presenting new toys or removing toys from reach. Competition over play with toys, 'bossing' the child or excluding him/her from games; inhibiting imaginative play)

BOOK-READING & JOINT IMAGINATIVE PLAY can expand teen/child's <u>shared world</u> (inventive use of clothes, boxes, packaging, furniture, etc).

VULNERABILITY

Play: a transitional state between 'me' & 'not me' inner & outer worlds, experimental activity & relaxed **defences**→players are **vulnerable:** *'Playing is always liable to become frightening'* unless it takes place in a protective area, like that initially shared with a trustworthy, sensitive m/other (Winnicott, 1971:58).

OBSERVATION: <u>Toddler & mother playing with shredded paper</u>. *Discuss possible reasons for her shut-down and its effect on the child. Is her reaction dissociation or a game? What is his reaction to the younger toddler? Watch it again*

Distinguishing reality/'pretence' depends on the child's clear sense of the carer's capacity to do so.

• For the child – a carer's distorted response breaks the 'frame' of expectations - creating confusion between play & reality
• Frightening when a carer projects his/her own disowned feelings into mutual play, or are too deeply affected.
For a troubled carer - unstructured play feels risky – it can unleash frightening ideas. Results in their dissociation or concrete enactments.

Leads to child's controlled repetitive play and impoverished or over-active frightening fantasy life.

TODDLER PLAY GROUPS provide a **safe** play place
• Encourage parents to **share** their toddlers' play
• child can use play to express excited feelings & to master anxieties; learn to communicate in words and distinguish fantasy & reality.
• Staff facilitate interaction among parents; support them in managing child's aggression/setting limits.
• Practitioners may speak directly **to** the child about what s/he is feeling, or **for** him/her, to make carer aware of the child's emotional state and enlist a contingent response.

SKILLS:

By naming and verbalising the child's feelings and supplying words to identify and legitimise his/her experience, practitioners help child & carer feel less overwhelmed, out of control and/or alone with unknown emotions

ROLE PLAY: Mother, Toddler & Play leader

CONCLUSIONS:

Imaginative play builds on interactions with internalised 'collaborative partners'. Teen parents so close to their own childhoods, may use play with the toddler a means of completing their own developmental growth; others find it challenging, threatening to arouse unresolved issues. Play also reveals interactive distress. Anxious or traumatised children who have not internalised a safe home display repetitive, monotonous play to defend against unbearable arousal, or chaotic enactments in an attempt to make sense of their predicament.

8. Skill Building Seminar
CONTEMPORARY PARENTOOD
Emotional Disturbances in Teen Parents:

YOUNG FATHERS *What is the paternal role?*
• Previously was seen as breadwinner. Often ignored or excluded by practitioners.
• Today, better support for young fathers (or couple).
• But most providers seem unaware that **80%** of the babies born to teenage mothers are conceived within **an ongoing relationship;** 78% of these young pairs register the baby's birth together
• However, practitioner's expectations of paternal involvement in pregnancy, in antenatal classes, labour and 'hands on' fathering are less likely to be met if the pregnancy was unintended, in a casual encounter.

CONTEMPORARY PARENTS:
Gender-convergence with sexual-equality in education & job prospects. Parenting roles are less polarised.
• In today's economic climate, men less employable than women→**more primary carer fathers**
• Previous research focused on parental **differences:**
Mothers seen to provide empathy, soothing, singing, emotional support while **fathers** worldy stimulation; concern with discipline, temper tantrums, sleep disruption & food fads. Contemporary research:
Similarity between the sexes: Fathers can be as nurturing & sensitive as mothers. **Parental styles** are not sex-related but a function of primary vs. secondary care. **Intimate familiarity improves cue recognition**

Boisterous play-style and realistic risk-taking
- encourages robustness
More **complex language** (less baby-talk) - encourages toddler's verbal facility
Focus on exploration & competitiveness boosts confidence in 2-3 year old child
Differences among fathers
…a father can be 'hands on' or defended against emotional arousal
ROLE PLAY: *5 minutes*
Tantrum throwing toddler; 'Escapist' absentee father. Concerned mother. Mediating Practitioner
After audience comments, ask players (still in role) about their feelings during this exchange

ADOLESCENT FATHERS >50% have ever lived with their child. *Non-resident biological fathers* at risk of losing contact: 20%–40% see their children less than once per week. 20-39% not in a year.
Research findings: under-involved teen fathers were brought up in stressful environments with insensitive, harsh or unpredictable carers (often in poor neighbour-hoods in large, low-socioeconomic status families with lone-mothers who have low educational aspirations). Compared to resident fathers: insecure attachments, low threshold for anxiety and anger; high alcohol and marijuana dependency. More often disabled by mental health or drug problems; engaged in illegal or abusive behaviour; more criminal convictions (Jaffee et al, 2001).

TRANSGENERATIONAL ISSUE: lone mothers are generally poorer, and more likely to suffer from depression, stress, and other emotional, psychological and health problems.

Children living without fathers are more likely to
• live in poverty and deprivation
• have more trouble in school & socially
• have higher risk of health problems
• run away from home
• suffer physical, emotional, or sexual abuse(O'Neill, 2002)
In father's absence another partner male/female, her own mother can co-parent.
Most important: The image of <u>Father in Mother's mind</u>

<u>Teens living without fathers</u> are more likely to
• become teenage parents
• suffer from long term emotional, psychological, general health & sexual problems
• offend, smoke, drink alcohol, take drugs,
• play truant, be excluded or leave school at 16 with lower qualifications, low income, unemployment or income support
• experience homelessness, to be caught offending and go to jail
• enter and dissolve partnerships earlier & have children outside partnership (O'Neill, 2002)

Girls who did not have a father are disproportionally represented among teen mothers. WHY?

INTERIM CONCLUSIONS:

Antenatal staff: in prime position to alert expectant parents to the importance of continuing contact.
• Practitioners receptive to the hardships of young couples can encourage them to maintain a partnership in parenting even if no longer together.
• Can serve as a sane paternal figure when a baby's father is unknown, an elusive gang member, in prison, violent or where no mitigating third in an enmeshed mother-child dyad.
• Can try to re-engage absent/ under-involved fathers recognising that positive fathering can take many shapes in our multi-factorial society.

Obama re fathers: "Our children don't need us to be supermen or perfect. They need us to be **present** and give it our best shot, no matter what else is going on in our lives..." http://www.youtube.com/watch?v=eRJBkoq1DXs

Emotional Experience & Timing of Disturbance reveal the **weakest links** of the adult's infancy & childhood. Traumatised people may seek out or recreate the form of relationship they had with their abusers. They try to avoid yet are drawn to re-traumatising situations (re-triggered and reenacted with their own children).

PERINATAL EMOTIONAL DISTURBANCE:

•13-20% of new parents meet diagnostic criteria for **clinical depression** [2-3 times higher in areas of socioeconomic adversity]. No single cause.
• Triggered by transition to parenthood + stressful **life events**: losing job; moving house; family conflict; racism, relationship break-up; death of a relative; worry about responsibility, a difficult delivery.
• Heightened by **socioeconomic deprivation,** lack of emotional and practical support; social **isolation** (which is exacerbated by own withdrawal).
• **Vulnerability factors:** Previous or family history of mental illness, PTSD, or abuse. Insecure attachment. Poor couple relationship or violent partner.

TEEN MOTHERS x3 risk of PND vs. older mothers. Many feel trapped with the baby or not doing as well as they had imagined. Humiliated by professionals. Little socioeconomic support.
Importantly, detrimental effects of PND persist long after disturbance abates

Boys, but not girls, of PND mothers had poorer GCSE results than control children. This was principally accounted for by effects of maternal non-interaction on early child cognitive functioning, which showed strong continuity from infancy. [for PND not later maternal depression]

Murray et al, Journal of Child Psychology & Psychiatry 51:10(2010), 1150–9

EFFECTS OF DISTURBED PARENTS

Children of PND mothers develop a hyper-sensitive stress response. A **three-fold risk** of emotional disorders in childhood. Anxious/escapist play. Greater risk of depression in adulthood
Children of angry parents: difficulties soothing self /others; anger control; understanding emotional states
Violent or **abusive parents** play out their **sadism** with the child, who projects it into toys which then become **hostile persecutors** rather than comforters. Play brings no pleasure. The child feels compelled to torment, destroy, 'kill their teddy bears' (Sinason, 2001).

Useful distinction:
PN DEPRESSION & PN PERSECUTION
DEPRESSIVE DISORDERS: [Failed Facilitator]
Behaviour - withdrawn, anxious, guilt-ridden. Less interaction with baby. Suicidal thoughts.
PERSECUTORY DISORDERS: [failed Regulator]
Behaviour - hostile, intrusive, suspicious.. seeing others/ baby or external events as dangerous: **Phobia** (irrational fears) **Paranoia** (unfounded suspicion & projections). 40% of PNP mothers: **intrusive thoughts** re harming baby. Obsessive Compulsive symptoms.
***Message to Practitioner**: Reassure the client that these feelings are common and rarely acted upon. Nonetheless, self/baby harm ideas must be explored and taken seriously, especially if there are 'visions' of intentions. Offer support & referral for counselling.*

SKILL BUILDING:IDENTIFYING DISTRESS

Clients may be on their best behaviour, hiding painful feelings. Practitioners can ask neutral questions **compassionately** encouraging the young mother to **voice** her experience:"Tell me about your nights"; "What are your days like?"; "What do you enjoy doing?"

If worried, screen using EPDS. Or ask the client:

1. *During the past month, have you often felt 'down', depressed or hopeless, taking little pleasure in doing things that usually make you happy? [PND]*
2. *Do you feel your baby does things just to annoy you?* [PNP] If 'YES' to either the GP should be alerted & client asked permission for referral to specialist help

PRECIPITANTS in ADOLESCENT PARENTS:

Immaturity, insecurity & low self-esteem;
Current and/or childhood abuse or trauma contribute to a greater sense of powerlessness, and inability to cope with everyday parenting demands.

• Family conflict, physical complications following the birth and/or problems with the infant increase stress
Discrepancies between AN expectations & PN reality

• Social isolation: loss of school friends & divergence between new lifestyle and previous peer-group.

DISCUSS: *How can practitioners reduce carer distress?*
Create support groups and friendships with other young parents, with encouragement to utilise some of the many possibilities offered by a variety of services.

POSTNATAL DISTRESS IS COMMON!

A COMPARATIVE STUDY of 15 centres in 11 countries found that **'morbid unhappiness'** after childbirth is widely recognised
Across cultures distress is associated with: lack of emotional & practical social support; crying babies, difficulties with feeding, tiredness, concerns about the baby's health in the context of isolation, poor relations with partner & family conflict & (Oates,2004)
Much parental disturbance is UNDIAGNOSED.
Maternal depression is the strongest predictor of *paternal depression* in the postpartum period (Goodman, 2004).

PATERNAL DISTRESS

A meta-analysis of 43 studies involving 28,000 parents from 16 different countries, incl. UK & USA:
Cohabiting fathers - happiest in the early PN weeks
By 3-6 ms 10-25% develop PND (Paulson & Bazemore, 2010). 40% of men living with disturbed partners.
Group Discussion: **Why are live-in partners more affected?**
Either due to the strain of living with an ill partner, or due to 'assortative mating' - choice of a similarly susceptible partner.
Conclusion: interventions should focus on couple

A very large UK study: **Paternal PND** has specific persisting detrimental effects on child's early emotional & behavioural development; increased risk of conduct problems in **boys** (Ramdachani, et al 2005).

WHAT MIGHT NEW FATHERS BE FEELING?
Participator feels left out; disappointed; envious of Facilitator mother; Previously 'spoiled' Renouncer feels jealous of the mother-infant closeness. The new baby can retrigger old feelings of 'sibling rivalry'.

INTIMATE PARTNER ABUSE:

WATCH: http//www.thehideout.org.uk/over10/whatisabuse/videos/default.aspa
Evidence of increased violence in the **perinatal** period
Reasons why a teen-expectant-father feels aggrieved?

• insecurity & sense of being **neglected**/overlooked
• **demasculating** effects of a low earning capacity + extra financial pressures.
• **alienation** of the non-cohabiting sexual couple, each living with their own parents.
• **detrimental effects** of binge drinking, substance abuse, belligerent mates, poor social skills, etc.
• **pregnant girlfriend's** emotional unavailability, introspective preoccupation or refusal to make love.
• defensive attempt to restore reduced **'masculinity'**
NOTE: *Many young women can be violent too, however, generally, they are injured more than men.*

SKILL BUILDING: PERINATAL VIOLENCE
Violence during pregnancy & early parenthood
must not be tolerated. It heralds **child abuse** in which
the parent identifies the child as **a despised/bad part
of his/her self** to be bludgeoned into submission.
How do we deal with intimate partner violence?
EXPLAIN the baby's sensitivity to an aggressive
climate and entitlement to security.
CHALLENGE macho stereotype: like rape, violence is
not a sign of manliness, protectiveness, or caring but
a coward's option of expressing feelings through
action rather than words.
REFER. The reasons for violence are deep and
intractable, necessitating specialised help/therapy.
Mother & child may need **sanctuary**

POST TRAUMATIC STRESS DISORDER **PTSD**
Young people who have suffered childhood trauma,
neglect, abandonment, violence or sexual abuse are
over-represented across a variety of **care facilities**.
1/5 care-leavers at 16 are mothers within a year!

**Cumulative experiences of trauma reduces the
capacity for mentalization:**
▶ defensive use **dissociation against**. terrifying internal
scenarios.
Parent may provide competent routine child-care but is
out of touch. Control over their own emotions means
little curiosity about the baby's inner experience

ABUSE: When parent is unable to protect child, or is a
perpetrator ▶ child experiences horrific happenings, in
or outside the family. This is more likely with violent,
drug or alcohol addicted parents.
CHILDHOOD TRAUMA results in permanent disorders,
developmental distortions & deficits which persist even
if the child is removed from the abusive household.
ABUSED CHILDREN tend to manifest low self-esteem,
shame, self-blame, guilt. Defences [denial, dissociation,
self-destructive behaviour, projection] undermine the
capacity for reality-testing & self-protection. Confusion
between love & sexuality; sadism & caring.
Experience: Involuntarily flashbacks, physiological
reactions, nightmares & repetitive intrusive images

CHILD PROTECTION ISSUES:
• **Greater Mental Health risk** to babies & toddlers
whose teen parent/s themselves experienced trauma,
stress, emotional abuse, discrimination, loss, poverty,
neglect, frequent relocation, trauma, exposure to
violence, parental alcohol or drug use.
Interdisciplinary multi-agency services are designed to
safeguard & promote child welfare: must find a way of
working/thinking together as **an integrated system**
• **Crisis measures** are fraught with stress, anxiety &
complex feelings for practitioners.
•Our subjective emotional responses & identifications
affect the decision making process.
•**TASK**: HOW DO WE GET TO KNOW OURSELVES?

SUMMARY:
Disturbances are interactive. The child's defences
and responses to stress reflect their own
adaptations to parental disorders which render the
carer more rejecting, hostile, inconsistent,
ineffectual or less responsive and poorly attuned -
all of which lead to cognitive and psycho-social
developmental deficits in the growing child.
Resilience is a protective factor, comprising self-
efficacy, security, and assets such as and
resources such as supportive care systems.
Conversely, risk factors are those that weaken or
threaten protective systems.

CONCLUSIONS:PERINATAL DISTURBANCES
PTSD, Childhood Abuse, Depression and Persecution
have high co-morbidity with anxiety, substance
abuse, psychosomatic & eating disorders
Disturbed parents are less responsive, less attuned,
rejecting or hostile, inconsistent or ineffectual
→leading to cognitive, emotional and social
developmental deficits in the child
Children and partners of a disturbed parent are
significantly more likely to be disturbed themselves
Perinatal therapy (individual, Parent-Infant, Couple,
Family) helps integrate contradictory forces

Adolescence as a 2nd Chance ©
devised by
Professor Joan Raphael-Leff

MODULE V
**FAMILIES, GROUPS &
ORGANIZATIONS**

9. Interactive Workshop:
Family Dynamics

OBJECTIVES:

To review the **crucial functions of a family**, and group dynamics in the context of contemporary psychosocial changes. By the end of this course you will have reflected on **interactive forces** in individuals, couples, families, small and large groups. The aim is to
• better understand interpersonal dynamics
• to deepen awareness of the effects of our own initiatives & counter-responses in work situations
• acquire **greater insight** into our own personal strengths, biases and blind-spots; and insight into habitual defence patterns.
• to promote better cross-agency and interdisciplinary **team work**, and understanding of institutional defences.

FAMILY FORMATION AND STRUCTURE

Worldwide over past decades, dramatic changes due to? [group discussion – 5 minutes]
• **Social forces** (Feminism)
• **Scientific advances** (the Pill, Reproductive
                          Technology)
• **Disasters** (population decimation: AIDS, war
                refugees, climate change migration).
In societies-in-transition (such as ours) contemporary family composition ranges from traditional structures to multiple **new socially acceptable patterns**, often coexisting side by side.

What family patterns do we see?

• **lone-mothers** by choice
• **partners** non-cohabiting or 'live-in'
• **composite** ('blended') step-families, cross-race, different fathers, mixed ethnicity/religion, etc.
• **same-sex** parents [gamete/embryo donors]
• three generational, or polygamous (several 'wives')
• **unrelated**: foster care/co-opted communes/gangs
• **no parental generation**: grandparent
  or child-headed family
•   **adolescent parent/s**

FAMILY FUNCTION: GROUP DISCUSSION:
What is a family? [5 minutes with flipchart]
• **Traditional families**: genetic kinship 'shared blood', & often, <u>arranged marriage</u> between families.
Today's family: not necessarily a **reproductive** unit to transmit **genes** (surrogates, gamete donors, adoption, fostering) &/or to bequeath **property**
So--what is it??
THE PRESENCE OF A CHILD FORMS A 'FAMILY'[?]
• Family=a regulating force & agent of society
<u>Boundary interface</u> between Social and Individual.
If too tight=constraint; if too loose=non-containment
No longer a single family-name marker.

AN 'EMOTIONAL FAMILY'

Idea of a family-group in the mind defined by each family member's notions of who it consists of (social or biological parents, siblings, friends or others).
• 'Family' members can be co-opted:
• share common values, linked 'destinies';
• wish to promote improved quality of life.
• relationship co-created in frequent exchanges
• varies within groups, and between cultures

FAMILIES: DISTINGUISHING FEATURES:

Protection: meeting members' basic needs for food, shelter, sleep, safety, (sex). **Defence** against external forces, perceived as hostile.
Family culture/ethos: offers i**dentity**: integral to that family (or genealogical lineage)
Cultural transmission: older, socialised members nurture & pass on skills, tools & understanding to younger or less knowledgeable ones.
Other features are **durability** and **continuity**: trust that despite failures, family members can **repair** and continue to negotiate **proximity**. [Some families fail to provide this - for instance Personality Disordered parents may 'dump' their children if something goes wrong].
· provides multiple perspectives

THE SOCIAL CONTEXT
includes which other institutions?
Health, Education, Social services, Religion etc with similar nurturing roles or even surveillance of the family on behalf of the State
• These also convey a sense of identity and of belonging to larger & unrelated groups.
• Institutions offer *a variety of perspectives* but in fragmented urban communities, may feel *alienating*.
• Societies vary in the **degree of freedom** allowed to families (China:one child policy; Romania:5 children)
•Families vary as to internal degrees of freedom/ obligations on individual members Authoritarian/Permissive

---

The safe family acts as a '**PLAYGROUND**' enabling play, illusion and fantasy to flourish: an experimental context to try out *different roles* and *imaginary states*. The child can play with different activities & identities (vs. set roles) to evolve a broad stable **self-structure**
• A well-functioning emotionally invested family provides a '**facilitating environment**' (Winnicott) so each member can reach his/her own highest potential.
• Children need a play-space with peers, to develop linguistic/social/gender skills **away** from close familial understanding. Individuation is repeated by teenagers
• Parents, too, evolve. Achieving a coherent internal organization constitutes **a life long process.**
Healthy family engagement = privacy+curiosity.
Respect for internal experience of all family members

FAMILIES generate/interpret **a range of emotional experiences** that provide meaning for each child. These vary with each family ethos & cross-culturally
• The **strong passions** played out in the family are the *seedbed* within which the **child** learns to understand the **meaning of basic feelings**: love, hate, anger, envy, jealousy, empathy
Given the close quarters, bodily care and intimacy in families, *boundaries become permeable* as through constant interaction *one mind enters another mind.*
Conversely, proximity & continuity can create *entrenched positions*, allocating each member a *designated role* in the family, affecting self/other reps

---

Finally, regardless of its composition, each family is a group of people linked by common '**Founding Myth**' Child's preoccupation with **genetic history**: *Who am I and were do I come from? How are babies made?* [Hurtful if teen parent answers *'you were a mistake'*].
• From early on infants have a capacity for **3-way** communication. This is more robust when 'scaffolded' by parental **coalition** ['2 for 1' alliance]. Undermined by parental conflict ['2 against 1'] (Fivaz-Depeursinge, 2008).
• Internalised **primary dyadic & triadic relational patterns** constitute the foundation for an expanding world of external relationships, and social structures.
•**Each child evolves a different elaboration of the 'primal scene'** (of parental sex & reproduction).
Michaelangelo Creation]

THE OEDIPAL PARADIGM: Freud believed that each child wishes for sole possession of the parent & elimination of rivals. But a toddler raised in a two parent family comes to recognise the father & mother's special connection. Coming to terms with **exclusion** from their sexual relationship ultimately motivates the child to seek a mate of their own, outside the family of origin.
DISCUSS: The importance of **triangular** contact - *'One looking in at a relation between two others'* can be applied to all triangles, including relations between siblings. 'Triangulation' gives the child a different perspective as a 'witness, not 'partici-pant' to another relationship (Britton, 1991). But resolution of Oedipal issues is a family affair – generated through interaction between **all** family members   Jocasta Mum jfa0497t

• **A strong couple relationship** ▶ **better prognosis for child.** Enhanced maternal caregiving. (**Non-resident fathers** must make extra efforts)
• Yet most relationships **deteriorate** when partners become parents (Cowans, 2002). WHY?
• High level of **family breakup in West.** WHY?
• Shift from sexual twosome to three: **triangular** relation – revived Oedipal feelings. Competition, jealousy - *one feels left out.*
•.

• The family confers *belonging* that promotes *a sense of identity* and (portable) *self-esteem.*
• Anxieties when this cannot be taken for granted
Problematic families:
• **Unsupportive families**
• **Families who abuse**, reject, eject or lose their members (i.e. children taken into care, abandoned street children, those institutionalised by over-burdened parents)
• **Secretive families:** child's ignorance about facts, *origins* (disruption to sense of historicity)
• **Chaotic households,**
Confusion=more disturbing than unpalatable facts.
A 'good' family is a place in which questions can be safely asked, even if unanswerable .

FAMILY DYNAMICS
Loss of traditional patterns generate **choices** – various parental orientations, many different life-styles, childrearing patterns practices & family forms
Internal family dynamics too vary as each child takes his/her place in the family, depending on the number, ages, gaps, sex, personality & parent's psycho-history
Family myths, secrets & non-conscious influences live on in names, emotional transactions, identifications, fantasies, projections, ascriptions …
A child unconsciously absorbs unvoiced parental feelings, and familial trauma such as perinatal losses, registering in a child's sense of shame, guilt, pride or triumph over unborn babies before or after themselves.
Only children feel they demolished all successors.

CONCLUSIONS: Teens renegotiate self-image, gender sexuality & generative identity **outside the family.**
• Like individuating toddler, teens rely on **expanded environment** and a **small group** of loyal friends.
• Non-committal **experimentation** with temporary roles & identities to cope with changes: body-schema, sexual/ aggressive urges, new social/psychosexual expectations
• Complications arise when pregnancy forces decision
• Demands of parenthood interrupt ongoing processes
• In violent families or no paternal figure, teens turn to **gang-related activity:** to belong to a <u>powerful social organization</u> with exciting 'phallic' activities, risk-taking, rebellion/vandalism. Violence may escalate into murder

---

10. Skill Building Seminar
TEAMS, GROUPS & ORGANISATIONS
We belong to multiple informal & regulated groups: WHICH?
Family, work, friendship circles, recreational or interest clubs, educational or religious groups. *Common aspects?*
• Interdependence of group members
• Shared representations of the world – tacit beliefs, values & social norms of mutual conduct.
• group identifications grow as members interact & communicate – cultivating & influencing connections.
• Groups promote new thinking in individual members reinforced by ongoing group process
• Groups persist/flourish; or disintegrate/dissolve. WHY?
Tensions *arise within groups due to?* internal conflicts (ideological shifts, conflicting aims, dissident subgroups), and/or external forces(altered circumstances, real or imagined threats)

ROLE PLAY:
*A **team** of 4-6 different practitioners (composition specified by the large group) meet to discuss a 'hot' issue (also chosen by the group).*
COURSE LEADER: After 3-5 minutes – STOP, 'REWIND' – and look at non-mentalising group process. Then START AGAIN.
MESSAGE: The Course itself reflects some of the large and small group dynamics

GROUP DISCUSSION:
Most practitioners work in teams:
'What kind of problems can arise through inadequate communication channels?'

TEAMS

In more formally structured groups, members work together as a TEAM. *What makes a good team?*
• Focus on a particular goal requiring <u>coordinated interaction</u>.
• may involve inter-disciplinary sharing of skills or forms of expertise.
• Team members may democratically select leaders to facilitate exchange and coordinate/delegate.
• Most teams confer a sense of belonging, self-worth & satisfaction on members.
• **group goals** and **individual rewards** often change after completion of specified tasks, bringing about a possible change of leader and membership sub-groupings or belonging.

When interrelated groups aggregate ► ORGANIZATION
• Common social purpose, collective goal & ideology
• Members/sub-groups accountable to the organization
Group classification: by *purpose?*
• groups (including teams), creative groups (bands, reading, writing or art), gratification groups (social recreation & sports), political (social-action groups)…
• <u>Degree of cohesiveness</u> (smaller size), loyalty (related to specified task, shared beliefs and values), explicit aims of the group & motivation to fulfil goals.
• *Group's emotional climate?:*
formality of organization, rigidity of hierarchical structure; authoritarian/democratic leadership style; voluntary/coerced participation; sharing of personal vulnerability

---

WORK GROUPS are evaluated by their productivity: does not reflect the group *potential* as the group process is subject to **resistances** & **unconscious forces** which undermine the work.
Cooperation arouses anxieties!

Seen *psychodynamically,* a unique '<u>group mentality</u>' composed of unconscious basic assumptions & more 'primitive' fantasies often operates in contradiction to explicit aims. A group's specific **ethos/culture** reflects this conflict between task & 'group mentality'.

Also, a conflict between individual participant & group aims. In most groups, including families, individuals must sometimes renounce or compromise some of their interests to achieve the collective aim.

The more powerful the group's basic assumptions and primitive anxieties ► the more trivial the conversation.
Action prevails over language
Loss of personal distinctiveness ► *depersonalization.*
The GROUP LEADER too, absorbs the frustrations, rage, desires & anxieties of the group. Unless can make sense of *counter-transference* s/he will get caught up in many transference attributions & projections of the group
These dispositions & dynamics found in *any* group situation, are best observed in work groups [See handout 5].
GROUP EXERCISE: *Small groups of 6-8.*
<u>**Task:**</u> *come up with **a name** for your group [5 mins].*
<u>**Feedback**</u>*: 1 min per group about group process: awareness of interactive group pressures, personal feelings & expectations during your own discussion (5 minutes).*

GROUP DYNAMICS: when individuals come together to form a work group → <u>2 levels of emotional activity</u>:
• a seemingly **rational, cooperative work group**
• alternating '**anti-growth' basic assumptions**:
1. **Dependence**: group members ignore each other and relate to the **idealised leader**: hunger for nurture, guidance & protection.
2. **Pairing**: unconsciously, the group has a different leader in mind:unborn messianic **saviour** from coupling of 2 group members co-opted to monopolise the group.
3. **Fight-flight**: group members seek instant satisfaction by a **substitute leader**'s uncontrolled **attack** to rid group of persecutory feelings; or his/her leading a panicked **escape** from a perceived threat (Bion, 1952)

INSTITUTIONS:

If organizations such as interest groups constitute **temporary** arrangements, <u>institutions</u> are a society's **permanent** *structures of social order* & *cooperation*
What institutions can you think of?
Religion; Education; Scientific institutions; Hospitals and other medical & psychiatric institutions; Military, Legal & Penal systems; Communication, Mass and News media; Factories & Financial Corporations, Marriage and the Family, etc.
Many of us work in an institution, but we do not often consider the **emotional forces** & **mechanisms** that operate within them.
Many policies are instituted to manage *anxieties.*
Which anxieties?

Many professions invoke anxieties, especially work with vulnerable, anti-social, addicted, predatory, needy, violent, mentally ill, poverty-stricken or suicidal clients. Also Institutional threats: uncertainty; diversity; conflict; tyranny, exposure, litigation: boundary violations, power abuse, incompetence. Closure, redundancies…

A study of nursing practices examined **unconscious dynamics** of a London teaching hospital (Menzies, 1960). **Findings**: the nursing system evolved care patterns to *distance themselves* from *anxiety-provoking work-situations* – from patients in pain, disfigured, terminally ill… Anxieties of administering unpleasant procedures, coping with physical intimacy exposure to disgusting bodily substances, fear of contamination, and of death *Examples of distancing procedures?*

[optional] **MIDWIVES:exposure to emotional threats**

Chronic tension of uncertainty; **Acute stress** of emergencies; **Maternal pain,** physical/mental illness, 'hot' feelings transferred from the past (idealisation/denigration) **Naked physicality and primitive emotions** [screams, curses - pain, fear, rage, eroticism]; Her own **dual identifications**: baby & woman; **Primal substances** [amniotic fluid, blood, meconium, vernix; **Birth complications**/deformity of baby; **Real dangers** of maternal or neonatal death

Mysteries of origins – where we all come from
EMOTIONAL NEEDS of midwives?

Staff support group; Training in psychological understanding; Individual/group counselling; Time to form warm human attachments - **continuity of care;** More job satisfaction: broad areas of responsibility (vs. tasks); **Debriefing** after traumatic births; Opportunities to grieve losses (NICU) ;Open communication channels; Confidential complaints procedure

---

INSTITUTIONALIZED DEFENCES

Impersonal approach - denying feelings in oneself or other. Aloof **professionalism** (task oriented, rigid rules, routines, box-ticking, no initiative) or hectic **over-activity** (performative 'targets) with *no time to contemplate.*
Examples from participants' workplace or elsewhere?
Avoidance, denial or distortion of unpleasant realities splitting, un/intentional deception or fobbing clients off. Stripping clients of their identifying characteristics; treating them as *interchangeable;* maintaining *a task oriented attitude* towards featureless people, 'sign-posting', treating separate body parts or needs = **avoiding seeing the recipient as a whole vulnerable person, as fragile and fallible as ourselves** [same projective mechanisms as we saw in prejudice]

CONCLUSIONS:

Institutions evolve **'Social Defences'** to insulate their workers *against experiencing doubts, difficult or unbearable feelings.*

These organised but often unconscious procedures *fragment care and ritualise practices to* **distance worker & users:** Clients: only minimal participation in decision-making. Practitioners insulated by non-continuous care from the consequences of their actions and effects on clients.

► low staff morale & poor job satisfaction, high burn-out; frustration if no space for self-motivated intiatives Increased reliance on technology, electronic monitoring & impossible case-loads detract from human-contact.

Anxiety in work situations creates *DEFENCES* which lead to an ineffective system geared to staff convenience over client needs (early morning floor polishing on hospital wards). Other examples?
In caring professions, to keep the client's mind in mind, we ourselves need time and reflective space for thinking & self-inquiry.
Despite **institutional resistance to change, w**ith greater understanding of organizational dynamics **transformations can happen.**
Last task: How can we improve job satisfaction & efficiency in our workplaces?
...and now to end...

Self-Study/Group Discussion: Underline What constitutes a good parting? *[flipchart, add points that have not arisen]*
• Achieving *a capacity for mentalization* – tools for thoughtful processing
• Better tolerance of anxiety, insight re internal conflicts, more coherent story, integration & self-reflection
• *Plan* ending in advance with the client
• *Remind* client before the termination date
• *Hear* client's views of your intervention to date
• *Review 'journey'*: were their/your objectives met?
• *Discuss* disappointments, frustrations, gains - how this separation reverberates with earlier losses
• *Acknowledge* mixed feelings - of pride, abandonment, anxiety, relief, sadness
• *Mark* the event. Discuss *Follow Up!* future contact?
• *Express your gratitude* for the mutual learning experience